MIND-BODY MEDICINE & HEALTHOLOGY

Body-Mind-Spirit Science & Practice

The Advanced Holistic Life Science
Secrets • Wisdom • Principles • Techniques

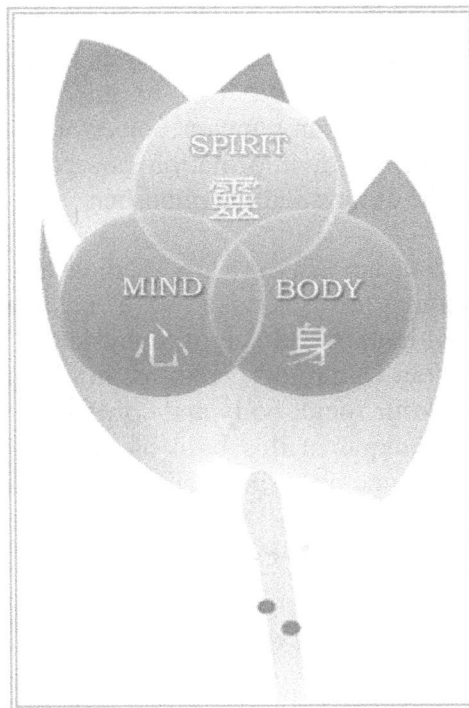

TEXTBOOK • HEALING BOOK • GUIDEBOOK

JASON LIU, MD/PHD

Professor of Mind-Body Medicine

Mind-Body Medicine & Healthology

Copyright © 2014 by Jason G. Liu

All rights reserved.

Publisher:
Mind-Body Science Publishing -
Mind-Body Science Institute, USA
ISBN-13: 978-0692257913
ISBN-10: 0692257918

The author of this book does not dispense any medical advice or prescribe the use of any technique as treatment or diagnosis of a medical condition, physical or psychological problem without the advice of a physician. The intent of the author is to offer general information of natural health as an alternative and complementary way to help you balance your mind, body and spirit for your well-being. Using any of the information or technique in this book is your constitutional right, and the author and the publisher assume no responsibility for your actions.

Library of Congress Cataloging-in-Publication Data:

Jason G. Liu, 2014 ~
Mind-Body Medicine & Healthology

July 18, 2014 published in the United States of America
Mind-Body Science Publishing
Mind-Body Science Institute, USA
www.mbmu.org

Available in Print Book (Paperback and Hardcover), Kindle Book and Audiobook
on Amazon.com & Publisher Website www.mbmu.org/books

PREFACE

In one lifetime, there's no way to master all knowledge that has been established throughout the entire history of human civilization and pre-historical civilization. You do have, however, the chance to gain the most precious and blessing wisdom from the higher divine teaching, with which to transform your life.

There's no one who can read all the books written by the countless number of geniuses throughout the entirety of human civilization, but you may wish you could and this wish has given you faith that out there somewhere, there may exist a text, from which you can learn and practice the most important and beneficial knowledge and skills for the improvements of your own life and your profession not only in the fields of conventional or alternative health practice, life science, *Mind-Body Medicine and Healthology*, psychology, family and marriage therapy, but also other fields of natural science, social science and practice.

This special faith could be what brings you to my book, which is trying to be such a book for you and others, although it may not be perfectly that way yet because myself as author is still a cultivator to be improved constantly, and plus our human language won't be able to perfectly reveal the complete truth we all quest with regard to the vastness and mystery of the universe and all the lives within it.

Yet, as a needle-free and drug-free alternative health practitioner and spiritual cultivator who is dedicated to helping people with difficulties in this life, I share my long years of experience, research, understanding, stories, techniques and cultivation energy to help you gain the most critical knowledge and useful skills for bettering the health of mind-body-spirit and life quality of yours and others through this book — the individuals from all walks of life, health science students, professionals, doctors, therapists, nurses, chronic condition patients, mind-body-spirit cultivators, self healing practitioners-centered learning textbook, teaching book, guidebook and healing book.

I very warmly welcome you and everyone from all walks of life to read this book. I humbly and honestly promise you this will be a book forever helpful to you.

Dr. Jason Liu, MD/PhD, author of Mind-Body Medicine & Healthology

ENDORSEMENT

I have read Dr. Jason Liu's book, *Mind-Body Medicine & Healthology* several times and will continue reading it many, many more times. It is a wonderful book that takes you on a compelling journey to the core of your Self.

Beginning on a path that zooms back through time to the first recorded texts of Chinese and Asian medicine and zooming forward into the cutting edge research of modern Western and Eastern sciences, Dr. Liu lays out a plan to keep you healthy and joyous and living beyond whatever you think is your fullest potential.

In his opening pages, Dr. Liu promises, "While you are reading, you will find that your health improves – you will look even younger and more beautiful, and some health issues you may be concerned about will also improve." In short, Dr. Liu asks three things of us in order to fulfill that promise: You have to be willing to change, keep and open mind, and believe that you can evolve to higher levels.

I wasn't even a ¼ of the way through the book, when I wanted to try some of its concepts. When I did, the result was immediate --- exactly as Dr. Liu had promised. I felt great.

Dr. Liu has written a remarkable and entertaining book on how we can employ the techniques of mind-body medicine to have a healthier, calmer, more satisfying and joyous life and help others do the same.

Mind-Body Medicine & Healthology is beautifully and compassionately voiced and will leave you feeling healthy, strong and inspired for many long years.

- Dr. Joseph Cardillo, PhD, author of *The Five Seasons*

ABOUT THE AUTHOR

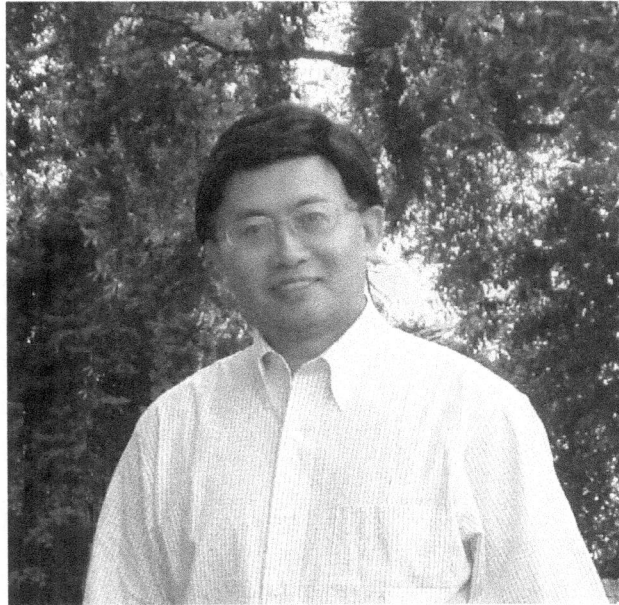

Dr. Jason Liu, MD/PhD, is the founding president of the Mind-Body Science Institute. He is a certified Alternative Medicine Practitioner, Drugless Practitioner, Clinical Hypnotherapist, meditation teacher, and neuron and muscular physiologist and scientist with quality research papers published on the top medical journals such as *J. Biol. Chem., Mol. Pharmacol.,* etc. [90-98]. Dr. Liu is a mind-body medicine practitioner and researcher [40-41, 88], and the composer/producer of *Energy Healing - Meditation Relaxation Music Series.* Dr. Liu invented Brainwave-Meridian Therapy, an application of mind-body medicine & healthology.

Dr. Liu has multiple academic education backgrounds and extensive trainings through his doctorate and postdoctoral programs in the medical schools of UC Davis, California, Miami University, Florida, and Nagoya City University, Japan, followed by the establishment of his mind-body healing and educational institution where he practices and teaches with colleagues. The fields he trained with and practice include quantum physics (his original bachelor education), neuron muscular physiology, biophysics, holistic psychology, hypnosis and meditation, eastern healing arts such as Chinese medicine, Qigong, Taiji, energy healing music composition and healing therapy, Chinese calligraphy, poem writing, etc. He is a certified Chinese Qigong master, but as he continued to search the truth and cultivate himself, since long ago himself has been humbly dedicated to mind-body-spirit cultivation as a lifetime discipline.

Acknowledgement

I am very grateful to my previous patients and clients who openly shared their healing experiences with BMT treatment and provided their testimonials to enrich this book with actual healing stories.

I would like to express my deep appreciation to Dr. Joseph Cardillo, Ph.D., best-selling author in the fields of health, mind-body-spirit, and psychology [83-87], for his excellent and passionate readings of this work as it took shape, as well as the great endorsement that he wrote for the book.

I am also grateful to my pervious professors who supervised me in University of California Davis, University of Miami Medical School, as well as Medical School of Nagoya City University, Japan, who greatly helped me in my academic learning and scientific research.

Deep appreciation to my spiritual teacher and master who gave me life-transforming guide and teaching of the truth, allowing me to deepen my understanding and explore my research and practice in mind-body medicine and healthology.

Finally I would like to deeply thank my loved ones in my family, dear friends, fellow practitioners, colleagues, patients, clients and students for their understanding, love, support, help, assistance, encouragement, and suggestions that greatly contributed to the accomplishment of this book.

TABLE OF CONTENTS

CHAPTER 11 311

ENERGY MUSIC THERAPY – AN APPLICATION OF MIND-BODY MEDICINE............................. 311

CHAPTER 12 339

BRAINWAVE-MERIDIAN THERAPY – AN APPLICATION OF MIND-BODY MEDICINE.............. 339

CHAPTER 1

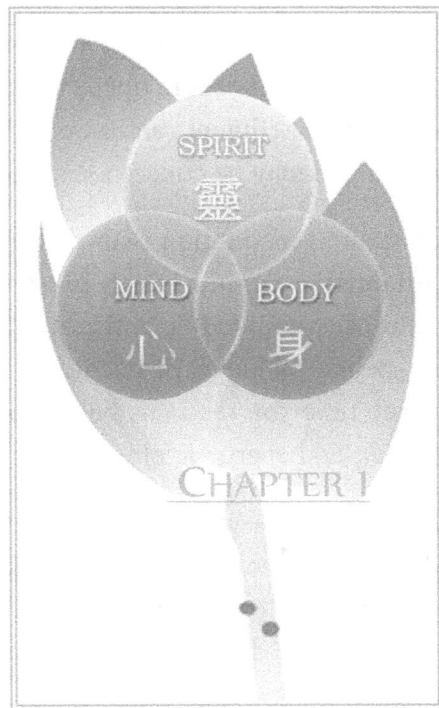

Open Mind to Learn Mind-Body Science and Practice

From the beginning to the end of this book, please read with your mind open and body relaxed, in a very quiet place, without interruption by anything or anyone. Read peacefully while naturally taking deep breaths, with calm and joyful mood, but never rush or in a hurry to read. To best benefit from the healing energy of this book, keep looking inwardly and humbly at your true Self at all times as you read and practice, so that you can absorb the meaning and energy of each word that is talking to you personally. You can also listen to this audiobook in the same way but sometime you can close your eyes in a meditative state with your conscious mind clear and focused while listening.

It doesn't matter if you are a mind-body healthcare practitioner, teacher, student, or an individual seeking self-improvement, you will benefit from this reading.

This chapter prepares you to get ready to read through this book and learn mind-body medicine and healthology. We will gradually build the strong foundation to help you get into this field. Please read with patience until we get into the actual depth of the central contents. This is a teaching book, an educational textbook, a guidebook, and a healing book. While you are reading, you will find that your wisdom opens up and your health improves – you will become more clearheaded and intelligent, and you will look even younger and more beautiful, and some health issues you may be concerned about will also improve.

I wrote this book in a deep state of meditation with wonderful energy and love. My sincere intention is to help you establish a natural health lifestyle for healthy, happy and meaningful long living, and to help open-minded scientists in different fields establish a new life science, which can help people achieve physical, mental, and spiritual health, beauty, happiness and longevity. Each time you read this book, you will feel more and more relaxed, clear-headed, positive, happier, and energetic physically, mentally and spiritually.

Mind-Body Medicine & Healthology is written for individuals from many different ways and walks of life, including everyday people in general, students and professionals in health science and practice and people in a wide range of other fields. Therefore, I have tried to write straightforwardly, clearly and simply as possible, so that its concepts and skills can be easily understood and practiced by all.

On the other hand, as a reader, you may also adjust your mentality as open as possible to accept new concept or old concept with new meaning. For well-trained professionals or well-experienced practitioners in the related fields, when you read those concepts that you have already known, please read with fresh mind, humble attitude and patience, so you can absorb the new meaning, deepen your understanding and insight. For the beginners or those who are not familiar with this field, however, when you read those contents difficult for you to understand, please read with mind open to build solid knowledge base and improve your understanding ability in the field of spiritual science.

In any case, because mind-body-spirit science is an extraordinary science and practice, you will need to open your mind, let go of some pre-existing notions, attachments, and rigid thinking, to study and apply what you learn within this field. This way you can explore and absorb the fresh knowledge and profound wisdom of this journey.

Throughout this book, at different places, the important concepts, ideas, principles, theories, practical methods, problems, solutions, recommendations, and suggestions are intentionally described and emphasized in different ways, from different angles and at different levels. The text was designed for different readers to read through sequentially upon your first reading. You may, however, wish to read it again several times, paying attention to specific parts that match your needs. Each time you go through the text, it will deepen your understanding, upgrade your ability to practice its many techniques, enrich your experience, and enlighten your spirit. You will, within this journey, fully learn and master a wide range of ideas and skills within the healing arts and learn how to cultivate the practice for your own true health of mind, body and spirit as well as for giving good energetic influence to people surrounding you.

If you are a professional or student in this field, while you learn the knowledge for your professional practice or research, please also consider yourself as a patient or an individual who needs to do self-healing and improve your own health of mind, body and spirit, this way you can understand your patient better with your direct experience. While if you are a patient or an individual who wants to improve health of mind-body-spirit, please also consider yourself as a health practitioner, so that you can better understand your doctor and get healed faster.

§1.1 MBM As Alternative Natural Health Science & Practice

Before we go any further, I would like to make a statement about this book as an alternative natural health scientist and practitioner. This will also help new learners and future professionals in this field have an idea to recognize and define your profession as mind-body medicine practitioner or scientist:

(1)   This book discusses approaches to health that are alternative, preventive and non-invasive. They are not the mainstream medicine, prescription medications, drugs, chemicals, needles, surgeries, or invasive treatments. Although we call it mind-body medicine, it is totally different from the meaning and approaches of mainstream medicine.

(2)   For this reason, I use a newly created term "mind-body healthology," emphasizing the science and practice that present a natural way to be healthy but do not intend to cure diseases.

(3)   I use terms such as medical, medicine, health practice, treatment, clinical, clinic, patient, doctor, diagnosis, oriental medicine, Chinese medicine, psychology, clinical psychology, etc. These terms from existing fields give readers immediate context and simplify understanding. But their meanings in this book

have been intentionally broadened in scope with the hope that they can serve as guideposts for individuals in these existing fields to further expand and develop.

(4)   None of the terms, however, conflicts with existing notions. An advantage of using these terms is that it helps the placement of the discipline of mind-body medicine within health science and preventive health practice. It as well incorporates mind-body medicine into mainstream primary healthcare as an alternative complementary health practice for the future. Such a natural mind-body holistic health system fosters the positive hope of prevention and self-empowerment, in our quest to live healthy and in the face of serious diseases and sicknesses.

(5)   Although we use the terms of oriental medicine or Chinese medicine, we do not use their actual tools such as needles, cups and herbs as treatment, only the principle and theory to understand the mechanism and apply them to noninvasive and nonphysical practices for mind-body-spirit health.

(6)   We do not claim to diagnose or cure any kind of disease, which is the business of mainstream medicine. Even though some people have been cured of such after following this model of natural health practice - e.g. meditation, energy music healing, hypnosis, etc., we believe the healing is due to the efforts of the person himself or herself. These are core objectives – to encourage everyone to practice preventive health on their own and health practitioners and scientists to be open minded when assisting patients and studying life science.

(7)   We refer to mind-body-medicine as science, but it is also different from the meaning of conventional science or modern life science, which are only based on laboratory experiments or evidence obtained through modern technology. We do refer to existing science and technology and sometimes also try to use them to study mind-body health science, but we do not limit our understanding to just these existing mainstream sciences and technology. We widely learn from all fields, crossing them and integrating them, combining with spiritual, psychological, mental, emotional, vibrational, energetic, and metaphysical practices to achieve the integrity of a new science that reveals or nearly reveals the truth about our universe and life within the unification, comprehension, and interactions of mind-body-spirit.

(8)   As this book discusses comprehensive, holistic and spiritual science and practice for mind-body-spirit health, we may at times point out some shortcomings or limitations of other fields such as within modern science, medicine, and pharmacology – some of which I personally also studied in the

medical schools. Note: By pointing out such shortcomings, I am not intentionally criticizing, discriminating or complaining against other fields or groups of healthcare practice or science. We are simply and objectively facing the fact and seeking the better solutions for whole being health and its science.

In addition to some existing terms in life science and mental health science, this book stands on an entirely new foundation at the edge of a new frontier, to establish a new science by using many new terms, concepts, and its own expressions. These terms will be defined in context.

Please be aware of the following notes, as well, when using any healing approach, idea or concept learned from this book:

All concepts and techniques taught within this text are alternative and/or complimentary and cannot substitute for your family doctor's diagnosis, treatments or therapies. You should make your own decision or consult with your family doctor or other mainstream medicine healthcare services on your health issue and treatment.

You may consult with your family doctor or other mainstream healthcare practitioner before using any methods in this book and openly let them know what you practice is self-healing learned from this book. You have the right and responsibility to make decisions on what personal health practices you wish to utilize, including any method discussed in this book.

Healing methods such as meditation, energy music healing, energy practice or mind-body-spirit cultivation practice are very natural, peaceful and have no side effects. If you experience any discomfort after using methods learned in this book, however, it must be due to another reason or may be the result of a temporary cleansing reaction (the emptying of negative influencers and replacement with positive energy)[1] and should be over shortly. Please be aware of this, and take your own responsibility for that.

If you are a healthcare practitioner and use any method or idea learned from this book, please take responsibility and liability in regard to your practice.

§1.2 Spiritual • Non-Spiritual • Religious • Non-Religious Readers

---

[1] Cleansing Reaction: a natural phenomena that may be seen sometime during the process of natural healing or energy healing; the symptom seems to get worse temporarily before getting better. The reason for this is the sick information or negative factors within the body and mind (physical toxin and mental toxin) are releasing and coming to the superficial level, resisting against, interacting with, and being replaced by, the positive healing energy. Therefore, rearrangements occur in the mind and body as an indication of improvement. Note that cleansing reactions are not necessarily seen in all patients.

This book is written open-mindedly and humbly by learning from a wide range of health sciences and knowledge, including ancient and modern, Eastern and Western sciences, practices, experiences, religions, beliefs, and philosophies, crossing many related fields. As a friendly mention, to spiritual or non-spiritual, religious or non-religious readers:

This book is not intended to promote any religion or belief system, and itself is not a belief system, but simply a vehicle for seeking truth and for learning and applying mind-body-spirit health as a health science.

When you read some terms cited from ancient or modern health practices, Eastern or Western medicine, philosophy or spiritual teaching, please be open minded.   Whether you are from an Eastern tradition or Western, from one professional field or another, just use your true Self and inborn wisdom to naturally understand what is being presented and look – beyond the superficial – at the whole issue and truth that manifests. For people with Western (or Eastern) backgrounds, please do not think the knowledge or ideas being shared belongs only to one particular group. In fact, this is the wisdom belonging to all of humankind. For modern science believers, please do not think the ancient wisdom is something out of date and ignore these precious teachings. For people who do not have a spiritual belief, please be open-minded and put your effort into learning and directly experiencing and practicing mind-body-spirit science as a special field, different from experimental or evidence-based, linear science.

Also, I would like to state to either spiritual/religious or non-spiritual/non-religious readers:

Although we cited or mentioned some belief systems or teachings in this book, it does not mean this book is the teaching of the system itself and nor does it intend to mix different spiritual practices. If you want to learn and practice the belief system or its teaching cited, you should read its specific and original texts and exactly follow its master's guide to practice. This book is simply and humbly learning from, enlightening by and sharing with the profound teaching, in order to broaden our mind and scope, helping establish the future mind-body-spirit science and health practice.

§1.3 This Book and Its Brief Summary

Mind-Body Medicine & Healthology covers mind-body medicine's most important original teachings, histories, theories, principles, concepts, ideas, secrets, models, hypothesis, methods, research and experiments, energy checkups and healing techniques.

Mind-Body Medicine & Healthology also introduces some mental and spiritual practices such as meditation, energy music and sound healing therapy, energy practice and spiritual cultivation, psychological healing, conscious and subconscious practice, healthy living lifestyle, brainwave meridian therapy, preventive healthcare, modern diseases (e.g., cancers, depression, anxiety, stress, etc.) healing and prevention, integrative care and practice, and a wide range of healing stories.

After laying out a strong foundation for *Mind-Body Medicine & Healthology* which includes principles, theories, ideas and methods, this book provides you with healing solutions and preventive care for some common and serious health problems such as stress, depression, anxiety, relationship problems, cancer(s) and other chronic health issues.

Chapters are arranged in an order that helps you understand step-by-step, so please read straight through the arranged order and do not skip around, read in part, or choose only titles that may superficially interest you at the moment.

Every chapter includes a meditation and energy music healing practice. Following instruction on their use and practice will help you understand the book much easier and joyfully.

§1.4 The Aim of This Book, Its Title and Readers

This book is published at this special time as we have entered a new era of spirituality. It is written especially to help nurture this transition. With such an evolutional science and practice, we can reestablish a higher quality, healthy, happy, beautiful, and highly synchronized and assimilated meaningful life of the body, mind and spirit. We can live into a brighter future. From the perspective of mind-body health science, an overwhelming material life, a tired and debilitated economy, anxious and fatigued emotions, depressed mindfulness and loss of spirit have driven people into a stressful, busy and Self-lost life for too long. As a result many have become unhealthy physically, mentally, and spiritually.

Modern medical approaches rely on drug treatment as their first choice and are often invasive (or disempowering) programs that rarely have an ideally desirable efficacy in dealing with these malaises. Such treatment usually generates a range of side effects, making the original condition even more complicated and difficult to heal. We cannot wholly rely on drug-based medicine and surgical medicine. Sitting back and waiting for sickness to occur and pharmaceuticals and surgeries to solve the problem isn't in anyone's best health interests and can have some catastrophic consequences. Way too often, all that kind of thinking does is rule out options of prevention and/or natural treatments. "What is the better way?" you may ask.

This question drills down into the heart of this book and will be answered in its subsequent pages.

Please note: I am intentionally using a new term Healthology both in the title and with these pages. Healthology uses "health" as its root and the suffix "ology" to create a new field of science, healthology, comparable to physiology, pathology, biology, etc. People are used to understanding medicine as a practice that treats disease, but this book emphasizes the concept of being healthy, not getting sick and healing the cause of potential sicknesses.

This, as mentioned above, was the philosophy of the original ancient medicine: "The superior doctor treats sickness before getting sick," (上工治未病, from Yellow Emperor's Classic of Internal Medicine, 475-221 BC) [1]. Such a science and practice that studies and teaches the way to be healthy is called healthology.

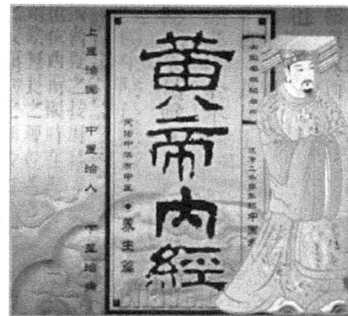

Mind-Body Medicine & Healthology is written for people from all walks of life.

You may be someone who wants to maintain your health (or that of others) or become healthy, beautiful and sustain a long life mentally, physically and spiritually and/or who wants to cultivate mind-body-spirit and have a meaningful, transformational and enlightened life journey. The following is an incomplete list of group categories of people who will most benefit from this book. In order to facilitate your reading and practice, please see where your interests match. For students or professionals in this field, the following will also help you broaden your compassionate heart to consider all kinds of people from different walks of life as your patients or subjects of your research.

1. If you have no health problem currently, but want to continue your healthy living, or become healthier, more energetic and balanced mentally, physically, and spiritually and stay clear headed, and work, study, and live with more life quality, efficiency and a more unified whole being of mind, body and spirit, then you can read this book and practice mind-body health daily by following this book's teachings.

2. If you want to look younger and beautiful and want to live a long life without sickness, stress, fear, worry, or weakness physically, emotionally, mentally, then read this book and practice as taught.

3. If you do not feel good and notice you are stressful, tired, anxious, not sleeping well, have low energy, are unhappy or depressed, or do not look as good, beautiful or young as before, or notice that you are aging faster, or have any specific health concern, then you can read this book and keep practicing its concepts and skills daily.

4. If you plan to visit any holistic health practitioner or mind-body healthcare practitioner, you can read this book beforehand, to help you better understand the doctor in the session, enhance your healing capacity and help engender positive results. You also can let your holistic doctor know you are reading this book, so he/she can make your session resonate more smoothly.

5. If you are diagnosed with a physical or mental health issue, then, you may wish to use the tools in this book or visit a mind-body medicine doctor to complement the mainstream treatment that your family doctor has established.

6. If you want to learn mind-body medicine to help family, relatives, or friends, then you will learn useful tools among these pages.

7. If you are a healthcare practitioner of mainstream medicine, mental health practice, psychology, or alternative medicine, natural medicine, or other therapies, and want to learn mind-body medicine to help your patients holistically, comprehensively, emotionally and spiritually, then you can deepen your understanding in health science and practice, and glean many ideas and tools from this book.

8. If you are a student or trainee in life science of either conventional or alternative medicine, psychology, natural health, mental health, nursing science, physical therapy, etc., then you can read this book.

9. If you are a college student, youth or teenager and want to have a healthy, meaningful, and brighter more satisfying future life, as well as improve your learning, relationships, work, communication, empathy, and physical, mental, and spiritual strength, then this book is for you to read and practice.

10. If you are a couple of husband/wife or boyfriend/girlfriend, or you are an individual with or without an intimate partner or soul mate, or who has difficulty in or has failed in developing such a relationship and want to develop a mutually trustworthy, honest, compassionate, passionate, transparent, communicative, sharing, attractive, personal growing and improving, healthy, beautiful, transformational, inspiring, spiritual, motivating, encouraging, energetic, positive, resonating, joyful, happy, understanding, tacit, cooperative, helpful,

comforting, nurturing, caring, considerate, giving, forgiving, loving and lovely, lifetime relationship (familial or otherwise) at all levels – emotionally, spiritually, energetically, physically, sexually, intuitively, intellectually, informatively, financially, then you should read this book and truly practice as instructed in this book.

11. If you are a middle age, busy parent with children, working hard with stress and want to be a good parent, employee, improve family and work relationships and learn how to make your entire family stay healthy, peaceful, communicative, and happy mentally and physically, have a happy working relationship, environment and stable job, then this book is perfect for you to read, learn and practice.

12. If you are a parent(s) and wish your children at teen or young age to grow healthy mentally, physically and spiritually, having a peaceful and happy quality life while becoming a good citizen to serve the society, but avoid troubles or problems in their life, then you and your teenager children should read this book.

13. If you are a business owner, involved in high-level organizational leadership or management and feel the stress, responsibility, and overload of job tasks and need more energy, freedom of mind, new tools and wisdom to work efficiently, then please read this book and practice its techniques.

14. If you are a senior and concerned about your health, and want to have a happy and healthy retirement life as well as enjoy longevity, more all-around energy and harmony, then this is the book for you to learn and practice daily.

15. If you are a scientist and study health of the mind and body, childhood development and health, environmental medicine, environmental toxicology, palliative care, mental health problems such as depression, autism, ADD/ADHD, anxiety, OCD, and other chronic health issues such as pain syndromes, fibromyalgia, multiple sclerosis, diabetes, high blood pressure, and other mental and physical health problems, then this book will be beneficial to your research.

16. If you are not listed above, but simply want to learn mind-body health science, you can read this book and practice as instructed.

§1.5 The Aim of Mind-Body Science

Throughout the long history of human civilization, the truth of life, health, happiness, emotion, mind, soul, spirit, sickness, disease, death, and the universe has always been a most profound mystery. Modern sciences, including modern life science such as medical science, are still not able to reveal this truth. Such truth is just what the mind-body science we are learning now aims to search for.

Almost all fields of our existing sciences search the physical realm from outside world of our human beings. When we study within the field of mind-body medicine, however, we have to look inwardly into our human beings own selves, broaden and deepen our searching scope to beyond the physical level and extend it to deeper levels, cross over different dimensions of time and space, break through the confines of modern science, let go of our rigid notions and conceptions, and use new wisdom and extraordinary ideology to explore the truth. I have tried to maintain a broad vision throughout the writing of this book, incorporating my many years of mind-body-spirit cultivation, meditation, education and research in both modern conventional science and traditional health sciences, healing work experience, personal direct experience, intuition and spiritual understanding. This process has been accompanied by my deeply inspired meditations and out of a pure intention and compassion to share my understanding, findings, and spiritual messages.

That said, *Mind-Body Medicine & Healthology* is not just a list of holistic medicine therapies, spiritual healing, or psychological healing practices. Rather, it is an integration of ancient and modern medicine, Western and Eastern healing arts as well as human nature. There is a word in original Chinese, *Wu Xing* 悟性 (pronounced like *Wu Shing*), meaning the intuitive, inborn ability or perception to have a sense and understanding about spiritual (not denominational) depth of truth. Directly connected to one's inborn true Self and experience of life as well as the capacity to live a life of purpose and satisfaction, *Wu Xing* is so significant in Eastern traditions because it allows you to access to your pure spiritual ability within your inborn Self. And this allows you to observe, understand and deal with fundamental issues of life in a wise way. Due to many individual's overwhelming material lifestyle at modern time, however, people often have lost touch with this inborn ability. In so doing, they are considered at serious risk on all of levels of living. This ancient concept – not often written about – is a core principle of all holistic arts. As such, this book is additionally intended to help you improve *Wu Xing*, so that you can re-open your mind and regain its inborn power, and then truly and directly sense, feel, experience and resonate with the energy and truth of healing, health, and life at multiple levels. You will be able to, then, integrate, inspire and enlighten your whole being of mind, body and spirit toward the best positive changes and transformations.

§1.6 Modern Medicine Mainly Focuses on Physical Body

Let's briefly review the development and history of modern life science (modern medicine, mainstream medicine, or drug and surgery based medicine and its associated biological science) by looking back several centuries.

Modern medicine essentially began with Dutch naturalist, Antoni van Leeuwenhoek (1632–1723) as recognized by Royal Society of London for Improving Natural Knowledge – the UK's version of the Academy of Sciences [2]. Leeuwenhoek is credited with developing the medical use of microscopes to study objects – e.g. red blood cells, muscle fibers and bacteria that were invisible to human eyes. Leeuwenhoek's work is considered iconic in that it brought medical science to the cellular level, even though the connection between bacteria and disease was yet to be made.

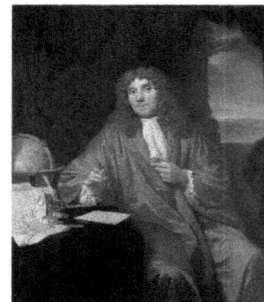

During the mid-1800s, French chemist and microbiologist Louis Pasteur proposed a hypothesis that germs cause diseases [3]. This theory is confirmed by his experiments conducted between 1860 and 1864 and by German doctor Robert Koch's research during 1880s   [4]. Throughout the next century, modern life science developed along with molecular biology, genetics, biochemistry, electronic engineering technology, computer science, and other modern sciences. Techniques such as X-ray (1895), Magnetic Resonance Imaging (MRI, 1952), nanotechnology (1959), CT (Computed Tomography or CT scanning, 1970s), functional MRI (*f*MRI, 1990s), DNA engineering, drug manufacturing, and all kinds of biotechnologies have been widely developed and applied to the modern medical research, diagnosis and treatment. All of this has given us the capability to see and work within the body at cellular level and molecular level [5].

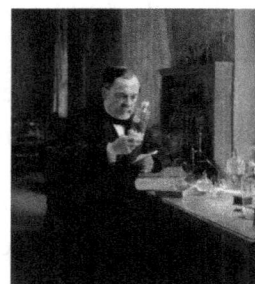

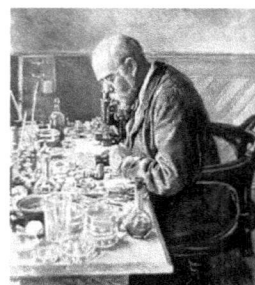

People are often fascinated with all these modern medical techniques described above because they enable us to see some detailed internal images of our physical body as well as to localize disease on the physical body. Such techniques have helped us deal with virus, bacteria, infections, tumors, and the like at the physical level. Many old-time diseases such as plague, fever, infectious diseases, epidemics, and tuberculosis (the list goes on) became relatively controllable.

Today, as human society develops with greater speed, however, an increasing number of new diseases and health problems have arisen. The most commonly known of these are: cardiovascular diseases, infectious and parasitic diseases, ischemic heart diseases, heart attack, cancers, stroke, respiratory infections, AIDS, digestive diseases, diarrhea diseases, chronic pain syndromes, fibromyalgia (FM or FMS), multiple sclerosis (MS), diabetes, high blood pressure, depression, anxiety, insomnia, imbalanced weight (e.g., obesity), attention deficit disorder (ADD), attention deficit hyperactivity disorder (ADHD), autism, and more and more newly developed modern diseases, including life-threatening viruses caused by genetic mutation – e.g. swine influenza (flu) virus H1N1~H7N9, and its series.

Unfortunately, the causes of many of these modern diseases are not clear when using only the "lens" of modern medicine, and many of them are not curable with modern medicine.

The World Health Organization (WHO) reports the number of cancer patients per year will increase by 50% to 15 million new cases in year 2020 [6]. The number of deaths per year due to cancer will increase from 6 million to 10 million. In the next 13 years, depression will become the second most common disease among humankind. 15-20% people of the world's population are already suffering from depression [7]. Leading science researcher Dr. Somnath Chatterji, from WHO (in Geneva), reported in HealthDay News that, "Compared to the chronic physical illnesses of angina, arthritis, asthma and diabetes, depression [now] produces the most decline in health" [8]. Disease knows no borders. Many people including the wealthy and the famous continue to suffer from so many physical and mental problems in spite of all of modern medicine's great advances. On the flipside, people do have good healthcare insurance that covers the mainstream medicine, the drug and surgery based medicine, and many individuals do have a very good material life as compared to ever before. But all of this data triggers many questions regarding our healthcare and well-being.

Why, for instance, with all the advancements in modern medicine, why is it that we cannot heal modern diseases? And why is it that we cannot help people achieve satisfaction in regard to their personal lifestyle healthcare needs? *Why with all of its enrichments has material life failed in providing good health, curing diseases and achieving the longevity people wish and hope for?*

The answer to the above question is obvious: modern medicine – as is – has been mainly or almost only focused on the physical structures, functions and biochemical processes of the physical body, but has not or has barely looked deeply enough into emotions, mind, spirit, belief, value system, personality, lifestyle, family and social relationships, as well as environments of growing, living, learning, education, profession and type of work, social system and social activities. These are all closely related with physical and mental health as well as character, emotions and spirituality. Modern medicine does not integrate the components and factors of the whole being as one unified life system to diagnose and treat. Modern medicine puts emphasis on what disease has affected a particular individual, more than on how and why a particular individual has contracted a specific disease?

Even when dealing with the physical body only, modern medicine is divided into so many meticulous fields, divisions, branches, clinics, specialties and subspecialties. For instance, internal medicine can have so many specialties such as cardiology, endocrinology, gastroenterology, hematology, oncology, nephrology, and so the long list goes on. A cardiologist, for example, usually only deals with cardiovascular system problems, and it is further divided into many subspecialties for specific areas such congenital heart diseases, heart failure, transplant, cardiac electrophysiology specialty, etc. Each of these deals with its own specialized field and related organ and system of the body, de-emphasizing the entire body and the person as a whole entity. Therefore, no matter how much advancement has taken place and no matter how much detailed knowledge about the physical structures, physiological functions and pathologic knowledge about the diseases it has acquired, modern medicine's understanding and treatment for the entire being (the mind, body and spirit) at multiple levels beyond the physical body is actually very limited. In fact the more detailed specialties within modern medicine are divided, the further away from the truth of whole being holistic health modern medicine delves into. This is because it has missed the most important key - the wholeness of the human being - the connection of all components of the life, mind-body-spirit. It is just like what the Chinese saying: "Pick up the sesame seeds, but overlook the watermelon," meaning one concentrated too much on trivial matters and neglected to pay attention to the much bigger and most important thing.

Despite the fact that modern psychology deals with the mind and emotions as a separate field from modern mainstream medicine, it is currently being driven by a tendency to rely on neuron science or brain science, which focuses on the emotional and spiritual behaviors and functions of the whole person as simply biological activities and biochemical/electrophysiological processes of the brain – the visible existence of the physical body. Some psychological practices even use n*eurological drugs* to treat psychological and emotional diseases as neurologists or psychiatrists do.

As such, modern medicine mainly or almost mainly deals with the physical body, but not all the components of the whole being of body, mind and spirit in an integrative way. It is not an exaggeration to say that modern medicine today actually should be called physical medicine or body medicine. Since the physical body is only the part of the whole being, it is not surprising that modern medicine has so many limitations in curing the whole person, especially in dealing with modern diseases that are caused by complicated causes at multiple levels such as those of the mind, emotions, and soul or spirit – as well as a person's environmental influencers, ranging from family/work environments to social and other life experiences and even, perhaps, within past lives [or other spiritual] factors [9].

To have a true healthy and happy life, modern medicine has to open its lens and deal more comprehensively with the entire being of body, mind and spirit and their inseparable relationship, which is what the mind-body medicine for [10].

§1.7 Mind-Body Science Deals with Your Whole Being

A human being is a living life not only equipped with the delicate physical body possessing complicated and well-designed structures and functions, but which is also mystically designed and equipped with a:

1) Powerful Mind – the set of cognitive faculties that enables consciousness, subconsciousness, perception, thinking, judgment, memory, emotions, feelings, will, desire, imagination, sentiment, etc. The mind is only partially facilitated by the physical brain, brain chemicals, nervous system and neurological biochemistries. It is also associated with after-born factors, e.g., family and social influences, education, spiritual inputs, etc.

2) Divine Spirit – the essential natures and vital principles of the human being; inspiring energy or animating energy within the being; soul thought, idea, creativity, character, manner, understanding, morality, passion, compassion, honesty, awareness of honor and shame, good and bad, caring, forgiveness, loyalty, tolerance, dedication, intuition, belief, spirituality, etc. at many levels.

The mind is established gradually. This happens throughout your entire life experience. The Spirit is a collective concept referring to the original natures of the human being that came from the original creature, the divine superior that evenly created all human beings with the same pure spiritual nature that is collectively called Spirit.

The Spirit exists in the higher spiritual dimensions beyond this physical realm where body and mind exist. The original natures of human spirit are never changed, but can be blocked, covered up, masked up, confused, temporarily or permanently contaminated, poisoned, distorted, or lost in this physical realm during this life or past lives.

The Spirit of an individual life after creation carries its own Virtue and Karma and passes on from one lifetime to another. A clear, unblocked and uncontaminated original spirit can lead the mind and body to grow in a healthy and beautiful way, resulting in a meaningful, healthy, spiritual, successful perfection of life. Such a mind bridges body and spirit in a comprehensive and cooperative way as a unified whole being.

The body, mind and spirit exist at multiple dimensions, associate with and influence each other. The key question is how are these life components associated and influenced by each other and integrated into one?

The connection of the body, mind and spirit is through a powerful energy field beyond the physical body and by a mysterious mechanism. The energy field crosses over all dimensions, from the spiritual world to the physical realm, and links the life components of body, mind and spirit together for their integration and synchronization. Although this is a hypothesis, it is suggested by ancient sciences, experience and practice throughout many thousands of years of cultivation, and can be supported by modern science. My personal clinical observations, over the years, within my private practice – particularly with regard to the positive effects of meditation, energy music therapy, and spiritual cultivation – provide further proof to the pudding, so to speak, and have increased my own understanding of this energy process and its finer (as well as truer) applications for healing, health, life transformation and enlightenment.

Energy is everything and everywhere in the universe in different forms, at different dimensions. It is like air or light that can pass through and cross over all different dimensions to unify the body, mind and spirit into one being. *Energy itself is the life within your life.*

Meditation, Qigong, Taiji (also spelled as Tai Chi), Yoga, religions, energy medicine, vibration medicine, human cultivation practice, and other spiritual practices are all working with this energy in their own way. This energy is a super-normal energy, with divine and spiritual characteristics and powers. To understand the truth about life and achieve true health, happiness and meaningful experiences for the whole being, we need to integrate, synchronize, harmonize and cultivate all components of the life, body, mind and spirit – as well as their sub-components – their energy, nature and character, through the process and approach of energy practice. As science or medicine, we call it mind-body medicine. And as self-healing and health practice, we call it mind-body healthology. This is the way that mind-body medicine and healthology deal with life, healing and health, as well as with research, diagnosis, treatment, practice, and cultivation.

§1.9 Energy of Mind & Spirit: Intellectual Living Matter & Energy

The energy we refer to in mind-body medicine and health practice mainly has two meanings: 1) energy in a form of ordinary matter such as biological substances in the body, nutrients in the food, environmental energies such as warmth, heat, coldness, oxygen, sunlight, radiation, magnetic energy, etc. 2) mental / conscious energy, spiritual energy and vital life energy, which are in higher dimensions, differing from the ordinary space-time dimension, not the ordinary matters, and can be tapped in many ways such as healing music and sound vibration, psychological and spiritual communication or conversation, family/social activities and influence, education, arts, relationships, hypnosis, biofeedback, meditation, other mind-body medicine treatments, mind-body-spirit cultivation, energy movements, other metaphysical, and spiritual practices, etc.

The first type of the energy is the relatively lower level of the physical realm that MBM gives attention to, but does not mainly focus on it. ***The second type of energy is the central focus of MBM.*** This second level is that of mental and spiritual energy. It consists of highly intellectual living matters and energies in higher dimensions. This energy is associated with the universe's natural law, spiritual natures, and energy process and mechanism. It pervades the universe, yet, exists in the background at other dimensions differing from this realm of space-time. To access and develop this energy, cultivation of mind-body-spirit is required. Only when a cultivator has reached a certain higher level in spiritual quality and energy will he or she have the power to enter other dimension(s) in the spiritual realms, connect to the higher spirit, and tap this energy. The cultivation of this energy is a process by which the cultivator returns to his or her original nature and simultaneously assimilates with that (the characteristics) of the universe.

§1.10 Intermediate Break: Story • Healing Music • Meditation

Before we end this chapter, let's read one healing story from one of my dear previous patients that will give you encouragement to get involved with mind-body learning and practice. Then we will pick one of our healing music CDs from the *Five Elements Energy Healing Series,* (can be found at www.mbmuedu.com/HealingMusic) and practice meditation for 30 minutes or one hour, whichever you are more comfortable with just now.

Brainwave-Meridian Therapy (BMT) Healed my Bladder and Kidney Infection from the Root [11]

- Mary A.

Nobody loves being sick. Especially, when you don't even know what the problem is, and neither do the doctors. This was my case. My journey to wellness began in late March 2003, when I began a series of illnesses that lasted for over a month. What began, as a bladder infection, or so I thought, then moved into a full blown flu, with terrible back aches and the list goes on, was really, in fact, a virus in my kidneys. I saw three Western medical doctors in three different areas of expertise. No matter what tests they did, they could not find something tangible to diagnose me with. Even the urologist that I saw, scratched his head and said, "You have had so many things going on, I don't know where to begin, so we will just begin a series of tests and go from there." This was in mid-April 2003. After my initial appointment with the urologist, I had to wait two weeks to see him again. Let's just say, that the idea of going through two more weeks of not going to the bathroom without pain and discomfort was not an option anymore! That's when I began seeing Dr. Jason Liu.

I never heard about Acupuncture-Music Therapy. I knew what Acupuncture was. But Dr. Liu's technique did not use needles. In my first session, he pinpointed my disease as low energy in my kidney meridian as well as in my liver. He even found out my physical illness was actually caused from stress and relationship related emotional blocks including anxiety, anger and depression. I was amazed at how clearly he was able to diagnose me by just listening to my pulse! From there the transformation began. The music was mesmerizing. It started with a guided meditation and then the music took over. Our sessions not only included the music and meditation, but Spiritual guidance. Each time, Dr. Jason Liu checked my pulse to see the progress. With each session, I was getting better and better. Little by little the pain was going away in all areas of my body, but the most amazing thing that I began noticing was how I was changing my perception of life, my thought processes, and how my focus shifted to bringing more peace and harmony to my Spirit. The physical challenges are only the manifestation of a Spirit's needs not being met or heard. I had no choice but to listen to my Spirit. What Dr. Liu did for me was heal me from the root. His Acupuncture-Music Therapy broke through the garbage of years of anger and negative energy blocks and cleared the path to the core so the Light could come in and heal me in mind, body and Spirit. I never met a Doctor or a healer that can do what Dr. Liu does. In my opinion, he does what a traditional Psychologist, a Massage Therapist, and Acupuncturist and Spiritual healer do all in one.

Dr. Jason Liu is also a warm and friendly man, who always emanates a positive energy, strong spirit and stable mentality. It is with these wonderful traits, that he has the ability to encourage people to heal and become whole again. I thank Divine Spirit for bringing Dr. Jason Liu into my life. You will too.

Music Healing Meditation for Chapter 1

If you have my energy healing music, you can use the following CD to practice meditation. If not, don't worry about that, you still can read the following instruction about the meditative image and meditate in silence.

The music is composed with focus on the relatively yang energy of water and wood elements to strengthen kidney and liver energy:

EHM01: Travel the Crystal Universe (Yang, Wood, Water)

However if you feel you are over heated, anxious, overwhelmed, have too much heat internally or feel too excited and ungrounded emotionally (yang type of condition), then you can choose the following CD (yin type of the healing music) to practice.

EHM02: Cultivate by the Quiet Lake (Yin, Wood, Water)

This one hour of energy meditation music takes you to the spiritual dimension and transforms your body, mind and spirit.

Sit cross-legged (if you can, otherwise just sit in a natural posture), or you may want to stand with relaxed posture if you sit too much over the day. And then, close your eyes and mouth, relax your entire body and keep your mind empty, peaceful and positive. Bring a peaceful smile to your face, and meditate with me (while listening to this healing music).

[*Play Energy Healing Music #1* while reading the following induction -] We are born from the beautiful, crystal, transparent universe. As a part of the vast cosmos, we have the same great nature of our divine mother of the universe. Now I invite you to join me and meditate with the peaceful, loving, compassionate, selfless, fearless, eternal, omnipotent, and energetic vibration of the universe. Please let go of all complicated thoughts and all stress from daily life, now you are a free spirit flying in the boundless cosmos. Its powerful super healing energy waves flow into your body, mind and spirit, bless you, heal you, purify you, rejuvenate you, energize you, and transform you to a totally new perfect being.

§1.11 Exercise Questions

1. For what purpose is this book written?

2. How do you understand the terms *mind-body medicine and mind-body healthology*? Please cite and define.

3. Who are included in the readership of this book? Are you in the list of readers and are there any other kinds of readers you want to add to the list?

4. What is the aim of mind-body medicine and healthology?

5. What does modern mainstream medicine focus on – the physical body or mental and spiritual aspects or both?

6. What does mind-body medicine and healthology focus on – the physical body only, mind only, spirit only, or all of them at the same time?

7. How are the body, mind and spirit associated with each other?

8. How do you understand energy or energy field as referred to in the mind-body-spirit connection and practice?

9. What has motivated you to learn mind-body medicine and healthology?

10. What is your goal in regard to leaning this field?

11. After reading the first chapter, do you feel your mind is opened or further opened than before, and you are ready for and interested in learning *mind-body medicine and mind-body healthology*?

12. Add our own questions to this exercise question list if you have any which help you summarize and extend the learning within this chapter.

SPIRIT

靈

MIND   BODY

心   身

CHAPTER 2

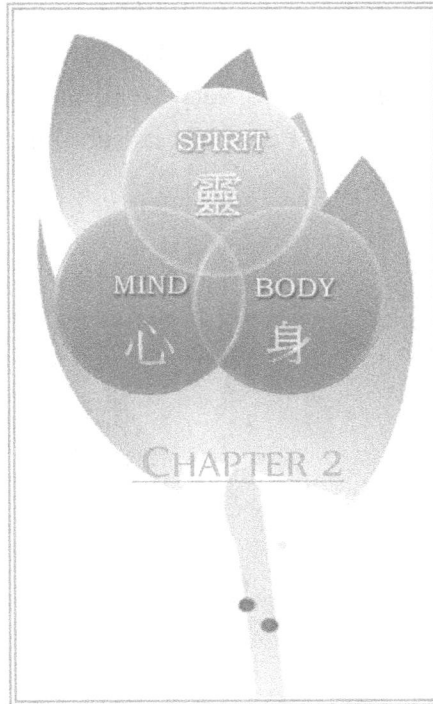

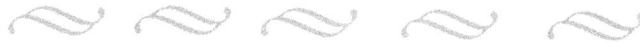

Definition • Ideology • Methods • Concepts • Practitioners

§2.1 The Anatomy of Mind-Body Medicine

MBM and MBH strive to make you more mindful of your life structure – the energy components that combined together to make your whole being. These are: Spirit, the fundamental life origin/essence; Mind, energetically your mid-level energy source; and Body, which is at the lowest level (superficial / physical realm) of energy. After becoming aware or experiencing each of these energy levels that are, in fact, your total being, you can learn to directly access them and how to use their influence to positively impact your life.

To do this, however, MBM drills into much more delicate and finer levels: from macroscopic levels, through the microscopic, cellular, molecular, and a subatomic particle level, as well as levels of composite particles and elementary/fundamental particles such as quarks, leptons, gauge bosons and Higgs particle, to the fundamental origin of living substances. Ultimately, this progression leads to the highest spiritual, intellectual matters and energy in other dimensions, which as we have noted differ in character from this space-time dimension. Therefore the life structure or anatomy of life in mind-body medicine is a very complicated system that is composed of multiple levels and components; from the physical BODY through the MIND, and finally to the SPIRIT. The physical body as treated by modern conventional medicine is only a very small and superficial part of life. Each component of the MIND, BODY, SPIRIT also has its sub-dimensional structures which are inter-connected and intra-interacted.

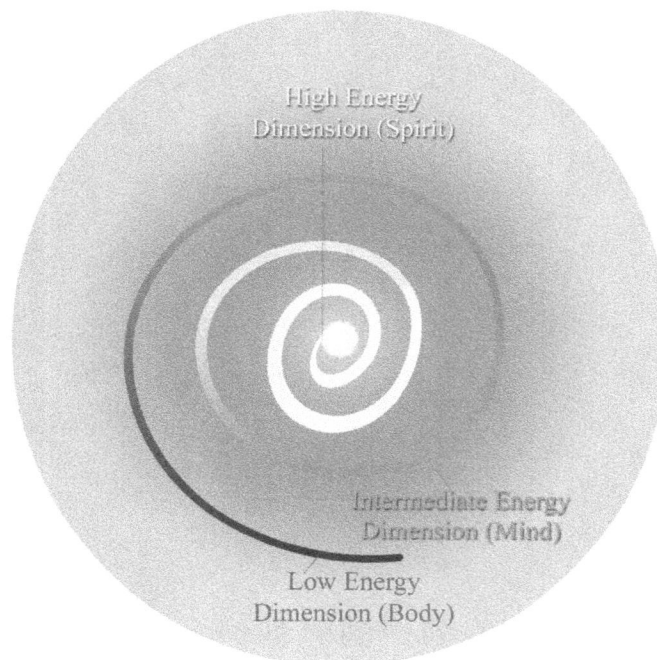

Fig. 2.1. BODY, MIND and SPIRIT are three primary components of a human being. They are one indivisible system connected together but at different dimensions - the physical dimension at low energy level (body, in darker red or darker black in black/white print), mental dimension at intermediate energy level (mind, in light red or lighter black / gray in black/white print) and spiritual dimension at high energy level (spirit, in bright yellow or light gray in black/white print). Each primary dimension also has many sub-dimensions. These primary dimensions as well as their subdimensions are connected through energy transferring and transformation mechanisms (*see* following sections and chapters for further discussions).

Fig. 2.1 uses an analogical image, a colored line, represents that the BODY, MIND and SPIRIT are an indivisible system but in different dimensions (*see* following chapters for more detailed discussion about the multiple dimensions of the BODY-MIND-SPIRIT). Differing from modern medicine, however, MBM integrates all these forms of energies and synthesizes all levels into one unified system.

In recent years, many scientists including mind-body medicine scientists and doctors have done a great job of incorporating brain science, neuron science, immunology, pathology, and other biological sciences with psychological science, behavior medicine, clinical psychotherapy, psychiatry, and mental health practices. They have established some new fields and created new terms such as psychosomatic medicine [2], psychoneuroimmunology[3] or immunopsychology, neuropsychology[4], etc. which are often called mind-body medicine. These fields, however, are mainly based on biological science at cellular or molecular levels (body science) and are rooted in the idea that consciousness, mind and spirit are functions of the brain – part of the body. However, not enough body-independent factors such as spiritual, mental, and energetic factors are considered within that outlook. With respect to these fields and opinions, in this book, we would like to break through the limits of body science, and provide essential informational additions as well as differencing viewpoints to these concepts, including ideas involving the origin of universe and its effect on life and living, characteristics of universe and lives, energy as a mechanism as well as a principle of the universe and lives, interaction and dependency between the universe and man, spiritual energy, mental energy, vibration frequency, frequency synchronization and distraction / disturbance, cultivation of mind-body-spirit and their energies, ancient and modern teachings on the mind-body-spirit connection from different sources and traditions, healing experiences, experiments, and research data with modern science and technology. And then, we can integrate all this knowledge into one simple and fundamental structure and model to understand, explain, improve, and develop the connection of mind, body, and spirit.

Our scope will include the biological science of the physical body (brain included), as well as opening our minds to the root connection of the body with the mind, spirit, and universe, including the more mysterious energies of other dimensions.

Experiments within the limitations of modern science and technology in this physical dimension may not immediately evidence this subtler, profound science. Yet, our fundamental structure and ideological model must work toward illuminating core truths.

---

[2] Psychosomatic medicine is an interdisciplinary medical field exploring the relationships among social, psychological, and behavioral factors on bodily processes and quality of life in humans and animals.

[3] Psychoneuroimmunology is the study of the interaction between psychological processes and the nervous and immune systems of the human body.

[4] Neuropsychology studies the structure and function of the brain as they relate to specific psychological processes and behaviors.

These must be correctly established without a narrow initial frame that could limit our scope, block our minds, and lead us to a very partial or even an erroneous conclusion that progresses us in the wrong direction.

§2.3 Inborn & After-Born Quality And Mind-Body-Spirit Energy

The quality and energy nature of a human being's mind, body, and spirit originates from two paths: past lives and this life. In other words, a human being has experienced (1) inborn (past lives) activities, which developed Virtue[5] and Karma[6] that passed onward to this life, and (2) after-born (this lifetime) activities, which develop Virtue and Karma. Virtue is good spiritual quality and nature that is recognized and blessed by the higher spirit and the law of the universe, while Karma is a sort of record created whenever the person acted out of accordance with universal laws (see later sections and chapters). The Virtue and Karma from an individual's past lives and this life together determine the quality and energy nature of the person's spirit, mind and body, thus determining the quality of the individual's current life and future lives.

In this life, the quality of the person's mental, physical, and spiritual character, their happiness or hardship, the good things or bad things, all are developed based on the Virtue and Karma generated while growing, living in family life, receiving an education, involvement in social activities, and the myriad of experiences throughout this life. An individual has consciousness and unconsciousness, emotions, feelings, thoughts, understanding, a value system, a belief system, moral quality, cultural edification, recognition, imagination, etc. Each person can have different inborn qualities and may have carried different energy in past lives, which can be passed to this life. Different experiences in this life can spark and develop different mental and spiritual energies, and corresponding consequences in Virtue and Karma within you. People may evolve different families, growing experiences, social environments, personal health practices, personal improvement

---

[5] Virtue: a good spiritual quality that carries good energy developed and accumulated through the past lives and current life, in accordance to the way one has behaved and cultivated by following the universe's law. Virtue appears as powerful bright substance in other dimensions. Virtue brings good life, health, happiness and fortunes. Sometimes Virtue is also called good Karma, but this book specifically defines good Karma as Virtue, and bad Karma as Karma.

[6] Karma: a bad spiritual quality that carries bad energy accumulated from past lives and current life due to one's actions and behaviors against universe's natural law. Karma appears as dark substance in other dimensions that brings difficulties, unhappiness, sufferings, sickness, and bad lucks in this life or future lives. Through cultivation with Universe's law, Karma can be eliminated and converted to Virtue. Note that sometimes people define Karma as good Karma (referred to as Virtue in this book), and bad Karma (just called Karma in this book).

practices, belief systems, and spiritual cultivation in this life through family influence, social influence, education, cultural activities, art learning and practice. All these make significant variations in their overall energy and spiritual quality (Virtue and Karma) and are related to the health and personal development of mind, body, and spirit. Some people may have such faith to have quality experiences and practice cultivation to improve mind-body-spirit natures that allow them to gain good quality of Virtue, but some individuals may not have these good experiences, and practice spiritual cultivation to improve themselves yet.

For now you can understand Karma and Virtue as bad and good energy, respectively. When one behaves by following the natural laws of the universe, Virtue is earned, resulting in good consequences to him/herself, while when one does bad thing against the natural laws of universe, Karma is created, causing bad results to him/herself. This is called Cause-Effect Relationship or Causality[7].

Here we introduce a non-leaner function equation to express this natural law:

$$R = F(x_1, x_2, x_3, \ldots x_i \ldots x_n)$$

Where R is the result, effect or consequence, and F is the function of factors or causes $x_1, x_2, x_3, \ldots x_i, \ldots x_n$, and i is an integer number of the ith factor (cause), and n is the total number of factors. A result can be a cause of another result, while a cause also can be the result of other cause(s). These results (effects) and causes (factors) are linked based on the natural law of Cause-Effect-Relation. In mind-body-spirit science, this is due to the mechanisms of inter- and intra- energy transformation and transferring within and between multiple dimensions in the universe (*see* following chapters). At human level, for instance, the following are some circumstances presenting the facts - some causes cause the results in our life, and these results become causes that further cause other results, and so on:

An individual has his/her specific inborn characteristics, Virtue and Karma genetically and spiritually, as well as particular growing environments, family activities, social activities, education, experiences, behaviors, activities and all doings in this life, which are causes (factors, $x_1, x_2, x_3, \ldots x_i \ldots x_n$). These factors form his/her specific mental, emotional and spiritual characteristics, manners, value system, beliefs, lifestyle, thinking patterns, conscious modes, ideas, notions, attachments, addictions, habits, mindset, temper,

---

[7] **Cause-Effect Relationship** (also called **Cause-Effect, Causality** or **causation**) is the relation between an event as *cause* (factor) and the second event as effect (consequence) of the first event. There can be multiple factors that cause one or more consequences. Causality is a natural law applying to common phenomena in the natural world, social world, and human life.

and behaviors, which are the results (*R*) of the causes. With all these influences (causes), the person thinks, behaves, and lives as a particular entity in the form of a whole being, body-mind-spirit (results, but also the causes for further results). All these physical, mental, and spiritual characters, activities, environments and experiences influence the person's mind-body-spirit health, personal development, growth, psychological or mental characteristics, behaviors, and daily performances, leading to all the outcomes of his/her life (e.g., life quality, health, relationship, financial, luck, difficulties, etc.) as final results.

Different from modern medicine that focuses on the physical body and its structures and which functions via the limited findings of experimental sciences such as biochemistry, physiology, biology or pharmacology, the mind-body medicine's methods, ideas, and procedures involve mental and spiritual energies from inborn qualities and after-born activities, experiences and internal (within one's self) and external (interacting with others and environments) energy processes. As such, an open-minded, spiritual and distinguished ideology, methodology, mindset and procedure in mind-body medicine help you glimpse into and better understand the inseparable interactions of your own (or another's) mind, body, and spirit, so that you can deliver the appropriate healthy energy and healing energy into its multiple dimensions.

§2.4 Different from Modern Science Ideology and Methodology

Mind-body medicine's focus and emphasis on the entire being determine its ideology and as such make its methodologies totally different from those of conventional medicine and modern life science. The understanding, study, diagnosis, treatment, healthcare practice and cultivation practice for a whole person of mind, body and spirit cannot simply rely on the biological, physiological, biochemical or other medical researches with laboratory experiments on the physical body, organs, tissues, cells, molecules and so on within the physical dimension. Indeed in mind-body medicine, we have to involve the mind and spirit, and their character, quality and energy as well.

Soul, spirit, mind, emotion, consciousness and sub-consciousness are in the energetic invisible dimensions that cannot be directly seen by human eyes, nor measured or detected by modern scientific tools, techniques or experimental methods in this physical dimension. It's true that we sometimes try to use the means of modern science and technology to demonstrate evidence that mental and spiritual energy can be transformed to physical, physiological or biochemical energy and improve health (see later chapter on some researches on MBM), but in most cases, the understandings and practices in mind-body medicine are not based on laboratory experiments or researches, but often obtained through (1) inspiration from divine spirits, (2) spiritual teaching, experience and traditional approaches taught by sages and ancestors, and passed down from generation to generation, (3) messages and energies from spiritual dimensions, (4) knowledge accumulated and developed and improved over history, as well as through personal experience, and cultivation. To continue its growth, open, intuitive, practical and inspired minds are necessary and must be extended to experience a newer, brighter and bigger picture. This will lead to a more complete vision and practice, better health on all levels, less suffering, and greater joy.

So, ideas and knowledge in mind-body health science are not "so much" or only based on laboratory experiment, biological research or modern medical research. On the contrary, most of the wisdoms in this field are obtained from mind-body cultivation practice, direct experience, messages obtained from higher divines and through the application practice. Although this book sometimes cites modern scientific research, in many cases, we address the same issue from different sources of wisdom such as teaching from ancient human cultivations and traditions, cultivation practice, meditation and clinical experiences. Part of the knowledge in this field is based on the modern science, yet in many parts, it may not have experimental supporting data. This is due to a few factors – but particularly because of the limitation of science and technology in this physical dimension. This is also due to traditional differences guiding the concerns of mind-body medicine throughout history. Traditional Eastern psychology and Western psychology, for instance, are quite different in approach. Whereas in the Western psychology there is emphasized interest into the difference between cognitive and emotional states, Eastern psychology is more interested in the difference between afflicted and non-afflicted states of mind and body, with its aim on putting an end to an individual's suffering by identifying and clearing its root causes crossing times from past lives to this lifetime at all dimensions of mind, body and spirit. As well, in Western sciences there is no notion of non-sensory cognition whereas in mind-body medicine and holistic psychology we place, as mentioned earlier, a lot of significance on *Wu Xing* (a kind of sixth sense plus self-wakening cognition from the original Self) which, again, refers to the mental and spiritual realm and includes intuitions, perceptions and conceptions. The problem is that modern medicine's approach often leaves out both MIND (the individual's subject experience) and SPIRIT. This exclusion, from the mind-body science point of view, limits its ability to identify "the root(s) of one's suffering and offers only partial relief. That said, an ongoing dialog between the two traditions could be helpful and valuable to all. This book opens the mind to bring both Western and Eastern traditions together in attempt to appreciate cognitive, emotional and psychological science (Western approach) and at the same time to explore the deep root causes involving man and universe at all dimensions and the entire lifetime (including past lives and this life), while seeking the fundamental solution through mind-body-sprit cultivation practice.

Hence, one who has a narrowed mind or has become skeptical and dysfunctionally analytical and hardened in attitude may not easily understand some aspects we addressed in this book. However, if you open your mind and read this book with a humble and positive attitude for discovering and learning how to practice a new and different field of knowledge, and if you are willing to directly experience its effects of actual practice in your personal life, then you can begin to reap its benefits.

§2.5 Fish-Water Model - Works with All Energy Sources

Hardware and Software – An Imperfect Analogy

As we have discussed, what modern medicine does is to deal with the ordinary matter or physical substance that is visible, measurable or detectable in this physical dimension including the physical body of human beings and chemical drugs. It uses chemicals and physical tools, within a range of technologies such as X-ray, CT scan (computed Axial Tomography / CAT scan), ultrasound, MRI (magnetic resonance imaging), *f*MRI (functional MRI), biotechnologies, bio-products, and so on. These tools directly or indirectly provide the information or images of the physical structure of the body. They tell us how the physical body's organs, tissues, cells, bones and blood vessels look. In terms of the chemicals or pharmaceuticals, these can make some biochemical modifications on these organs, tissues, cells, nerves, genes and their molecules as chemically reacting targets, isolated from the mind and spirit. They do not, however, make fundamental improvement on the vital life force or energy, the person's feelings, emotions, thoughts, personality, character, spirituality, life-style, or other psychological and spiritual factors, or how these factors affect or interact with the physical body. This emphasis on the physical body alone, at best, blurs the majority of the whole being, which is integrated with other dimensions (to which you will be introduced in the next chapter).

Consider this: Figuratively speaking, the body alone can be likened to computer hardware, the metal part, which has no intelligent functions, and cannot do anything without software. Yet, modern medicine's typical approach is to recognize only the hardware. It deals with your physical body alone and doesn't put much care into emotions, mind and spiritual characteristics. This analogy, granted, is not exactly the same situation (the body is with the mind and spirit as one system so it is not like the hardware and software as separate parts), but the point holds.

Fish-Water – A Model to Explain the Mechanism

As shown in Fig. 2.5.1, imagine the pond with fish swimming inside – the fishes are the physical body, including the organs, tissues, cells, hormones, bloods, etc. The water and plants are the mind, consciousness and subconsciousness, spirit, emotions, environments (e.g., family, society, etc.), energy field, the universe, and other psychological, emotional, spiritual and energetic elements. These comprise the environment, conditions, and energy source in which the fish live. Carrying the analogy further, modern medicine deals with the fish but not the entire pond. Mind-body-spirit medicine deals with all these components, including the fish and all their surroundings as well as invisible energies from the universe which are affecting them.

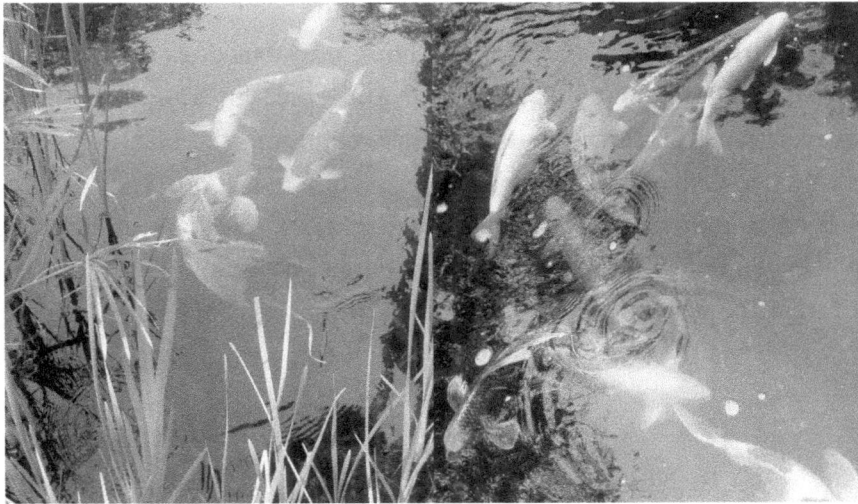

Fig. 2.5.1. Fish-Water Model explaining the whole being mechanism of mind-body-spirit medicine.

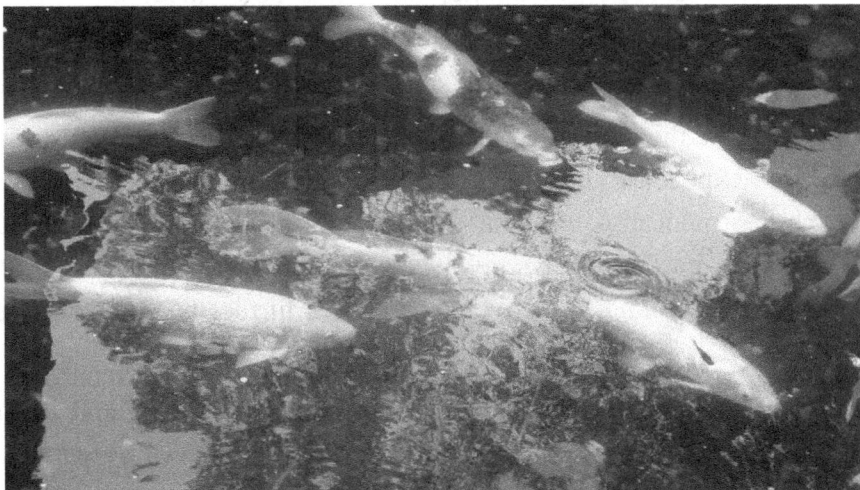

Fig. 2.5.2. In this Fish-Water Model, the water is poisoned with toxins, and fish are sick. Mind-Body Medicine as a whole being practice deals with cause of sickness and works to purify the water (mind, spirit and energy) as well as the fish itself (body), while modern medicine's focus deals only with the fish.

Of course, this is still not a perfect example because there is no perfect form with which to liken mental and spiritual energy in other dimension(s). Nonetheless, I believe the visual helps us better appreciate the point.

When the water became poisoned with toxins (Fig. 2.5.2.), the fish got sick. Focused only on the fish, modern medicine's first and only treatment was pharmaceutical. It did not deal with the water (emotion, mind, spirit, energy, surroundings, and universe) beyond the fish (body). In fact, the contaminated or poisoned water (energy field) was the actual cause of the fish's sickness. The point is that treating only the fish without cleaning and detoxifying the water (energy field, mental and spiritual elements and living environments), will never heal the sickness from the root. This is the way of modern medicine that uses drugs to treat the physical body only but does not attend to the energy within and surrounding the body – the mind and spirit in all dimensions. Mind-body medicine, however, puts all components together, including the body, mind, spirit, energy and environments (the fish, water as well as the plants, fish foods and all things inside the water), to understand and treat the causes of the sickness. We look at the integrated whole and consider the mutual influence and deep connections and relations between these components to treat the whole being and restore health from root.

Different Treatments - Modern Medicine & Mind-Body Medicine

Let's take cancer treatment as a specific example to further explain what is different between modern medicine (body medicine) and mind-body medicine (mind-body-spirit medicine).

Chemotherapy and radiation treatment for a cancer patient are aiming to kill cancer cells with attempt to cure the cancer. In fact as the result of the treatment, good cells (non-cancer cells) are also exposed to the cancer drug or radiation and become damaged during the treatment. The treatment also weakens the patient's immune system. This is why after the treatment the cancer patient always gets very weak and life becomes difficult in many aspects, often taking a long time to recover. Sometimes further health problems are caused by the treatment.

In mind-body medicine, however, we consider the cancer itself and also consider the cause, environment, energy field, and mental and spiritual factors that may cause or trigger the cancer condition. We involve a wide range healing resources, including the healing power within the patient – his or her own life force, as well as that found within nature and that which can be cultivated from the universe, divine spirit, mental and/or emotional energies, and so on.

The methods can be psychological, spiritual, energetic, and may include conversation, music and/or sound therapies, hypnotherapy, meditation, Qigong, energetic exercises, nutritional and therapeutic diet, natural herbs, acupuncture, mind-body-spirit cultivation, self-healing practice, spiritual and mental supports from relationships, families and communities, etc. These approaches produce a powerful healing energy field and vibration frequencies that go deeply into the body to strengthen the immune system, enhance the microcirculation, and cleanse cancer cells' microenvironment, restoring and re-harmonizing the healthy condition surrounding and within the cancer, as well as inhibiting the cancer's growth and further spreading. Although this is a hypothesis because modern science is not yet able to perfectly approve it, this hypothesis is suggested by existing researches [12].

Cancer scientists believe that cancer could originate from alterations in intercellular signaling through gene that resulted in the transformation of cells, their uncontrolled proliferation and metastasis. There are increasing evidences that demonstrate that the surrounding matrix and cell-matrix interactions are the major players in this process, involving cells adhering and receiving signals from various extracellular matrices via transmembrane receptors, such as the heterodimeric glycoproteins, integrins and others [13, 14].

"In the last ten years, a more holistic understanding of cancer slowly emerged, stressing the importance of interactions between neoplastic and various stromal components: extracellular matrices, basement membranes, fibroblasts, endothelial cells of blood and lymphatic vessels, tumor-infiltrating lymphocytes, etc. Nevertheless, the commonly held view is that changes in tumor microenvironment are 'soft-wired,' that is: epigenetic in nature and often reversible. On the other hand, there exists a large body of evidence suggesting that well-known mutations in cancer genes profoundly affect tumor milieu. In fact, these cell-extrinsic changes might be one of the primary reasons such mutations are preserved in late-stage tumors." by the author of *Cancer Genome and Tumor Microenvironment,* Thomas-Tikhonenko [15].

Regarding the microenvironment of cancer genome (set of chromosomes containing all of an organism's inheritance traits) or cancer cells mentioned here, there are many layers of meanings. Besides the meaning addressed above by the scientists of cancer genetics, here in mind-body medicine we do refer to a much deeper meaning. The microenvironment of cancer genes or cancer cells means not only the surrounding substantial contents of the cells or genomes, but also the energy field, and spiritual, psychological, emotional, conscious and subconscious energy filed within the microenvironments.

In mind-body medicine, we believe that the subtler energies we attend to, which operate as mysterious particles with vibration frequencies spreading within – surrounding and beyond the physical structures of the body, the cells, genes, and all other cellular, extracellular, molecular, atomic, nucleus and particles' contents and structures play into the picture. An idea we think of, an emotion we feel, a word we talk, an action we take, a thought, notion, habit, attachment, addiction, and lifestyle, all of these actually produce vibration frequencies that carry energies. These energies can be bad or good, positive or negative, healthy or unhealthy, healing or disease causing. In addition, all of this can affect the physical body, including microenvironments of all internal contents and structures. For instance, if using cancer development as example, we believe that the mutation or alternation of the genome that causes cancer is probably initiated or triggered by the process involving an emotional, mental, spiritual, and subtle energy disturbance, imbalance, stress, or disharmony. This process may occur through a series of unknown stages in any possible period during this life.

Many researches indicate that the stress of modern life is most likely the cause of cancer. Stress can be caused by many factors such as psychological (e.g. negative emotions such as worry, fear, anxiety, depression, etc.), physical, living or work environments, quality of relationships, lifestyle, habits, inborn character, attachments on life issues, job nature, financial, and stresses of unknown causes as well as stress with combinations of all or some of the factors described above. Such stresses can cause cellular, molecular, genetic alternation and disturbance, thus resulting in cancer or other diseases. Therefore, in mind-body medicine, we use different approaches to produce powerful and profound energies or frequencies to deeply permeate the whole being, connect the mind-body-spirit, and restore the harmonious life force, purify the molecular and cellular microenvironments, restore the healthy microenvironments, and rectify the alternation or mutation of the cells, genes, or other cellular or molecular sickness factors, and, as a result, heal the disease.

Of course we do not refuse drug, surgery and radiation treatment, especially for a disease like cancer at its late stage or early stages, but from the point of view of mind-body medicine, we believe that a holistic approach can efficiently heal the disease and maintain daily health from the root, by treating and preventing the causes.

In the fish-water model described in this chapter, the water and surrounding environments of the fish do not only represent the visible surrounding environments of human living conditions, but also importantly represent the universe's energy, vibration, spirit, and characteristics – the individual's energy, emotions, mind, soul, character, lifestyle, and so on as the energy sources of life. The principles, concepts, ideology, methodology and practice of mind-body medicine and healthology adhere to and work within this holistic model. The healing energy is in an invisible form, but permeates the entire body and body-mind-spirit unit. It heals and energizes the whole being of life by treating the all-in-one life system as a synchronized energy form. This energy practice of harmonizing, balancing and rejuvenating the life force is the key focus of mind-body medicine and healthology.

§2.6 Methods, Truth & Integration

Some of the energy models employed by mind-body medicine include Qigong, Taiji, energy movement, meditation, hypnosis, visualization, music sound vibration, arts, psychological conversation, brainwave treatments, biofeedback, neuron feedback, muscle tests (applied Kinesiology), acupuncture, herbs, nutrition, healthy diets, environmental healing, natural health, herbs, spiritual cultivation practice, etc.

As a science which reveals and explores truths in other deeper energetic dimensions, the limited instruments and tests commonly employed in this physical dimension do not always allow us to perform experiments confirming the total results of these techniques, nor give a logically perfect explanation of their efficacy. Nonetheless, MBM demands exploration and the extraction of information and wisdom from these areas within which we cannot always demonstrate evidence. However, this does not mean we cannot find the truth. There is no such rigid logic that insists only technique-proven-truth is the truth or it is not the truth. If restricted by existing science and technology, the science and truth of mind-body-spirit and universe will never be achieved.

Some skeptical people, including some scientists, may say if there is no way to experimentally demonstrate the evidence, then you should not refer to it as science. I disagree with such a comment or statement although I do understand why they think that way. However, if you very rigidly define the science as the knowledge that is only based on the evidence obtained from laboratory-based experiments, which is designed and performed by humankind's limited ability and tools, then such so-called science or knowledge will be also very limited, and far away from the real truth.

The truth exists out there no matter if you discover the evidence for it or not. The nature and principle of the universe exists out there no matter if you have evidence for it or not. The cosmos is operating all the time and beings living within it are following comic law no matter if you have evidence or not. We can discover and know truth from an experiment that we can design and perform under existing laboratory conditions, or from existing knowledge that we can use to explain, but we can also know truth from all other possible pathways if our minds open to the broad cosmic and profound spiritual realms through a highly cultivated state and wisdom.

These pathways include direct and indirect experiences, facts, teachings, inspiration, wisdom, intelligences, linear or nonlinear logics or even from the imagination or intuition (with careful confirmation by combination with other facts), and messages from the spiritual world (with good principle guidance and clear mind) in the deep spiritual cultivation state, as well as from ancient sages, higher divine spirits, and our own Selves - our direct experiences and practices in the past, throughout history, and today.

Therefore, when we study mind-body medicine and healthology, our methodology and ideology must be changed and extended to many ways that are not relying on or not only relying on laboratory experiment or existing science or knowledge. We must be fully open-minded; take a special path to maximize our learning, understanding and ability to discover and optimize all possible resources available throughout human civilization. All these together will help us paint the picture of the truth and establish the fundamental principles, structures and practical skills of this profound and mysterious science and practice: the spirit-mind-body (words intentionally reversed) medicine and healthology. The special path we mentioned here means anyone of us, as a learner, teacher, doctor, practitioner, therapist, patient, or any everyday individual interested in this field must be an actual cultivator of mind-body-spirit, so you can gain the direct experience by yourself, connect to the higher spirit, obtain the divine wisdom and extraordinary inspiration and knowledge on mind-body-spirit cultivation and enlightenment science (the truth), and reach a higher level of life – spiritually, mentally and physically.

Our resources include ancient teachings on human cultivation, philosophy, energy healing and longevity, Eastern and Western traditional medicine, classic books and scripts, stories of the grandmasters of ancient physicians or cultivators, and principles and techniques of natural healing and spiritual healing modalities, modern science of mind-body medicine, mental health, psychology, immunopsychology, neuropsychology or psychoneuroimmunology, neuroscience, energy medicine, quantum medicine, other fields of science including natural sciences, arts, religions and spiritual beliefs.

All these fields reveal truth at different levels and from different angles. An ultimate principle is needed to provide an overall guidance and integrative connection between all these fields.

Many scientists, doctors or researchers in all these fields are trying to tell their findings about mind, body and spirit from their point of view in their fields. Such a wide range of knowledge bases or fields of sciences provide a great reference resource. However, it does not mean all these theories, understandings or findings tell the fundamental truth and ultimate integration of the mind-body-spirit.

Here in this book, however, we are trying to establish a "science" (new science in different definition as mentioned above) regarding the mind, body and spirit we are going to learn will be a core truth, original teaching, faithful inheritance and comprehensive integration based on the ancient wisdom and modern science throughout the thousands of years of human cultivation. Rather than simply packaging each of these knowledge and understandings together into the areas mentioned above, we will try to draw a clear and simplified picture about the mind-body-spirit by using some basic concepts such as supreme universal laws, energy principle / mechanism, energies in different dimensions, intra and inter-dimensional energy transformation, energy generation and energy consuming models, etc. This picture, in which some mechanisms and principles are presented, will provide a practical guide for the mind-body science and its practitioners, doctors, patients and any individuals who want to learn, practice, study or research in this field or simply want to learn this practice to improve own health or help others. We will address these fundamental concepts, theories and models, and then integrate them and apply them in the following chapters.

§2.7 Consider All Factors of Surroundings And Beyond

In mind-body medicine and healthology, we extensively consider a human being as a part of the universe and rooted into the original spirit or spiritual nature of the universe. Born from the universe, we carry, within us, the universe's characteristics – our spiritual root. This root is what we rely on as fundamental life force during this entire lifetime.

At the same time, we consider the human being in this physical life, as the genetic, biological and psychological being birthed of his/her parents and as part of the family in which the individual grows up and lives with. We consider the human being as a part of the school in which the individual is educated, as part of the company or organization for which the person works, as a part of the society in which the person involves himself or herself, and as a part of relationships in which the person engages. We think that all these elements contribute to and determine how the particular person is and behaves – his/her personality, character, behavior, lifestyle, customs, habits, emotions, thoughts and ways of thought, manner of communication behavior, beliefs, value system, notions, and understanding regarding the meaning or purpose of life – as well as his/her body type, nutrition, condition, living and working profession and environments, family and social relationships. All these factors produce energy vibrations in different dimensions from higher spiritual levels to lower physical realms, resulting in his/her health condition and mental and spiritual state and behavior physically, mentally, psychologically and spiritually as a whole being. Sometimes this information and other factors surrounding the person in this life are yet not enough, so we may have to go beyond this life and further to learn about the person's past lives that can carry forth previous messages, characters, faith, spirituality, Virtue, Karma and energy vibrations resulting in a certain impact to this life.

In mind-body medicine study and practice, we do not only access broadly all these surrounding factors in this life and past lives as mentioned above, but also most importantly we open up all these areas for the person to access, understand, experience, develop, synchronize, unify, assimilate and practice with, and finally be one with all these factors and the synchronized energy vibration based on a simple core principle - the ultimate law and energy mechanism as the standard or principle to follow and practice (see ongoing sections and chapters). As a result, the true health and integration of mind, body and spirit are achieved.

It is not easy to reach all areas and understandings about mind-body medicine as described above. If a doctor or practitioner of mind-body medicine does not practice cultivation of mind, spirit and body, and does not have such a broad, profound and extraordinary sense, intelligence, wisdom, energy and as well as such direct experience by his/her self, it is impossible for him/her to have the broad view and access to all these areas and dimensions, and to lead others into this field or help patients to heal and improve their health and life. The practice of mind-body medicine is not based on the human logical understanding, analytical thinking or human level of efforts, while it needs to work with, behave and function at, high level of energies in other dimensions where the mind, spirit, soul and emotions exist. The practitioner has to let go of human mind, narrowed thoughts, attachments, and cultivate mind nature and spiritual quality to assimilate with the universe's spiritual energy vibrations, and then obtain higher energies from other dimensions, spiritual and mental dimensions, and higher divines while he or she practices spiritual cultivation and elevates his/her Virtue energy level.

§2.8 Core Principle - Being One with the Universe

Throughout its long history, mind-body medicine deeply originated from ancient divine teaching though it named differently within different historical periods in which it had been enriched with different connotations and forms. Its teaching provides humankind with a way to practice understanding, staying with, and connecting to the profound and powerful energy source and spirit of the universe in order for human beings to be synchronized, unified, harmonized, integrated, balanced and assimilated with the universe's characteristics and energy vibration frequencies.

This teaching was initiated by Lao Tzu (~? 600 BC - ?) in his book *Tao Te Ching* (*see* details in next chapter). Confucius (551-479 BC) was Lao Tzu's student who met Lao

Tzu often to learn *Tao* during the same period of history (Fig. 2.8). The central point of Tao Tzu's teaching is called 道（*Dao* or *Tao*）in Chinese, which means the way, the truth, the origin, the mystery, the energy and the super power for the universe to operate, and for lives including human beings to stay healthy, balanced and transformed physically, mentally and spiritually.

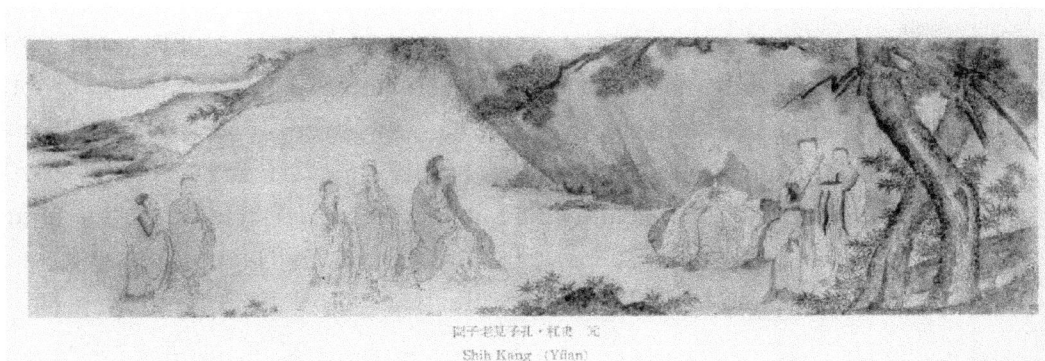

孔子老見子孔·紅畫　宋
Shih Kang (Yüan)

Fig. 2.8. Confucius visited Lao Tzu to learn *Tao* (孔子問道).

As such, the purpose of practicing Tao is to live in harmony with the universe as the life origin, its true Self, of which human beings were born and stay within, thus becoming a unified whole being of body, mind and spirit. This fundamental principle is called *Being ONE with the Universe* or *Man and Cosmos are ONE* (天人合一 Tian Ren He Yi, in Chinese), or called *Heaven-Human Induction* (天人感應，Tian Ren Gan Ying) / *Interactions Between Heaven and Human.*

It remains unclear when and who originated the concept of *Heaven-Human Induction*. But so far most ancient history and philosophy researches believe that influenced by Lao Tzu's thought of *Tao*, the ancient Chinese scholar, Dong Zhongshu 董仲舒 (179-104 BC), was the one who first *initiated* this thought: "Heaven also has joy, anger, sadness and happiness, which match with human beings. Heaven and Man are One." ("Spring Autumn Fan Lu · Yin Yang Yi") [16]. In fact the ideology of "Heaven and Man are One" or "Heaven- Man Induction" had been the most fundamental and central concept and practice in ancient life cultivation systems, philosophic systems, and ancient science systems including *I Ching*, Confucianism, Taoism, medicine, and longevity practice.

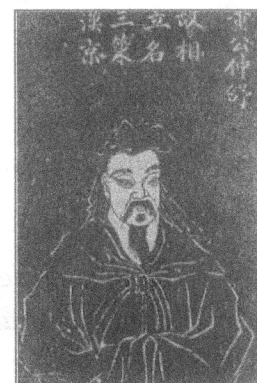

Nowadays many people cannot understand the true meaning of this concept, and think that Dong Zhongshu just simply personified and humanized the heaven, and made an anthropomorphic description about heaven based on human emotions. But in fact Dong Zhongshu was a Tao practitioner and longevity cultivator. By following the principle of Heaven-Man Induction, he cultivates Virtue with respect of Heaven's nature and cultivates energy (Qi or Chi) by directing it throughout the body via the feet (天氣常下施於地，是故道者亦引氣於足). His ideology teaches the secret that human beings came from the universe and they have the same character and spiritual nature as the universe has, both can mutually interact and influence to each other, and heaven governs everything including the human world. Therefore mankind should learn, follow, practice and assimilate with the universe's nature in order to live healthy and in harmony. His Heaven-Man Induction theory was applied to ancient social science, politics, social and family relationships, and greatly influenced medicine and healthy longevity practice.

Achieving the *Oneness with Heaven* is the true meaning and goal of life. Therefore when a human being returns to the original true Self and becomes one with the universe, his/her mind, body and spirit are integrated into a perfectly unified whole being - the same characteristics as those of the universe – thereby achieving an eternal life.

Today "Being One with the Universe" is still the most fundamental principle of the mind-body-spirit medicine / healthology and life cultivation. It is also the main goal and practice of human life. Therefore, the science of mind-body medicine or healthology is not just a life science or medical science, while it is indeed an extremely profound study and practice, most meaningful lifetime learning, practice and cultivation. Learning in this field is a fantastic life path of truth searching and a joyful journey of health practice and life enlightenment. When we learn mind-body medicine, we need to set our thinking mode and mentality in an open-minded state, letting go of human notions, attachments, rigid logic, narrowed thinking, ideas or skeptical attitude, experience, social influence, and preconceived notions which have been formed in this lifetime, and block your way to step into the profound kingdom and discover the golden treasure, the higher truth and life enlightenment.

No matter how many different techniques, modalities and concepts mind-body medicine teaches and practices, Oneness of Heaven and Man as the core principle of the mind-body medicine and cultivation system will never change.

To be one with the universe, a practitioner must learn, practice and assimilate with the characteristics of the universe. Only when being one with the universe and synchronized with the universe's characteristics, can the practitioner obtain the divine power and energy of the universe to sustain good health at a high level of life - as a whole being, the body, mind and spirit. This principle will be applied throughout the entire teaching and practice of the mind-body medicine and mind-body cultivation. In the following sections and chapters we will further explore and practice this principle.

§2.9 MBM Is Mind-Body-Spirit Cultivation Practice

Different from other fields of modern science, mind-body medicine is not just a pure theory, principle, logic, concept, hypothesis, or idea. It is actually a cultivation practice for the quality and life force energy of body, mind and spirit. The energy cultivated is an invisible energetic substance originated from spiritual divine essence, profound wisdom, true nature, and character of the universe. The energy is carried by and within each of living being itself, and can be felt, benefited from, obtained and elevated only when one directly practices the mind-body-spirit cultivation.

A student, healer or doctor of mind-body medicine should actually practice the techniques of meditation, Qigong, Taiji, hypnosis, visualization, imagery therapy, acupuncture, acupressure, energy music therapy and sound healing, herbs or other practices, but also cultivate the nature of mind and spirit to assimilate with the character of universe. These modalities are not just practices to heal others, but also self-healing and cultivation practice towards higher levels of body, mind and spirit for clients as well as practitioner.

Note: Within the history of ancient times, there were many masters, physicians and healers who achieved high levels of healing and possessed miracle power such as Hua Tuo, Bian Que, Zhang Zhongjing, Sun Simiao, Shen Nong, Li Shizhen, etc. They were actually Tao cultivators with super normal ability and great compassion to reach deep energetic dimension and heal people.

§2.10 The Earth Family Needs to Cultivate For Peace & Health

Every individual comes from the universe. And although we have within us the great nature of the universe, we also have to deal with the lower levels of the human mind - dysfunctional thoughts, actions, and feelings and even evil. Cultivating the good energetic characteristics and eliminating the bad is the way to achieve a higher quality of life and health. It is the natural law of the universe. However, it is totally up to each individual whether or not to wake up his or her true spirit, cultivate and assimilate with the great spiritual nature of the universe, and achieve the Oneness. But no matter what we choose, the consequences of our choice will affect our own life, health, peace, living quality, and living environment and can extend its influence to each individual human being.

If the whole of humankind, of course, is not cultivated well, the mind rather than evolving upward will decline. Then the entire human race will be in a very dangerous situation of sicknesses, distractions and disasters.

What emerges without healthy cultivation is a collective (and individual) mind of lower capacity and punctuated by selfishness, strong ego, and carelessness to self and others within the world.   This then manifests into conflicts between the whole of humankind and the universe. And the effects of that can be dramatic: the sick vibrations of moral crises, environmental crises, economic crises, health crises, political crises, human right crises, etc. which are actually going on over the world now. Such a downward spin can bring catastrophic consequences. Like an easy to miss computer virus, these frequencies will poison everyone – personally as well as a whole – and continue the downward cycle. The result is a loss of peace and harmony for the individual and all individuals worldwide – as well as a decline in health, life quality, happiness, longevity and life-purpose.

From such a point of view, world peace, and responsible effort for the peace of world and every country, community, and individual is the most important element of a healthy environment because it is physically, mentally, and spiritually affecting all of us, our development and capacities before we are even born, present time and ever future.

To foster, improve and protect such peace within the world and our community, the entire of humankind on the earth needs to cultivate and follow the concept of The Oneness with the Universe, and let that flow into all we do together as an earth family. This may, at first, appear to be a social issue, but it is actually a fundamental humanity issue, a law of nature, borne within everyone's life, health and happiness. From the perspective of mind-body science, this understanding that we are now talking about is extremely important. It is vital to mind-body healing and practice.

We as holistic health practitioners already often see so many negative impacts of disharmonious, immoral, unjustified, and overwhelmed materialistic social environment on the mental and physical health of the entire humankind throughout the world. These unhealthy impacts are not only caused by each individual's own lifestyle, but also by the entire world, the society, country, social system, community and family. These bring much emotional, environmental, interpersonal, economic and political stress to everyone, which results in serious sick and diseases, both mentally and physically. Everyone's cultivation of mind-body-spirit, from the top to the lowest of our society on the earth, is the urgent task.

Otherwise the health problems and associated humanity issues will not get better - only worse and worse.

Pass the message on to your families, friends, coworkers, and everyone surrounding you. Help as many people as possible learn and practice mind-body cultivation, so you can start to create a peaceful and healthy environment for yourself and your family.

§2.11 To Be a Mind-Body-Spirit Healer

As healers, therapists or doctors in the field of mind-body medicine, we are required to have both higher qualities of inborn natures and after-born education, training, learning, practice and cultivation. The following is a suggestive list of such qualifying characteristics:

1. You are a compassionate person with a kind heart to help others. You are a godly spiritual person, and heavenly connected with the divine spirit. You detached from the human ego and selfishness, stubbornness, narrowed mindedness, superficial notions, rigid thinking, skeptical attitudes, rejection and ignorance. You are fully open to spirituality, divine power, higher spirit, and super-normal ability.

2. You have great passion, broad interests, endless curiosity, and put tireless effort in spiritual cultivation, healing, mind-body-spirit improvement and growth.

3. You have excellent talent, knowledge and skills with which to communicate with people in flexible dynamic ways and from deeper / higher dimensions in understandable ways for all levels of people from low to high, not just verbally but also sometimes intuitively, emotionally, spiritually, energetically, musically, artistically, and silently.

4. You have a well-trained daily health and spiritual cultivation practice with a higher and clear guide – spiritually, mentally and physically; and you have a clear understanding in your mind and are taking it into daily personal cultivation practice based on the natures and laws of the universe. You are a truthful, compassionate, patient, tolerant and forgiving person with peaceful, gentle, harmonious, respectful, wise, warm, clear-headed, and spiritual natures, talents and personality.

5. You have a clear understanding and righteous thoughts about: good and evil, good and bad, right and wrong, beauty and ugly, the good and bad value system, moral standards and characters, personalities, lifestyles, habits, tempers, emotions, and social justice, so that you can guide yourself and patients to follow a good practice

of mind, body and spirit. Additionally, you are able to guide individuals to be good cultivators, let go of negative personality elements, as well as human attachments, notions, desires, and emotions that cause mental and physical problems. You cultivate yourself and have good energy to help people heal and upgrade cultivation – your own and other's. You can generate a healing energy field, help patients resonate with energy vibrations, and heal their condition mentally, physically, and spiritually. You can guide them to practice self-healing, self-improvement and spiritual cultivation based on the higher principle (*see* next chapter).

6. You are multi-talented in arts, music, philosophy, communication, and healing as well as flexible and creative in your rapport with people.

7. You are a humble and sophisticated practitioner and cultivator who keeps his or her mind open, learning about others, cultivating Self and helping people.

Your cultivated energy, wisdom and personality are the most effective powers with which to heal, influence and enlighten people.

§2.12 Intermediate Break: Story • Healing Music • Meditation

A fibromyalgia patient in San Diego who was healed by brainwave-meridian therapy provided this chapter's healing story. The story is dramatic and will help you keep an open mind to learn mind-body-spirit science and health practice.

BMT Ended My 8-Year Illnesses - Fibromyalgia

-Rose R

"Rose, you are really looking different now." All my friends have been telling me this for the last week, especially my husband, who was out of town for one week and called me: "Honey, you sound happier now." Yes, I do look happier and feel a lot happier, for the first time in years. I am sure the positive changes occurred because of Dr. Jason Liu.

I had been seeing different doctors and hospital staff for the past 8 years. I started with high blood pressure, developed fibromyalgia the same year, and the list continued: high cholesterol, amnesia, diabetics, tension, insomnia, depression, abnormal liver function, weight gain, 24-hour pain, swollen feet, fear, worry, anger … I had 18 things on my list before I went to see Dr. Liu. I had 13-14 pills to take every day. I knew these drugs had many side-effects and made me sicker, but without them I was unable to control my high blood pressure and couldn't sleep. Doctors told me walking would be good for my diabetes, but I could only walk 10 to15 minutes due to lack of energy. I couldn't have a normal family life with my husband, we wanted to do things together, but I was always telling him, "No, I am tired; I have pain in my body." He worried about me and our family a lot. I couldn't even drive from Chula Vista to San Diego because of the pain in my neck that prevented me from seeing straight. I had to ask for people's help all the time ... This was torture every moment, and I was constantly in a bad mood, and I would fight with everyone around me.

Thank God for helping me find Dr. Liu who took away my pain and all my pills! I would like to emphasize that Dr. Liu's healing does not involve needles or medicines, only his composed brainwave-meridian music, which is customized for each individual. All I needed to do was to lie down and enjoy his beautiful music. I could feel dramatic changes after the 3rd session. After 6 weeks, I stopped taking all medications except vitamins. I was able to walk 40 minutes every day last week; my blood pressure is 117-78 after walking, which is normal! I can now sleep 8-9 hours, but before I could only sleep 1-2 hours. I feel more energy during the daytime; I lost 8 pounds during the past 2 weeks, without the burning stomach caused by the medicine I was taking. My swollen feet became normal, and I can drive by myself now, without having to bother others. The most important thing to me is that I am able to calm down and handle daily things, and able to talk to people without fear, and have no worry about my kids. My husband is very happy to see these changes in me; we now can go out and enjoy activities together. Everything has changed, and so dramatically that I can hardly believe it; it seems like a dream! I am telling everyone what Dr. Liu has done for me, how great this therapy is and how lucky we are in San Diego. I owe it all to Dr. Liu, who took away the pain I endured for eight years, and all my medication without needles or surgery. He did it just with his music. Thank God for Dr. Liu's knowledge and compassion.

Music Healing Meditation for Chapter 2

Use the following energy healing CD to practice meditation. This music is composed with focus on the relatively yin energy of water and wood elements to strengthen kidney and liver energy:

EHM02: Cultivate by the Quiet Lake (Yin, Wood, Water)

However if you know you are relatively weak, cold, have low energy, or are unhappy, unconfident, or at a low mood emotionally (yin type of condition), then you can choose the following CD (yang type of the healing music) to practice.

EHM01: Travel the Crystal Universe (Yang, Wood, Water)

[*Play Energy Healing Music #2* while reading the following induction -] This one hour of energy meditation music flows like cooling soft mountain water into your body and mind, cleansing heat and fire, soothing mind and body, healing the entire you. Sit cross-legged (if you can, otherwise just sit in a natural position), or stand with relaxed posture if you feel you have sat too long during the day. Close your eyes and mouth, relax your entire body and keep your mind empty, peaceful and positive. Bring a peaceful smile to your face, slow down your breath, calm your mind, and meditate with me while listening to this healing music.

§2.13 Exercise Questions

1. What are the differences in ideology and methodology between mind-body medicine and modern mainstream medicine?

2. How do you understand the new concept Anatomy of whole being mind-body-spirit and how do you explain it with the Fig. 2.1?

3. What is the Fish-Water Model and how do you explain the fundamental differences between mind-body medicine and modern mainstream medicine with the Fish-Water Model?

4. Why is it that sometimes mind-body medicine works and at other times it does not?

5. What is the law of Cause-Effect? Can you explain with a daily life example?

6. List as many factors (causes) as you can that are related to the way mind-body medicine deal with health and well-being.

7. What are the fundamental laws and core principle of mind-body-spirit medicine and its practice?

8. Why should mind-body medicine practitioners or individual mind-body-spirit cultivators directly experience cultivation practice?

9. What are the qualification requirements for a mind-body medicine practitioner, doctor or therapist?

CHAPTER 3

~ ~ ~ ~ ~ ~

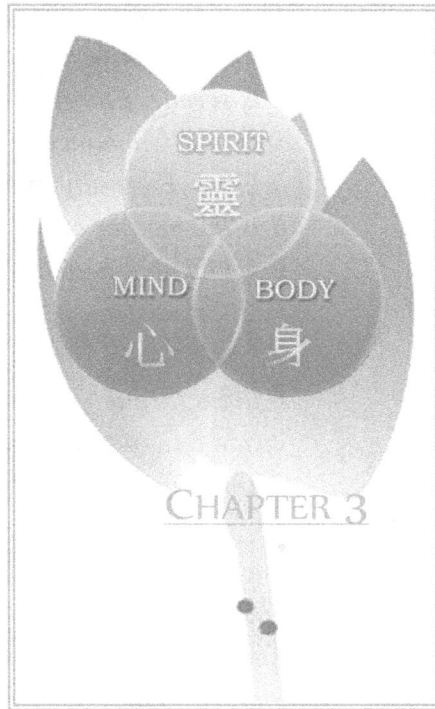

Universe • Lives • Energy • Vibration • Spirit • Dark Energy

Ancient Wisdoms – Tao, Medicine, Buddhist & Christianity

To know about the truth and natures of lives and the universe, as well as our relationship with the universe, we need to know the characteristics of the root from which the universe was born – its origin – which we can think of as holding the core nature or fundamental law (principles) of the universe and hence – of all lives.

The ancient sage Tao master, Lao Tzu (or Lao Zi) tries to help us understand this root nature in his classic text, *The Tao Te Ching* (sacred guidebook of Taoist practice). Lao Tzu wrote:

45

有物混成，先天地生。

寂兮寥兮，獨立而不改，周行而不殆，可以為天下母。

吾不知其名，字之曰道，強為之名曰大。

大曰逝，逝曰遠，遠曰反。

故道大、天大、地大、人亦大。

域中有四大，而王居其一焉！

人法地，地法天，天法道，道法自然。

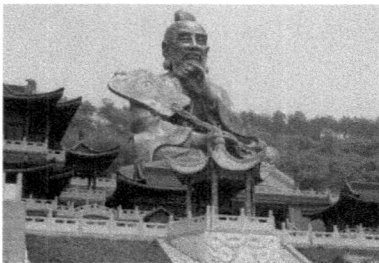

*There was something formless and perfect
before the universe was born.
It is serene. Empty.
Solitary. Unchanging.
Infinite. Eternally present.
It is the mother of the universe.
For lack of a better name,
I call it the Tao.*

*It flows through all things,
inside and outside, and returns
to the origin of all things.*

*The Tao is great.
The universe is great.
Earth is great.
Man is great.
These are the four great powers.*

*Man follows the earth.
Earth follows the universe.
The universe follows the Tao.
The Tao follows only itself. [17]*

The Tao (pronounced Dao), of which Lao Tzu writes, is in Taoist tradition (and other traditions) considered the highest origin of all things in the universe, earth and man. It is characterized as having the wonderful natures of peace, goodness, compassion, power and energy.

Importantly, half of the *Tao Te Ching* (In Chinese also spelled *Dao De Jing*) teaches about the Tao/Dao, which translates, in its basic understanding, to "The Way" as a direct superficial meaning of the word, conveying the way to reach the divine origin of universe, while its extensive meaning implies divine force, power, mysterious and profound truth. Another half of the text teaches about Te/De, which translates to Virtue. In the original order of the script, in fact, the Te/De was the first part and Tao/Dao was the second part. So in concept, the *Tao Te Ching* is to guide humankind to cultivate Virtue first and then be aware of the truth of universe and life, and finally reach the Tao, the divine force, power and eternal life in the heaven.

Lao Tzu instructs sentient beings to cultivate and improve Virtue. This, according to his teaching, must be done in order to reach the Tao or as the expression goes: "to tap in." The point is that cultivating Tao and Virtue is the Way to perfection – including the perfection of: morality, spirituality, energy, mind, body and spirit, as well as longevity in this life interwoven with a high-level spiritual life.

It is important to understand that: "perfection," in this sense, is not compulsive, competitive, or ego-driven. It is just the opposite. In Taoist tradition, perfection is a very high level of self-awareness, as well as the empathetic, compassionate awareness of others, all beings, matters and the universe. It is ultimate harmony. It is about how you become a perfect person like a master level composer or musician with your own notes and melody – completely unified or being one with all the elements of art vibrations – reaching the oneness. It is being fully aware and in control of your song and fully part of everyone else's, a perfectly harmonized part of the whole and fully your individual Self simultaneously. It is the ultimate going with the flow – doing things, in essence, that are core to your nature and core to the nature of the universe for the sole reason of doing them perfectly, no expectations, no rewards, no ego.

To help you understand, consider the following analogy:

Imagine the construction of the human body – from its first cells – each doing what it does to build the whole body – one synchronizing with others to build a heart valve, another constructing an eye. Yet, together they are "building" the human body. They are each moving to perfect what they do and as they do, the entire body is built. Although they are of a subtler energy, Mind and Spirit operate similarly. This is because the original creature designed the system in this way precisely.

Let's look, for a moment, at another significant Chinese text that emerged during the same period of time in Chinese history *as the Tao Te Ching*, in the West Han Dynasty. Influenced by *Tao Te Ching*, this book, *The Yellow Emperor's Classic of Internal Medicine* (Huang Di Neijing or Neijing for short) taught the precise and profound science of medicine and healing, from the scientific perspective. It is significant to the worlds of history and medicine in that it is the first, oldest and utmost medical classic recorded in China (as the oldest record entirely exists today). From its appearance on, thousands of texts have recorded clinical medical experience in China – **all emphasizing the incorporation of life experience and science into traditional frameworks – the *Tao*.**

So whereas the *Tao Te Ching* historically provided the substantial and seminal Way for balancing, synchronizing, and harmonizing the Mind-Spirit, *The Yellow Emperor's Classic of Internal Medicine* historically set the foundation for doing the same with the Body-Mind – only now, and for the first time, from a scientific point of view. Ultimately both of these iconic books, however, attributed true human empowerment as coming from the same source: the *Tao*.

Similarly, *The Tao Te Ching* and *Yellow Emperor Medicine* taught that (1) all material substances in the universe have the natures of Yin and Yang: complementary life energies, often understood with descriptors as dark, female, intuitive (for yin) and light, logical, male (for yang), and (2) they (the materials of the universe) are made of the material energies of Five Elements: Water, Wood, Fire, Earth and Metal. Both books highlighted the idea that balance among these energies is essential to sustain in the universe as well as to live a healthy, functional and happy life. Let's look closer.

One day at the ancient time, The Yellow Emperor asked a famous physician of that period by the name of Qi Bo, why it was that people of the "old days" lived to be one hundred years old and without showing the usual signs of aging. "In our time, however" said The Emperor, "people age prematurely, live only about fifty years." What The Emperor wanted to know was if this shift was caused by environmental factors or by the more philosophical changes in values and attitudes that determine "how" people's life-styles trend [1].

Qi Bo told him this, "In the past, people practiced the Tao, the Way of Life. They understood the principle of balance as represented by the transformations of the energies of the universe. They formulated exercises to promote energy flow and harmonize themselves with the universe. They ate a balanced diet at regular times, arose and retired at regular hours, avoided overstressing their bodies and minds, and refrained from over-indulgence of all kinds. They maintained well-being of body and mind; thus, it is not surprising that they lived over one hundred years." [1]

All of this aforementioned history became important to the development and continued refinement of what we now call mind-body medicine – its Way and goals. We had the philosophy. We had the initial and subsequent texts of medical concept. The underlying mechanism(s), however, by which the universe works and how exactly human beings can cultivate to be in harmony with the universe and importantly, how to bring all of this to bear on keeping ourselves healthy and happy in mind-body and spirit and as a world people collectively was still to emerge. But it did. Let's look at what occurred.

Historically spiritual teachings, metaphysics, philosophy, mysticism, ancient medicine, Eastern and Western religions, and then, modern sciences, filled in the gap while other information was yet to come forth. The guiding posts for these concepts were established by the teachings of higher spirits such as Lao Tzu who taught the Tao, Shakyamuni (Buddha) who taught Buddhism, and Jesus Christ who taught Christianity. These teachings passed on the important concepts and methods of life cultivation, and revealed some of basic natures about the universe in a sort of implicit way. It laid out important foundation for humankind to cultivate and remain necessary moral, mental and physical quality in the human society. It's why after a long history, today we human beings still have the will, idea, belief and faith to cultivate and improve, although some of people have forgotten or lost such memory after many past lives.

However, there was no such information that clearly teaches what are the exact natures or characteristics of the universe (and lives and all contents within it) and what are the specific mechanisms for accessing the root natures or characteristics of the universe. The complete core characteristics and mechanisms by which the universe works had not been the focus of these traditions. The universe's root characteristics and its operation mechanisms were not systematically linked as one life cultivation system.

Blessing Message - Almost Get There but Still a Gap To Fill

From the perspective of mind-body medicine, the additional missing information and integrative insights remained essential for us to understand. "What are the fundamental characteristics and actual operation mechanism by which the universe operates?" This sounds a cosmological question or philosophical question, but in fact it is also an important question in mind-body science.

Knowing such fundamental truth will help us find the healing power and tool, and understand the healing mechanism, from the universe, within our own selves, and between the universe and mankind. This is the way and goal the mind-body science and healthology study and practice. It will also help humankind return to the original Self and resynchronize with the original life force (energy frequency), which is the final goal of mind-body-spirit cultivation practice. As a scientist of mind-body-spirit healing and spiritual cultivator, this question naturally came to my mind when I reached a certain point in my practice. Since then I have been searching for the answer for a long time. Many students I told in the Qigong class also often asked these questions in our open discussion.

During 1990's, I was in Miami, Florida where I taught a Qigong (originated from Tang Dynasty physician Sun Simiao) in combination with my self-composed Energy Healing Music. One day in my meditation, when I got deep state with completely emptied mind, I felt a strong energy wave, from all the way up to the heaven, flowing into my Bai Hui point - the point on the top of the head. The energy wave was a beautiful blessing light beam connecting to the heaven all the way up. I followed the light beam flying up, passing through many layers of cosmos, flying through many stars, galaxies, and finally reached a big light source. The light source is somehow like a huge living spirit. At the same time a word came to my mind, said "Universe's Spirit Center" in the form of virtual message but not writing words. It was a very interesting (soul/spirit) Out of Body experience.

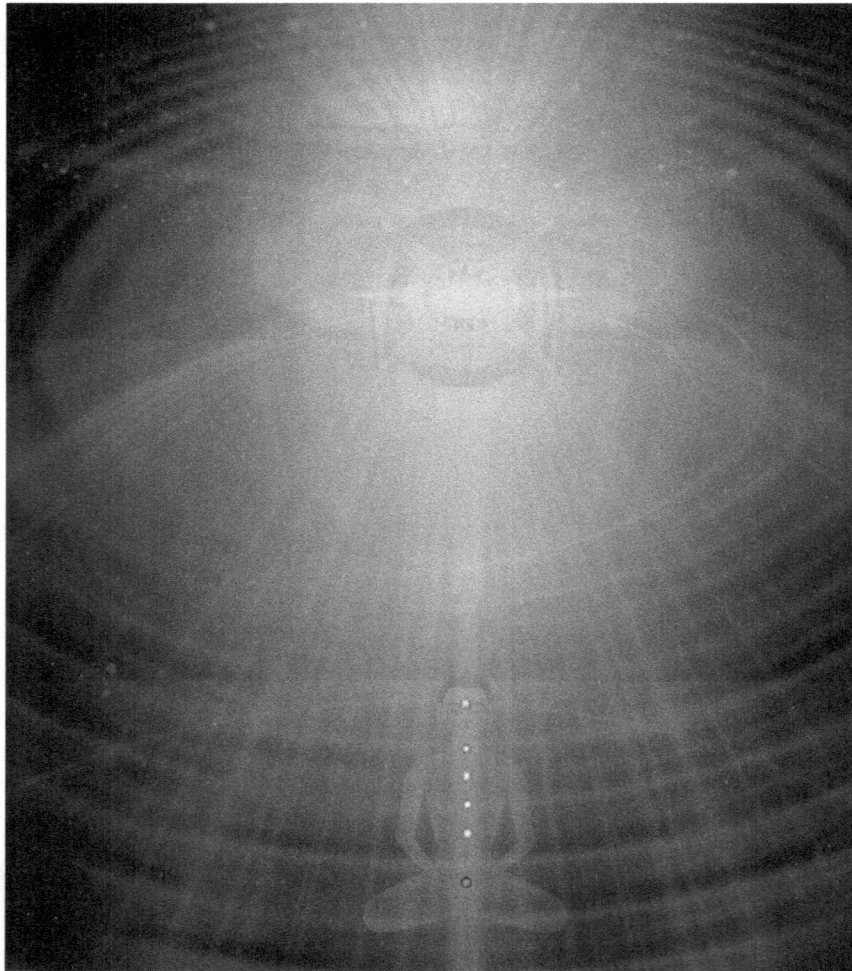

This happened quit a few times in the same pattern of image and message as described above. I knew it was an important spiritual message that teaches me something meaningful. As we study spiritual science, sometime we learn from the super intelligent spirit of the universe in this way. A good cultivation meditation in an emptied state of mind sometime can allow you to naturally access the higher divine that teaches you something meaningful. Often the message is helpful to improve cultivator's mind nature and *Wu Xing*, encourage your practice, increase cultivated Virtue, but it should not stimulate human desire and selfishness. If the message is the later, you should be careful: it must be the bad spirit from other dimension interfering your cultivation or testing your mind.

As a scientist, we want to understand something clearly and logically, or even want to build a model by which we can explain the mechanism of life and universe. Based on the blessing image and message about the universe Spirit Center, I proposed the following model and presented to the Qigong group I taught at that time:

(1)   The universe has a Spirit Center that has spiritual wisdoms, super intelligences and power to govern the entire universe.

(2)   When a meditator goes deep in meditation and let go of the human mind, then we can connect with the Spirit Center

(3)   The Spirit Center has some characters that require humans to follow. Otherwise it is not easy for us to get connected with it.

(4)   If we meditate, cultivate and let go of complicated human thoughts, be a kind and peaceful good person in everyday life, and then we can receive the blessing energy from the Spirit Center that can heal our problems in all aspects of this life and energize our mind-body-spirit.

I felt one step progressed in spiritual growth, teaching and study. But it triggered me to think: It seems everything makes sense, but one thing I still don't know, "What is the Spirit Center's character or criterion that requires our humans to behave, how can we connect to it, and what is the exact mechanism that operates the universe?" I wanted to meditate and further find the answer. I thought I almost get there, but there is still a gap to be filled.

For a while after that I tried hard in my meditation, but I realized one important fact: if I pursuit for it or attached on it too much, not only I could never get it but also my meditation quality becomes bad. Sometime I even could not relax well during the meditation because I attached on it too much. Therefore I know the higher truth cannot be obtained by human desire, instead it is the combination of the faith, fate and quality of mind nature (Virtue) cultivation.

The Higher Spiritual Teaching Helped Find the Answer

51

Around the same period of time when I had such blessing experience in my meditation and teaching, on the day of May 13, 1992, a remarkable event occurred in China and then spread across the globe. This is the date when Master Li Hongzhi began his teachings of the revolutionary and visionary practice, which he called in Chinese Falun Dafa or Falun Gong / FLG (In English meaning: *The Universe's Great Law*) [18]. In the 1990's, this teaching became a very popular spiritual movement that spread across China, reached over million practitioners, and improved their mental and physical health, and brought them spiritual enlightenment [89].

In the western world, however, we did not notice this event that time. What it really started to call our attention to the event was around July 1999 when the Chinese government started crackdown on this practice. In the west, we have all kinds of natural health and spiritual practices such as Christianity, Buddhist, Taoists, Qigong, Taiji, Martial Art, meditation, Reiki, and other mind-body practices. Myself as a certified Qigong master taught in the field, and also involved in "pure land" Buddhist and Tao temple activities in Miami, FL at that time. I heard people were talking about the crackdown on FLG in China.

Spiritual practitioners could easily sense that it is a sign that this practice must have a strong spiritual message that triggered the communist's anger and fear. Otherwise, they won't bother. Many types of medical Qigong that only focus on health were fine with them. Atheism ideology is fundamentally different from that of GOD believers. The crackdown tells that FLG teaching must be something very spiritual, so that it has a fundamental conflict with the atheism philosophy. Therefore, this brought a lot of attention to the western spiritual practitioners. As we read the FLG teaching book, *Zhuan Falun*, we understood what was really happening there. What it surprised me yet interested me was that the book answered my question, which I kept searching for a long time, especially during that time period.

As spiritual scientists in the west who used to appreciate and enjoy the freedom of belief and open-minded social environment, if something opens our minds, triggers our thoughts and helps progress our research and understanding in our field, then we will take it into reference for our study. Especially in the field of holistic science[8], it is very important to widely learn from all sources in order to advance our study.

---

[8] Holistic science (or Holism in science) is one of the categories of science that uses an approach called Holism in science. The research approach of holistic science emphasizes the study of complex systems and uses multiple theories, principles, methods and tools from different sources to gain a holistic and comprehensive understanding with focus on the subject's integrity and inner and intra connectivity. This practice is in contrast to a purely analytic tradition (sometimes called reductionism) that aims to gain understanding of systems by dividing them into smaller composing elements and gaining understanding of the system through understanding their elemental properties, piece by piece, but not the entire whole integrity.

Before we get into the actual answer for our question, let's review a little bit background information and my personal overall understanding about the teaching.

Trained by Buddhist and Taoist masters, Master Li Hongzhi's teachings provided the most profound guide, principle and practice of life cultivation from the point of universe's characteristics, the fundamental Buddha Law. Although originally his teaching itself is not primarily for the advance of science, but from point of view of life science or mind-body science, his teaching actually helps our scientists see through the truth of lives and universe, directing us to advance science in the right direction ultimately.

The teaching provides a link of the life (mind-body-spirit) cultivation principle and method with the core natures or characteristics of the universe. It provides a cultivation mechanism or a cultivation system for us to establish the technical links and core practices of mind-body-spirit, which indeed lays the foundation of mind-body medicine and Healthology from our point of view as mind-body science.

Master Li Hongzhi is iconic in that he delivered on that day in May, 1992, the piece of the total picture that mind-body-spirit cultivation practitioners had, for long years, been interested in nailing down, yet had evaded them. Not only that, but he used the shared tools of Buddhism, Taoism, and science to help us understand and "get to" the "mechanisms" we sought. These tools were, for example, meditation and movement exercises, moral philosophy, mind nature and longevity health Qigong (energy science, mind-body-spirit whole being cultivation), inner-look technique, main consciousness (true Self) cultivation, and so on.

Through his teaching, he kindly corrected many mistakes and misunderstandings in the fields of Qigong, energy healing and spirituality. Master Li also voluntarily (without charge of money) helped many practitioners or students clean up confused thoughts, mixed energy fields and sicknesses in the mind-body-spirit to prepare them for a pure high level of cultivation. His teaching books and meditation/exercise audio / videos are even offered for free on the Internet. These are very kind blessing and valuable teachings that we do not often receive from anywhere.

The holism-reductionism dichotomy is often evident in conflicting interpretations of experimental findings and in setting priorities for future research. Mind-Body Medicine and healthology is a sort of holistic science.

Different from many other Qigong masters, Master Li focuses on teaching the complete cultivation to improve the health of mind-body-spirit, but not just simply healing the diseases without teaching the truth and improving the whole person. It is very touching to me because we all know, as a spiritual teacher and healer, that changing the person is the most difficult thing to do, and also the most energy consuming work, which is only a Grandmaster at extremely high level can conduct such task. Many medical Qigong masters and spiritual healers felt tired, sick or even get severe disease after giving energy to heal others. I had such experience too long time ago when I conducted Qigong workshop. It is very grateful that Master Li revealed the secret about this and helped many Qigong healers understand why and how to avoid the problem.

Breaking through Chinese medical history as over five thousand years ago other texts did, and incorporating brand new vision into traditional frameworks, Falun Dafa advanced mind-body medicine, again – although as we have said, it itself was originally not for scientific advancement. However, it did, in fact, advance our science to a whole other level in its quest for better health and, ultimately, spiritual enlightenment. Falun Dafa is a significant component to activate and upgrade mind-body medicine beyond ideology. It advances MBM's mechanism and application. But what was it exactly that Falun Dafa so poignantly delivered?

The Characteristics and Mechanism of The Universe

What Master Li Hongzhi presents in his book of Falun Dafa teachings, *Zhuan Falun*, is a description of the characteristics of the universe *and* the life cultivation mechanisms. The following is a list of major concepts within:

- "The universe's most fundamental nature is to be true, good, and endure (Truthfulness, Compassion and Tolerance). This is the highest expression of Buddha Law. It is the essence of Buddha Law.

- Buddha Law is expressed in different forms at different levels, and at different levels it acts as a guide in different ways, with its manifestations getting more diverse as the level gets lower. Air particles, stone, wood, soil, steel, and the human body - all matter has this nature, to be True, Good, and Endure. In ancient times they believed that The Five Elements form all the myriad things of the universe. And they, too, have this nature - to be True, Good, and Endure.

- A cultivator can only know the specific manifestation of Buddha Law at the level he has cultivated to, and that's his Cultivation Fruition, his level. If you spell it out in detail, the Law is huge. But when you reach its highest point, then it's simple, because the Law stacks up in a pyramid-like shape. Up at an extremely high level you can summarize it in just three words: True, Good, Endure. But as it manifests at each different level it gets extremely complicated.

- Let's use human beings as an analogy. Taoists consider the human body as a small universe. Human beings have a material body, but just having a material body doesn't make somebody a complete person.

- It takes a human temperament, personality, traits, and a soul to make up a complete and independent person with individuality. The same goes for this universe of ours: there's the Milky Way and other galaxies, and also life and water, so the myriad things are its material side, but it also has its nature, to be True, Good, and Endure. The particles of every single thing have this nature, and extremely small particles have this nature, too." [18]

In the same text, the Master taught the cultivation, of not only "Triple-World-Law" (physical realm … more in upcoming chapters) but also "Beyond Triple-World-Law" (out of the physical realm), to the level beyond the Five Elements. These ideas and mechanisms also contribute to our discipline of mind-body medicine in practice and application and help explain how and why systems of energy medicine work and so we need to, as well, carefully examine and explore the following points:

- "Going beyond the Five Elements only happens in a practice that cultivates both your nature and longevity. It's not part of practices that don't cultivate both nature and longevity. They only grow the gong (energy) that determines levels, and they don't cultivate longevity, so they don't talk about going beyond the Five Elements. In practices that cultivate both nature and longevity, a person's energy is stored in all the cells in his body. The energy that an ordinary qigong practitioner gives off or that somebody who's just started to build up gong gives off, that gong has large particles with gaps between them and low density, and so it has little power. When a person's level rises, it's possible that the density of his energy will be 100 times, 1,000 times, or 100 million times higher than ordinary water molecules. That's because the higher the level, the higher the density, the finer the grains, and the greater the power. When that happens, the energy is stored in every single cell of the body, and it's not just in every cell of the body in this material dimension of ours, but in all the bodies in other dimensions—the molecules, atoms, protons, and electrons, and all the way down to the extremely microcosmic cells, they're all filled with that energy. So over time the person's body is completely filled with that high-energy matter.

- High-energy matter is an intelligent entity, and it has power. When there's more of it, when its density gets high, and after it fills all the cells in a person's body, it's able to suppress his flesh cells, those least capable cells. And once they're restrained there isn't any metabolism, and at some point it will completely replace the human flesh cells. Of course, this is easy to say, but cultivating to that point is a slow process. When you've cultivated to that point all the cells in your body will have been replaced by the high-energy matter, so think about it, is your body still made up of the Five Elements? Is it still matter that belongs to this dimension? It's made of high-energy matter collected from other dimensions. Note: The components of Virtue are also matter that exist in other dimensions, and it's not restricted by the time-field of this dimension we're in." [19]

- After a person goes beyond the Triple-World-Law he has to cultivate all over again. The body he has is like what I just talked about, a body that's gone beyond the Five Elements. It's a Buddha-body. Wouldn't you call that kind of body a Buddha-body? That Buddha-body needs to cultivate all over again and bring abilities about all over again. But those aren't called abilities; they're called Buddha Law's divine powers.

- Their might is infinite, and they take effect in every dimension - they are what really have an impact. So tell me, what's the use of wanting to get abilities? All you people who want abilities, isn't your intention to use them around ordinary people, to show off around ordinary people? If it's not, what do you want them for? They can't be seen and they can't be touched... If you're saying you just want to use them as decorations or something, wouldn't you be better off finding something that looks nice? I can guarantee that subconsciously your aim is to use them. They can't be sought after like skills of ordinary people. They're altogether a higher thing, and you're not allowed to go and show them off around ordinary people.

- For starters, showing off is a strong attachment, it's a character flaw, and it's a desire that a cultivator should get rid of. If you want to make money with them, if you want to get rich off them or achieve some worldly goal that you strive for, then that's even worse. That would be using higher things to upset the way of things in the ordinary world, to damage the ordinary world.

Those thoughts are even worse. So they can't just be used whenever you want." [20]

As we can read from this teaching, Falun Dafa associated the previous teaching in the history about the energy mechanism (yin-yang and five elements and the concept of Oneness of Cosmos and Man) closely and directly with the characteristics of the universe. This helps us understand that only when assimilating (resonating) with the universe's characteristics (the spiritual frequency), the energetic unification and balance will occur. It answered the question why some practitioners cannot get the connection with the higher divine, cannot get healed or cannot reach the enlightenment even though they seriously practice all kinds of physical forms. Knowing the core law of the universe and practicing it by following the energy mechanism are extremely important.

Complete Model – Spiritual Character & Energy Mechanism

Now after a long history, we have a unification of both philosophy and mechanism. The spiritual characteristics of the universe as the supreme law at the highest level, along with the principles of Yin and Yang and Five Elements (Or Beyond) as the energy mechanism (nature and principle) of the substantial world combined with supreme law, establishing the most fundamental basis and underlying guide for mind-body-spirit science, practice and cultivation.

Following this supreme law and energy mechanism (or energy principle), a human being can cultivate to higher levels of spiritual character and energy quality. When the cultivation practice reaches the highest level of triple-world (material world, the physical space-time dimension which is made of ordinary matters that are visible, detectable and substantial physically), it can further reach the level beyond the triple-world: out of The Five Elements of material realm.

After the long darkness we have undergone in the scientific journey for truth searching, this, as mentioned above, gives us and entire humankind tremendous blessing light and hope as well as tool to grow towards the best life quality and future destination. As scientists, this is our day that we need to appreciate this and celebrate this as it gave us the ultimate guidance and finally turned on the light shining on our future path, the scientific truth-searching journey.

As a spiritual scientist and healer, in the past we often said something like this, "Be one with the universe. Synchronize with the universe's vibration frequency," but we could never clearly tell our patients, clients, students and audiences in our healing lecture about what is exactly the universe's frequency, and how to synchronize with it. Now we are finally able to say it and actually practice it.

As a part of the universe, we human beings originally came from and live with these characteristics and energy natures as the universe has. Although humankind's spiritual quality dropped down dramatically after a long history of life journey, if we cultivate and assimilate with the vibration waves of these spiritual (in human language, Truth-Compassion-Forbearance, but can be in varying forms in other dimensions), and energy natures (yin-yang and five elements), we can return to the original Self and stay in harmony and peace with the universe, therefore achieving true health as a whole being of body, mind and spirit.

Everyone has such power to heal and stay in true health with his or her original Self. The father of holistic medicine and the most documented psychic of the 20th century, Edgar Cayce said: "I do not believe there is a single individual that does not possess this same ability I have. I am certain that all human beings have much greater powers than they are ever conscious of -- if they would only be willing to pay the price of detachment from self-interest that it takes to develop those abilities."

To detach from "self-interest" and to be a truly unified being as a part of the universe, the person must assimilate with the universe's characteristics of truthfulness, compassion and tolerance and cultivate mind nature. This is the most fundamental law of the universe and also the natural law of human life. These characteristics of the universe are in their barest essence *spiritual energy vibrations* with creature-created characteristic frequencies that characterizes the spirit and energy character of the being (*see* ongoing sections of this chapter), the original inborn spiritual characteristics at the time when created. These are expressed in non-mathematic analogy, using human language: truth-compassion-tolerance (forbearance). Note: A human being is a part of the universe with the same characteristics of energy vibrations as the universe has, therefore a human life, its life phenomena, behaviors, and activities must conform to the energy frequencies - as they will unify and harmonize our lives, as well as keep us healthy. Deviation from these original energy frequencies or imbalance or disharmony with these energy vibrations is a Self-distracting and Self-destroying condition, which leads to sickness and disease.

As we alluded to earlier, under the supreme law of the cosmic spiritual characteristics, the universe is also an energy system composed of Yin and Yang and Five-Elements. When a person assimilates with the same characteristics as the universe, then he/she is in harmony with the universe as a unified energy system of Yin-Yang and Five-Elements or beyond the Five Elements when the spiritual energy goes beyond the material realms.

At this point in our discussion and leaning, we can look back on an earlier statement of "Being One with the Universe" or "Human and Heaven Merged As One" or "Heaven and Man Are One" (in Chinese: 天人合一 *Tian Ren He Yi*) with greater understanding and depth, philosophy and mechanism.

The Heaven and Man Are One *is the goal in perfecting the whole being, the body, mind and spirit. But what and where is the Heaven, and how to be one with it?*

We understand now that "Being One with the Universe" is actually to assimilate to the universe's spiritual characteristics and then the whole person of body-mind-spirit will be able to stay in harmony with the balanced energy system of Yin-Yang and The Five Elements or even beyond The Five Elements, the higher level of true health. Please be aware that further definition and potential implications of these terms will appear in forthcoming chapters.

Rightfully understood, such universal law along with the energy principle was originally taught as a belief system. From the perspective of mind-body medicine as science and practice, however, we recognize this significance. Yet, for human life science they are a blessing. They have carved an inspirational and enlightening path for the teaching, study and practice of health and life quality improvement. Revealing one of the greatest secrets about its own character and that of all lives, the universe has gifted humankind with a key to resonate and synchronize with the very original and most beautiful life frequency from which we have come into this world, giving us, as our birthright, the power to heal, live and flourish our body-mind-spirit in peace and health.

As such, we bring these spiritual teachings (the universal law and the energy principle) to mind-body-spirit health science, and put efforts in their study, research, practice and cultivation. We are aware that this is a revolutionary transformation from laboratory experiment based science to integrative holistic science, from local linear deterministic science to universal nonlinear comprehensive science, and from rigid logic science to a dynamic flexible science. Our mindset, however, is that there is a better way to forge forward than having to rely solely on test-tube lab proofs for every step we must take. Instead, we encourage and incorporate into our vision and mechanisms learning from the great wisdom of the universe, divine spirit; the teachings, inspirations, experiences, intuitions, common understanding and inborn nature; different fields and paths, no matter whether it is ancient or modern, direct or indirect, East or West. From all of this, we establish our model to guide our practice and further experience, benefit from it, as well as prove and advance it.

We will address, in coming chapters, specific Mind-Body-Spirit techniques as they are aligned with the universal law and the energy principle for these are our highest teachings and guide. These techniques include meditation, energy music, brainwave-meridian therapy, spiritual conversation, energy healing, energy exercise, mind cultivation and healthy lifestyle practice. We include their experiments (evidence based and empirical/self-experiential) and healing applications.

Our spectrum includes learning, study, development, research, cultivation and experimental application over years and under the universal law and the energy principle, which truly opened the door that allows us to explore the study and practice of mind-body-spirit health from a broader scope for future medicine and life science. As such, we can and will cross over the limits of conventional modern science and religion beliefs to explore with deeper insight and to establish the basis and further development of mind-body-spirit science.

Note: The universe has its spiritual nature, energy field, physical form and structures crossing many dimensions. How these are associated is the key to understanding how they work, their capabilities and uses. Mind-body science believes that the spirit, mind and body are associated through energy. Energy is the medium crossing all dimensions from physical realms to spiritual worlds. In the following pages, we will further discuss this topic from several different angles.

§3.2 Traditional Energy Medicine

Now we come back from the higher spiritual teaching to medicine – understanding will be clear and deeper.

Traditional Energy Medicine, including all kinds of mind-body healing arts and human cultivation practices such as Traditional Chinese Medicine (TCM) or Traditional Oriental Medicine (TOM), Tao and Buddhist cultivation practices, meditation, Qigong, Taiji, Yoga, Indian medicine, western ancient practice, hypnosis and other energy medicine and spiritual healing modalities always introduce the concept of energy as the central focus when dealing with the whole being of the mind, body and spirit. This is because these practices believe that (1) the universe is made of energy and (2) the balanced energetic state of the living being is the most important vital life force in accordance with the same natural law and principles of the universe. In other words, the human being is considered the same as the universe in terms of spiritual characteristics and energy natures. This means a human being was originally a unified and harmonized energy system of the Yin-Yang and The Five Elements or beyond The Five Elements, with the same spiritual natures as the universe: truth good endurance or truthfulness compassion and tolerance.

The human being resonates and emerges to the universe through the same spiritual characters and energy vibrations in the same universal system under the same supreme law and mechanism. The following chapters of this book will further discuss the detailed aspects of this energy system and its application to human life phenomena and healing process.

Original mind-body medicine was developed from a long history of ancient wisdom and the advanced human cultivation teaching in modern times. After we learned the universe's spiritual characteristics and energy mechanism, the energy that energy medicine deals with, is not simply the energy substance in the physical form or specific form or body practice, but actually it is also the living spirit possessing the spiritual characters expressed in all dimensions of the mind, body and spirit. Therefore in our new mind-body medicine we deal with energy at all different levels at the same time.

§3.2.1 Quantum Mechanics and Wave-Particle Dualism

We in mind-body medicine enjoy the modern quantum science implications that a living being is also energy formed as part of universe as this supports the principle and practice of ancient and modern energy healing science described above. In addition to the understanding from the pure quantum physics that treats the quantum particle as a substantial object or energy wave with or without mass but with energy force, now we understand the particle much deeper by involving its spiritual characters into consideration.

A little background: Quantum physics (quantum mechanics) known as Planck's Law, was initiated by Max Planck in 1900 [21] and further developed by Albert Einstein [22] and other physicists. The theory believes that the universe is made of fundamental particles at multiple quantum energy levels and these particles have their particular nature with substantial energy (E), and at the same time, they are also characterized by the form of a wave with a certain characteristic frequency (f or v). This is called wave-particle dualism. It means that all particles exhibit properties as both wave and particle.

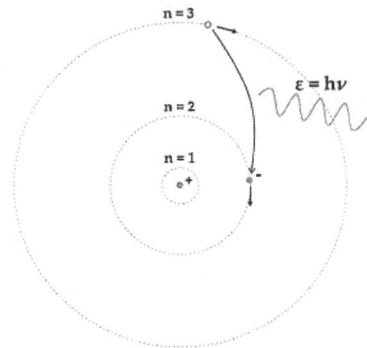

This central concept of quantum mechanics explains the fundamental property of the Universe from the point of view of quantum physics. In other words, the universe is composed of particles that behave as an energetic particle (energy property) and also as a vibrant wave (wave property). Since the particle is in the form of a vibration wave, the particle is also called an oscillator. The particle property and wave property are related; its characteristic Energy *E* and wave frequency *f* (or *v*) are associated mathematically. The quantum energy *E* for each oscillator is proportional to the frequency *f* (or *v*) of the oscillator through the proportionality constant (e.g., *h*, Planck constant for the case of photon) known as the Planck constant, *h*, having the value 6.63×10^{-34} J s.

$$E = nhf, \text{ where n} = 1, 2, 3, \ldots$$

The energy state that a particle most possibly stays must be one of a sequential quantum levels, rather than any level in the continuing gradient. Therefore, the energy carried by each particle can be interval (integer) *n* times of an energy unit *hf*, that is, *nhf*.

The universe consists of uncountable particles spreading over many dimensions from the highest dimension (spiritual), through intermediate levels of dimensions, to the lowest dimension (material or physical). The highest energetic spiritual dimension is the realm where the lives of origin, the most fundamental elements of lives, exist. The intermediate energy dimensions are the realms where microscopic particles exist. The lowest energy dimension is the visible physical dimension where human beings exist physically, and as well as the other visible macroscopic realm where planets and its clusters exist.

At the low energy dimension, the matter vibrates at low frequency, so it behaves more like matter than energy waves, therefore appearing as visible objects in this macroscopic physical dimension or visible material world. At the higher energy dimensions (the microscopic space, such as the realms where mind and spirit exist), however, matter vibrates at higher frequencies, so it behaves more like energy waves instead of substantial matters; therefore its characteristics are more like energy vibration waves, spiritual and mental energies. Those higher energy vibration matters or energy waves may exist as dark matter or dark energy because they are not easily detected, measured or visualized like ordinary matters in this physical dimension by modern science and technology.

Although we described the energy forms of a particle, an object, or a living being, exist in multiple dimensions from low to high levels, separately, but in fact they exist in all dimensions in different energy forms at the same time as one system. For example, a human being has a physical body in this physical dimension, but at the same time he / she has many layers of sub-structures inside the body, which exist in different dimensions: an organ has the organ's dimension, a cell has the cell's dimension, a cellular component has its component's dimension, a molecule has the molecule's dimension, and so on. But all these are at physical dimension and their corresponding physical sub-dimensions.

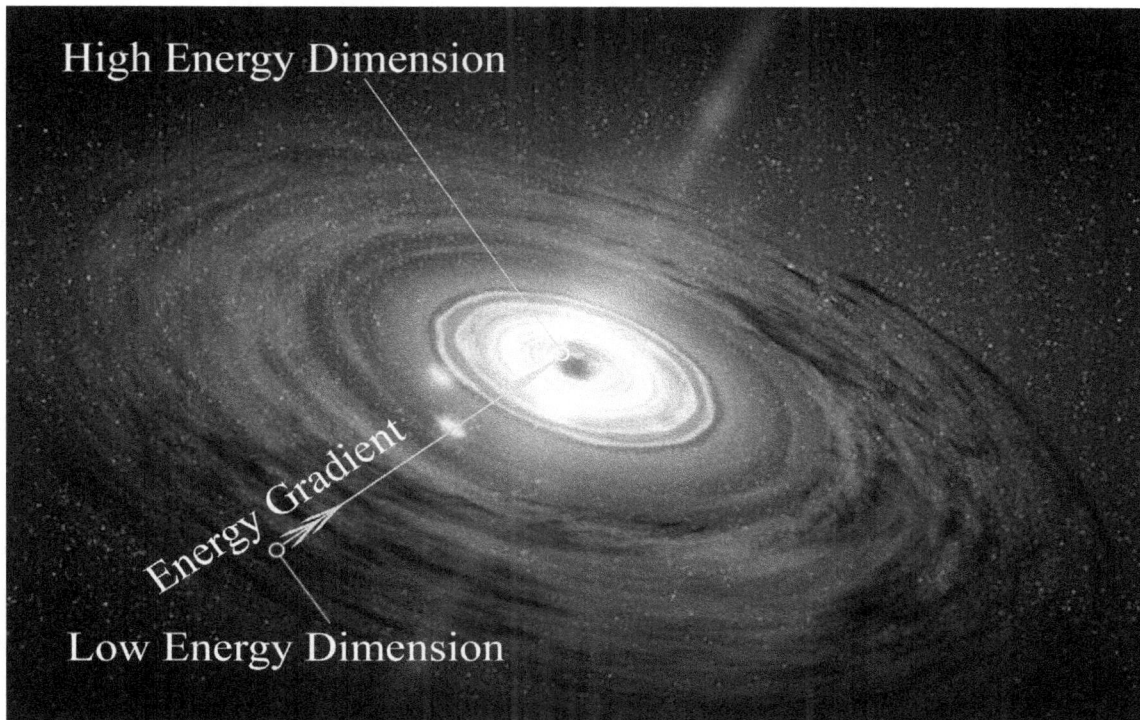

Fig. 3.2.1. The universe is made of energy at levels from high energy dimension to low energy dimension. The physical dimensions are at the lower and lowest energy levels and spiritual dimensions are at the higher and highest levels. This image is only an analogical figure that illustrates the multiple energy dimensions by using the astronomical image but cannot exactly present the actual multi-dimensional system of the universe.

At the same time, the body and its all sub-structures also have their mental and spiritual forms in the mental and spiritual dimensions, respectively. These mental and spiritual forms are at higher energy dimensions, expressing their properties of energy vibration in different frequencies. Furthermore these physical structures, sub-structures, mind and spirit are all governed under the spiritual law and energy mechanism at the corresponding levels. The physical body and its sub-structures appear more like a substantial (physical) particle, while the mind and spirit appear more like energy vibration waves, which can reach higher dimensions, even connect to the universe's spiritual origin.

From our perspective in mind-body medicine, the physical body, in this visible physical dimension, is only part of the whole being, and it has lower vibration frequency and appears as a physical object/body, but the mind and spirit behave more as energy waves in the higher energy vibration dimensions.

§3.2.2 Dark Energy Everywhere Dominating Universe

In modern science we know much more about physical matters (ordinary matters) than their mental and spiritual aspects. We used to conduct research, experiment and measurement in this physical dimension to characterize the natures, and quantify the size, mass, weight, structure, form, shape, motion, biological functions, electronic and magnetic fields, etc. of the physical substances (including human body). We use animal body to study human body by assuming the biological body is everything, so the functions of the animal are equally the same as that of the human body. Is our physical body is everything of our human being? Are the visible physical matters are everything of the universe? If not, what are the other parts of our body and the universe, and where are they? This is not just a cosmology problem or philosophy issue, it is the issue of mind-body science.

In fact, ordinary matter is indeed just a very tiny fraction of the entire universe. Modern astronomers and cosmologists have discovered that the universe contains about $22.4 \pm 1.4\%$ of dark matter and about $73.0 \pm 1.5\%$ of dark energy, both of which, 95.4% in total, are mysterious, invisible and remain unknown and secret to humankind. The ordinary matter is only about $4.6 \pm 0.15\%$ of the universe [23]. This means that, so far, all human knowledge, including science, has been limited to the universe's superficial layer that is a very small proportion of the whole universe. Nearly all the books carried by all the libraries over the whole world together regard ordinary matter on the surface of the universe, a very tiny part of the entire cosmos, but there is not much written about the majority of the universe. So, our existing knowledge base is very limited.

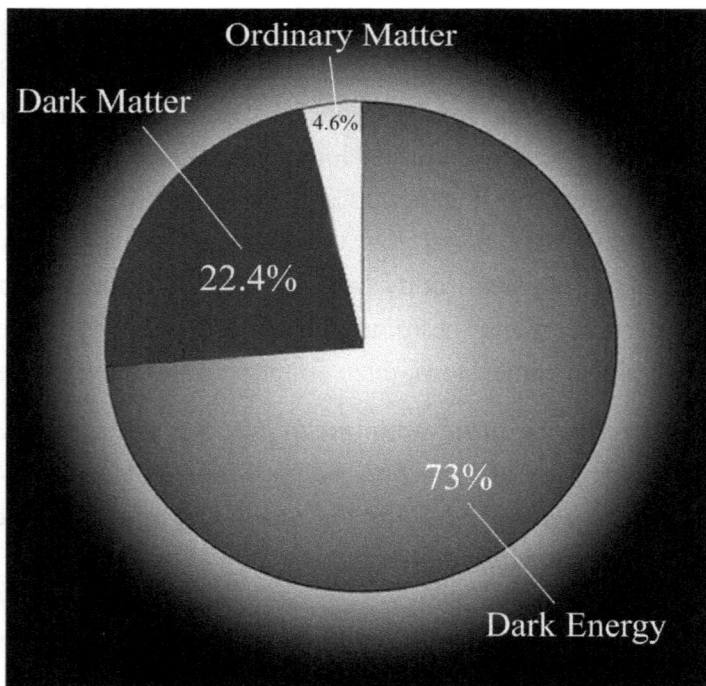

Fig. 3.2.2. The universe is composed of 4.6% ordinary matter, 22.4% dark matter and 73% dark energy.

Let's zoom back for a moment to the 1929. This was the year Edwin Hubble first observed the universe's expansion [24]. Since then, so much interest from cosmologists and astronomers has been focused on how and why the universe is expanding. The Gravitational Lensing Experiments (to seek dark matter) discovered that the universe is expanding at an accelerating rate of 74.3 ± 2.1 kilometers (46.2 ± 1.3 miles) per second, per mega parsec (a mega parsec is roughly 3 million light-years) [25]. This means its hundreds of billions of galaxies are outwardly moving away faster and faster, the distances between galaxies becoming bigger and bigger, the spaces within galaxies becoming colder and colder, but the relative distance or the size of each galaxy remaining unchanged [23]. One may ask why? What is going on with the universe? The answer is completely out of humankind's imagination and intelligence.

The secret must be in the dark energy. Otherwise, think of this, why is it that dark energy dominates the universe and constitutes the majority of the universe? At this point, however, the only thing cosmologists understand is that the mysterious, dark energy pervades the cosmos and contributes the force to accelerate the universe's expansion.

This then is just an understanding from the perspective of gravitational force based on Einstein's general relativity. But begs the question; does the dark energy do anything else?

It seems not so simple. Think of this, why does dark energy outwardly pull the galaxies away continuously and where is the universe going? And why? Will this accelerated expansion have a termination or it will go forever like this?

From the perspective of a spiritual practitioner, we look at all things as living lives with spirit, wisdom and intelligence (at different levels). This, of course, includes the 95.4% content of the universe: dark matter (22.4%) plus dark energy (73%), which is everywhere spreading out all over the universe.

There must be a significant reason for the existence of dark energy and dark matter. Just like there are no useless anatomical parts in a human body, it is impossible that the creator created more than 95% of the universe's content as useless. Even if the universe becomes nothing more than a vacuum, this dark energy and matter are still pervading the entire universe in the background. As such, sometimes scientists refer the dark energy itself as vacuum energy. This means the dark energy and matter are like a background medium behind the ordinary matters. Those ordinary matters make up only about 4.6% of the universe and are just like the reefs and islands exposed on the surface of the vast ocean. The vast secrets hidden deep within the ocean, however, are often doing their business under our radar, or, more often than not, we are simply ignoring it, never giving it enough attention and study, so that in the end we know very little or almost nothing about it.

Where are the 95%+ of the mysterious matters and energies? For what reason do they exist? The advanced modern technology cannot find it from this physical dimension just like we do not find mind and spirit on our physical body, so, isn't it suggesting that there is a fundamental problem in our ideology and methodology or we need to take different approach?

To understand and benefit from such secrets of the universe and the lives within it, including the full dimension of our own human life, we need to open our mind, awaken our spirit, and develop special *radar* in the deeper and higher dimensions with much more sensitivity and broader reaching power.

Such radar must be in other dimensions in order to reach the mysterious place. Our adventure journey to search the mystery is still far away to the destination. Keep your curiosity and never give up until you find it.

§3.2.3 An Inspiring Experience: Elastic Energy Force

I would like to invite you to join me in a small meditation practice and enjoy an interesting phenomenon you may never have experienced. If you are an experienced meditation practitioner, however, you may already know this. In either case, let's practice a few minutes of meditation together by following my instruction below, so you will be inspired by what you will experience during the practice.

Sit on the floor or bed, and cross your legs in a lotus meditation position if you can. Don't worry if you cannot cross legs exactly in the lotus meditation position, you can sit in regular cross-legged position. It will be fine.

Relax your entire body and mind completely. Empty any thoughts in your mind and keep it as empty as possible, so you can truly enjoy the relaxation and peace. Then try to slow and deepen your breathing. Let any images that come into your mind float across it like reflections on water. Don't cling to any. Just try to be very still, relaxed and quiet physically and mentally - you go deeper and deeper … into the stillness. Remember to relax your arms, shoulders and hands during the entire process.

Some minutes later (3 minutes or so, but no need to be exact at all), still in the meditation state, move your arms and hold both hands in the front of your abdominal area like you are holding a basketball. Leave some space between your upper arms and upper body (armpits are open) and relax your arms and entire body. Keep your fingers are naturally apart with a little space between. Stay still in this posture and continue to meditate.

About one minute later, still in the meditation state but slightly with your conscious mind, gently and slightly move both hands – palms open – toward each other (about 1 inch at most) and then back, while relaxing your hands, arms and shoulders during the entire process. Do this a few times. Don't push your hands together, but rather undulate back and forth.

If you physically really push, then you "wake up" from the meditation and come back to this physical dimension. It is not what we want. Keep in the meditative state as you move your hands like this. Then you will probably feel something (a pressure of sorts, as if the "skin" of the basketball had disappeared but the air has remained intact, still in the shape of the ball) between your hands. This "pressure" you feel presents a slight resistance when you try to move your hands closer (you just try to move but do not really physically move, or move a little bit). It can feel like an elastic gel surrounding your hands and in between them. You can try to gently push your hands toward each other (not really push that much but try to push) for a second then release, and again, push for a second then release, repeat this (not too fast though): push and release, push and release ... Enjoy the feeling of this mysterious resisting force between your hands.

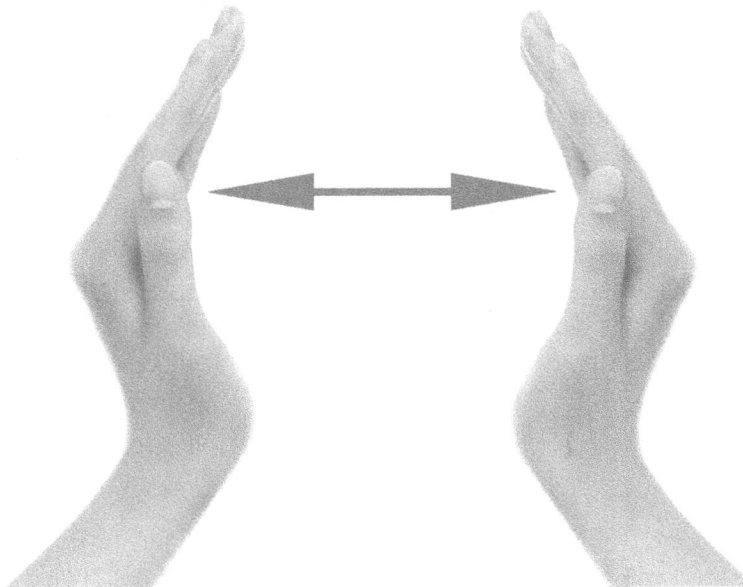

You also can try to slowly move your hands apart (pull away) each other, still in the meditation state. Try to pull for a second and release, then again pull for a second and release, and repeat this (not too fast though): pull and release, pull release. Again, you will notice something between your hands creating pressure and resistance as your hands move apart.

Now you can try pushing for a second then pull for a second, and then repeat this (not too fast): push and pull, push and pull … Soften and relax your hands, arms, shoulders, body (and mind). This will make you more sensitive and capable of feeling the energy. Try to increase your sensitivity to this force between your hands that acts like a sticky invisible gel that has some elasticity between and surrounding your hands. You can feel it as you push them together or move apart.

Most people can feel it even upon their first attempt, but sometimes you may not. If you cannot, don't worry. As you practice your meditation more, your mind will become quieter still and then the energy will naturally come to you and you will feel it.

Also you should not get attached to this phenomenon by making yourself feel you "have to experience it" or else. Otherwise, like so many things we force; it may never show up or disappear after you have experienced it a few times. This is because letting go of attachments is essential to opening the mind and keeping it open and is key to sensitivity and connection to more subtle energy sources.

In actual practice, you do not have to hold your hands in the exact way mentioned above at all; as other ways or positions are just as good. You can also feel the same energy without using your hands – as long as you are in a meditative state, you can feel it, although the feeling and strength may be somewhat different when not using your hands, perhaps just feeling it upon or along your skin.

Sometimes (for instance when you meditate in a standing position) your entire body can feel it, too, as if the energy is holding you in posture. When you practice movements in this mindset, the energy is like a sort of sticky liquid surrounding your body and flowing around you. During energy movement practices such as Qigong, Taiji, etc., you can receive and feel this amazing energy from other dimension(s) with even greater sensitivity.

If your mind is open and pure, sometimes referred to as "beginners mind," new and simple, pure, transparent, clear and open to the beautiful universe and its spiritual characteristics, this powerful energy can always be felt surrounding you and within you. You can luxuriate in it. You can live this way. You can. You can live in the safety and comfort, ease and generosity of this great restorative energy every moment if you choose. All you have to do is turn on the switch and make yourself aware because after all, no matter whether you physically feel the sensation or not, this mysterious energy from another dimension is with you and within you, to bring you peace, calmness, happiness, clarity, wisdom, health, beauty and longevity. Mindfulness is, then, your first step.

So you may be thinking, what kind of energy is this? Where does this energy come from? Why does the mind have to be quiet, in the meditation state or cultivated state (such as peaceful, no attachment, anxiety, worry, busy mind, impatience, etc.), otherwise it is not easy to feel it? Why is a well-experienced meditator or spiritual cultivator able to immediately feel it without even trying or even with his or her eyes open throughout daily events? Is this implying that the cultivator's mind has to stay in a spiritual cultivation state in order to connect to the energy source in the other dimension? Is this telling that good cultivator is always having such blessing energy within and surrounding him/her, so he/she always feels energetic and clear headed, and performs daily tasks efficiently, but never get tired?

We cannot directly say that this energy we just felt between hands during the meditation is simply the dark energy. We can't say it – at this point. It is too early to say it. But this energy is really there as we felt it. It is not anything like a regular gravity force, electromagnetic force, or any ordinary kind of force. So what is it?

We do not have a direct experiment to testify this energy because it is not something we can measure directly at this point. However, we applied this energy to a biological system, such as cardiac cells in the physiological condition and measured the biological activity such as the cardiac cells' contractile force (heart beating), and we saw the contractile force of cardiac cells was increased significantly (for details, see experimental research in the later chapter). As a control experiment, instead of experienced meditator, a non-meditation practitioner could not generate such energy to increase the contractile force of the cardiac cells. This implied that the energy on our hands generated during a quality meditation can react with the biological tissue and be converted to biological energy form: the contraction force in this particular case. We have more such experiments that will be presented in a later chapter, suggesting the energy during the meditation is invisible in this physical realm, but can come to this physical dimension to do something. In other words, this energy is real, can be transformed into this physical dimension and react with the biological system in addition to our hands-felt physical force generated during the meditation.

This makes us think – just an idea or hypothetical idea: Is this energy something like the dark energy that exists everywhere, even in vacuum space, and has a sort of force but not necessarily the same as the gravity force or the same gravity force but other additional effects on our biological body? Of course, the strength of the force we felt on hands is not comparable to the gravity force that pulls the supernovae away to accelerate the universe expanding. This can be simply due to the disparity of their masses in these two cases. Or perhaps because we human beings are ourselves passengers on the huge celestial system that is being rapidly pulled away outwardly, therefore we are not able to notice by ourselves that we are under such strong pulling force and in the process of rapid cosmic acceleration. But the energetic force we felt during meditation or Qigong or Taiji movements may be something additional to the gravity force, and it can be even more critical and interesting as a nature the dark energy may have.

Of interest is that this energy is not just a force we felt on hands, and that it does something with the biological system and physical and mental health as we mentioned above, and will be also addressed in details in the following chapter. As well, it seems to involve the spiritual aspect because it appears within a meditation cultivation mindset, with the mind kept empty and clear of human thoughts as we mentioned above. Otherwise, it is not felt nor does it have any effect(s) on the biological tissue and health of the body and mind.

Is it an intellectual power behind this physical realm that provides this energy with a precondition requiring a higher standard of human mind quality and nature? Is it possible that the human mind in the meditation state passes a pure spiritual message to the higher intellectual energy source (higher spirit) and gets connected with the higher spirit, so that as a result the energy comes to this physical dimension? We cannot say anything about these possibilities yet, but it is truly inspiring for us to further consider the possible relationship between the cosmic dark energy and spiritual energy, their association or identity.

If this energy we felt during meditation cultivation is something related with the dark energy or maybe just the dark energy from the vast compassionate universe, it will be a great golden key gifted to us to open the blessing path to the truth of the universe and life even wider, encouraging us to cultivate spiritually for the higher life destination. Just as a **hypothesis**, we may say it this way:

> ***The spiritual energy generated during meditation cultivation could be the force or one of the forces (powers) that transports the cultivator to the higher dimension to heal and eventually to the heavenly place as the final goal of spiritual cultivation.***

§3.2.4 Missed Point: Intellectual Spirit In Science

Please keep in mind that the reason we are talking about universe or cosmos is not just because of our curiosity about the cosmos like cosmologists do. In mind-body-spirit science, what we are interested is to interact with the cosmos and learn the knowledge about its energetic nature and spiritual character, with which we can activate our spiritual ability and sensitivity (*Wu Xing*), open our mind and enlighten our spirit to connect our true Self with the universe's spirit and energy source, achieving the complete healing, health and enlightenment of mind, body and spirit. Below please read with your opened mind and maximized imagination.

So far, the overwhelming majority of our understanding about the universe stems from our understanding of ordinary particles such as atoms, protons, electrons, photos … quarks, … etc. We have ignored the majority of the vast cosmos and its characteristics and functions, perhaps its most important part, dark energy and dark matter, completely different new "particles" (if it is particle) from ordinary particles. Our knowledge is thus very incomplete, only a drop of the ocean.

The cosmologists consider dark energy based on gravitational force, which is simply a mechanical or physical force. Conventional science thinks the universe started 13.7 billion years ago from a Big Bang and then exploded, expanding and accelerating continuously due to gravitation. The standard model of cosmology basically considers everything about the universe – its origin and dark energy included – from the understanding of mechanical or physical interaction forces (attractive and repulsive forces). Yet, it never considers factors in any spiritual force, intelligent energy or wisdom behind or within visible matter in the universe.

Think of this: When we as a living spirit drive a car, we drive with a mind that knows clearly how to drive, where to go and for what – e.g. going home, going to work, attending an inspiring discussion forum, or visiting a fun place, etc. From the surface, the car is moving physically due to the mechanical driving force generated by the burning gasoline and/or mixture with electricity, but in fact the car's entire moving process involves the mental and conscious energy of the driver.

Imagine we are inside an airplane. Before landing we are overlooking the freeways steady stream of vehicles coming and going. Isn't it just as we look up the night sky – where the stars, planets, and galaxies float in the sky of our vast cosmos? We all do know the vehicles are not just moving mechanically by themselves due to the physical force from gasoline and electricity, but also driven by living spirits, and therefore they are very organized on their way, each with its own driver, with

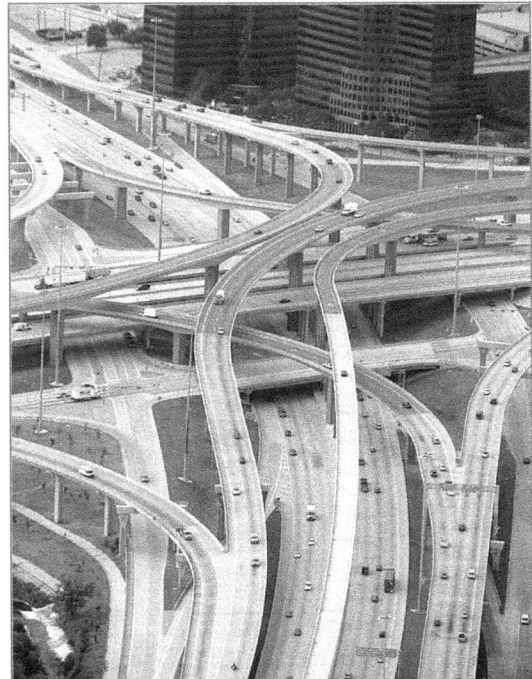

driving skill and knowledge, following driving rules with care of others and without hitting each other (in fact, not only driving, but also carrying on all other phenomena of the lives within, all involving intellectual spirit). Yet, we never think of the stars, planets, and galaxies (or other atomic objects) of also having spirit operating them, moving them along their way, providing order, destination, and purpose. Of course, it won't be that simple that the astronomical objects drive themselves as human beings drive the cars. What I mean it is possible there is a super powerful intellectual spiritual force and wisdom behind the objects (for instance, the dark matter and dark energy or their supreme force behind) is operating all these in the way our human beings cannot imagine yet.

Human beings have the tendency to study something in the world outside of ourselves, the objective world, by assuming everything (except ourselves) is an inanimate thing. With such assuming, we try so hard and precisely to establish theories, techniques, and equations to calculate, measure, quantify, explain, guess or infer how the universe or the matters (including lives) will behave.

Think of this, if we consider only the mechanically based current moving status of each of the vehicles on our freeway, can we possibly know, analyze, calculate or guess where each of these vehicles will go? Of course we can't tell. This is because that information is in the minds of the drivers - the souls driving the cars that we don't know about and is never taken into account by the mechanically based science.

The purpose of this simple analogy is to help clarify: When we study anything in this universe, we should not forget that in addition to our human beings, other things, objects, matters, including small particles, bigger planets, stars, galaxies, or supernovae in the universe, and the universe itself, as one entity can also be alive with wisdom or intellectual soul. Of course, we cannot use human's idea to understand the soul of the universe and its sub-layers although they could be originated from the same core characteristics. Without introducing the factor or parameter of living spirit or intellectual soul

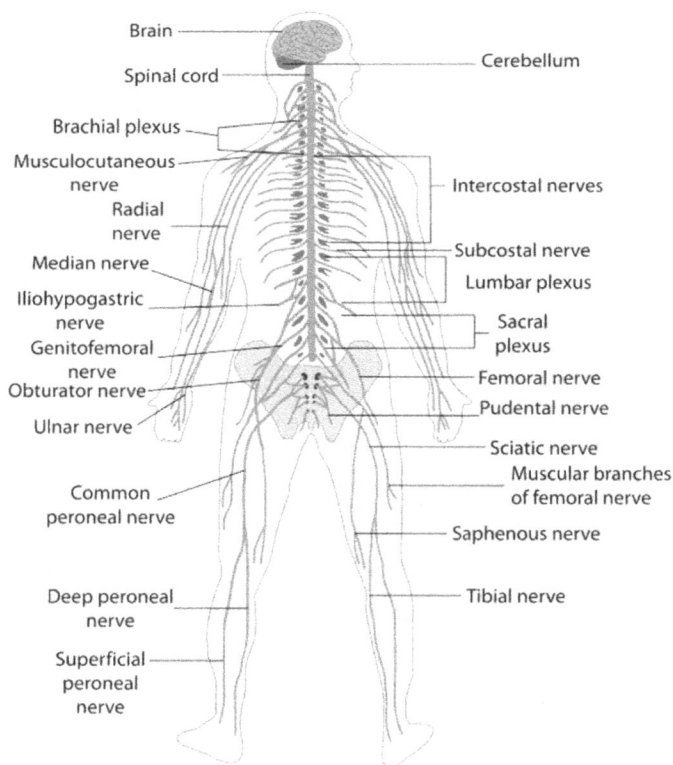

Brain
Cerebellum
Spinal cord
Brachial plexus
Musculocutaneous nerve
Radial nerve
Median nerve
Iliohypogastric nerve
Genitofemoral nerve
Obturator nerve
Ulnar nerve
Intercostal nerves
Subcostal nerve
Lumbar plexus
Sacral plexus
Femoral nerve
Pudental nerve
Sciatic nerve
Muscular branches of femoral nerve
Saphenous nerve
Common peroneal nerve
Deep peroneal nerve
Tibial nerve
Superficial peroneal nerve

(including that of humans but it is not necessary that all of them are like that of human beings), our study of the universe and life will be forever too difficult to reach the truth.

If the entire universe is a huge living spirit, why can't we think of the matters (including lives we have so far defined) in the universe as having consciousness or spirit to operate itself locally and individually under the supreme spirit of the universe and by the mechanism originally installed by the supreme spirit?

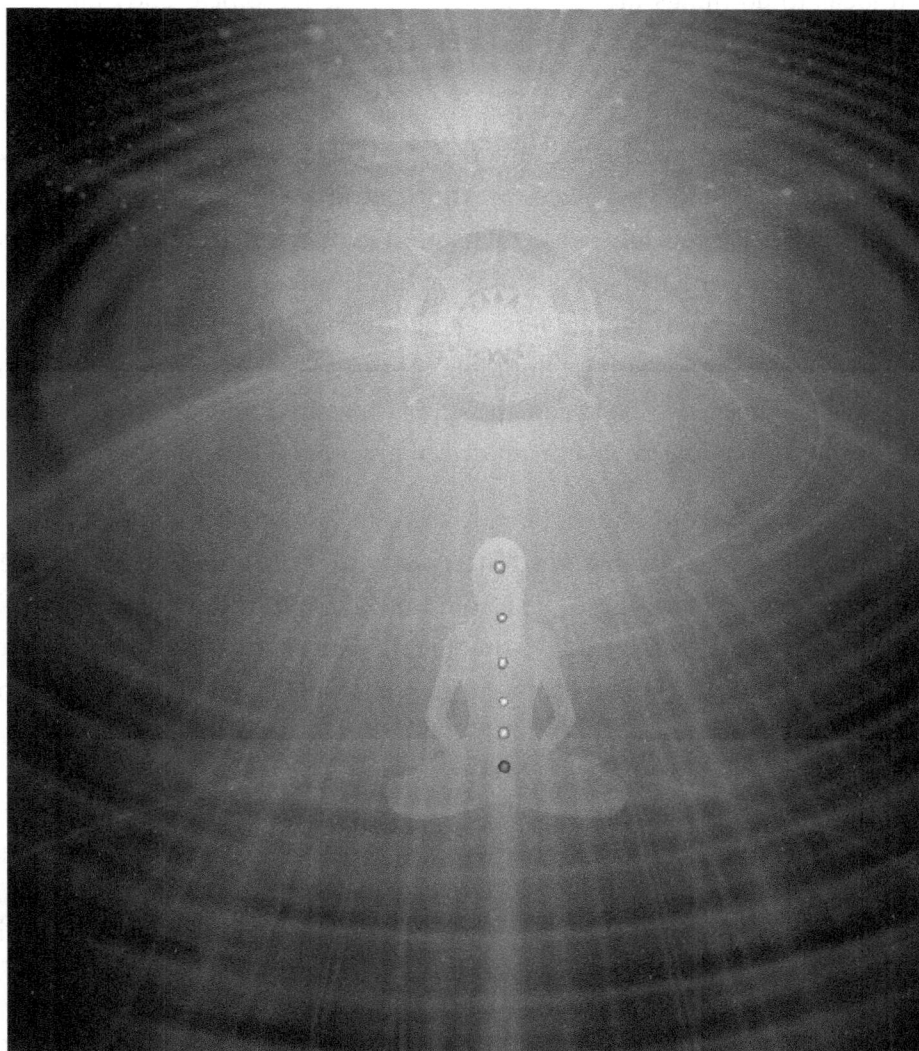

Isn't it possible that universe, the stars, planets, galaxies, all lives and objects in the universe have their own spirit (at different levels and in different forms) inside of themselves (1) that was installed by the creator originally, (2) that knows what to do, how to do it, where to go, how to live and how to behave, and that (3) that are operating with the internally preinstalled intelligent spirit and under the ultimate supervision of the universe's supreme spirit?

Isn't it possible that all these objects and lives in the universe and the universe itself are in a similar way to human beings which have a brain to operate the entire body and each of the organs, tissues and cells which also have their natures, characters, feelings and behaviors to live?

If simply thinking of this way, don't we have reason to say that the spirit of the universe has spiritual energy just like our human minds have spiritual and mental energy, thoughts and ideas to do things including influencing the biological body and sustaining all components within the body (organs, tissues and cells, etc.)?

Aren't all objects and lives within and under the universe like the organs, tissues, cells, genes, and molecules inside the human body which are cooperated with each other, and harmonized, guided and organized by the central neuron system, mind and spirit? Aren't they all designed precisely with such intelligent spirit installed at different levels with (1) Independence in order to operate at their level, and (2) Connectivity with the whole in order to keep the oneness of the universe and cooperativeness between each party of the universe, and (3) Belongingness to the Supreme Spirit in order to be operated and guided by the Supreme spirit? Otherwise how can the entire universe and all forms of objects and lives operate, develop, live and behave in an extremely precise order and process?

Of course, compared to human beings, the universe's spirit is much more powerful, highly intellectual, has unbelievable wisdom, energy and profound characteristics such as compassion, peace and righteousness – all based on the law of the universe, which creates all things in the universe with the same characteristics originally. It is then later, over time, that these shared characteristics may drop to different levels as an individual's behavior and spiritual quality may change.

If above hypothesis is true, then it will be extremely helpful and critical for us in order to establish the fundamental principle, theory and practice of the mind-body-spirit science. It means, as a part of the universe, a whole human being with mind, body and spirit is directly related with the universe, its spirit, and its mechanism by which lives were created and operated.

As scientists, we need to open our mind, to use all our knowledge not only the knowledge given to us in schools or textbooks (that are very incomplete and not always correct or sometimes actually wrong, as we already know), but also knowledge embedded in our true Self, our own common sense, intuition, inborn ability, spiritual *Wu Xing*, daily observations, experiences, and importantly spiritual teachings from higher masters.

Among all these, the first, simplest, and most important knowledge, logic and fact we have is: We human beings are living spirits. And this is simple for us to know, sense, and prove. We see fishes are swimming under the water and birds flying in the sky as living lives. Why can't we think the stars, planets, galaxies and all other matters in the universe are also living lives? When, where, why and who defined organics as lives, but inorganics as non-lives?

If we know a car cannot appear and move on the earth all of sudden by itself without design, creation and operation by human beings that have higher spirit and intelligence than the car, how can the universe and lives, including human life, appear, exist, move and live all of sudden without higher intellectual spirit to design, create and operate them? Here we are not talking about any belief system or religion concerning believing in GOD creature or not. As scientist of mind-body science when we cannot scientifically explain something such as acceleration of the universe's expansion, which is unexpected by our model, we have to think again and ask ourselves: did we miss something fundamental from the very beginning? Is the science we are using for definition looking too far from the truth and too narrow-mindedly so that it restricts us from a much more open, wider path toward discovering the real truth?

Personally I think it is the time we have to introduce the concept, factor or parameter of spirit – an intellectual energy - into the science of the universe and life and broaden the scientific ideology and methodology from only conventional mathematics, physics, and experimental testing and measurement in this physical dimension to include other spiritual dimensions. Otherwise our study will be difficult to progress or will even fall into a wrong direction.

§3.2.5 Supreme Spirit and Its Energy Carrier & Operator

So where is the universe's spirit located? Isn't it everywhere? It is very possible. This spirit has such energy intellectually operating the universe, including accelerating the universe expansion. If this is true, it is possible that dark energy can be the carrier, operator, and entity of the spirit of the universe in a form invisible to humankind but existing everywhere as background within the universe at other dimensions different from this space-time dimension to operate, take care of, protect and supervise everything of the universe such as all galaxies, planets, stars, astronomical objects, particles and lives, of course, including human beings, human societies on the earth planet.

This is a hypothesis at this point without evidence from conventional science. However, it can be reasoned after putting together conventional sciences, spiritual studies, and teachings from higher masters, blessing enlightenment messages from cultivation, long years of spiritual practices, experiences, common observations, common logics, and intuition. As a hypothetical model, the dark energy (or part of it if conservatively speaking) may be an Intellectual Energy (IE) or Spiritual Energy (SE) that pervades the universe everywhere, forming an Intellectual Energy Field (IEF) or Spiritual Energy Field (SEF). This energy is part of the Supreme Spirit Power (SSP)[9] of the universe, so it is operated, taken care of, protected, supervised, and controlled by the Supreme Spirit (SS), and at the same time it also has its Local Intellectual Powers (LIP) or Local Spiritual Powers (LSP)/Energy to lead, supervise, operate, take care of, interact with, serve and provide needs of, the individual celestial objects, galaxies, stars, planets, particles, and lives (including human beings on the earth) in the universe.

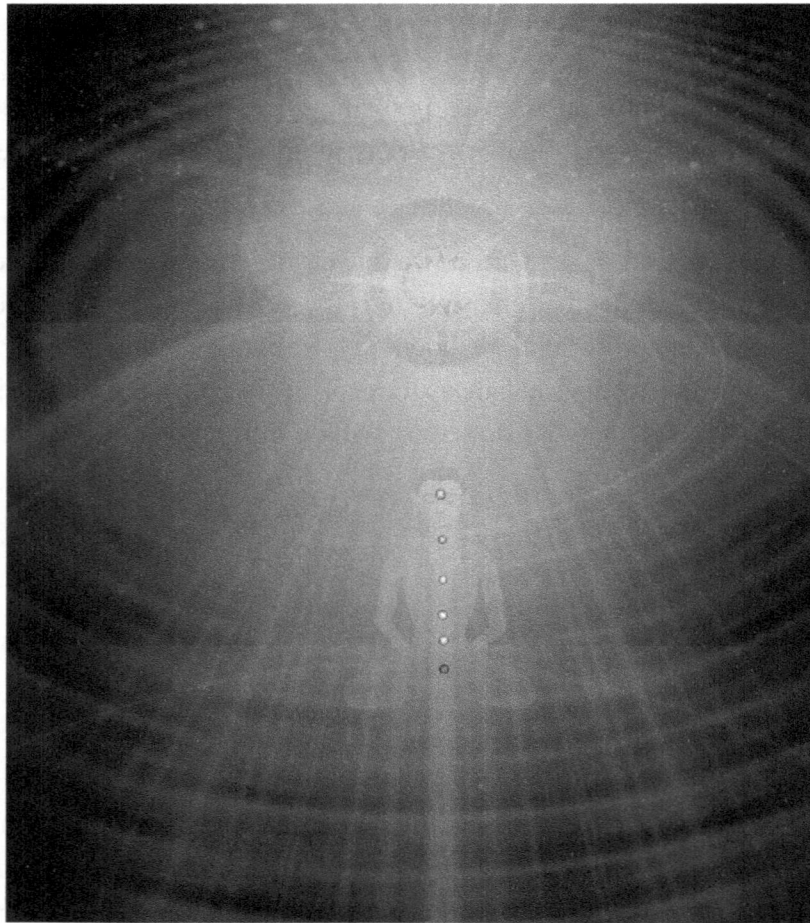

The force to accelerate the expansion of the universe is perhaps just one of the Supreme Spirit Power / SSP, a macroscopic expression as a repulsive force of the dark

---

[9] The Supreme Spirit Power (SSP) of the universe is defined as a hypothetical idea that the universe itself is the greatest spiritual being that possesses an intellectual spiritual Supreme Spirit (SS) blessing, operating and governing the entire system. Sometime we also refer this SSP as Highest Spirit / HS or Highest Energy Source / HES.

energy, but not the sum of the powers. Although this energy field is everywhere in the universe, maybe operating the universe and all things within it uniformly independent upon the distribution of ordinary matters but maybe regionally dependent upon distributions of the ordinary matters. The outcome or effects of the Spiritual Energy Power on each individual, objects, or lives in ordinary matter's space-time are not uniformly the same because it is depending upon the spiritual quality or energy nature of each individual, objects, or lives, in the way that SSP's natural law operates and governs the universe. For example, a person with good Virtue (e.g., truthful, forgiving, caring others, loving and compassionate), and cultivation energy often leads to good health, happy and long living, gain good social reputation, honor and respects, while a person having bad personality, character and behaviors often leads to health problems or difficult life. This is just an example that the Supreme Law or SSP takes effect on human beings based upon the individual's Virtue level or amount of Karma.

The reason that dark energy is named "dark energy" is that it does not emit light nor reflect light and is totally invisible to humankind. However, from the perspective of spiritual understanding as described above, dark energy is not termed well because of the negative connotation of the word, *dark*. It is dark to the human being at this lower dimension, but it is bright and powerful in the higher spiritual dimensions. We really want to call it Intellectual Energy (IE) or Spiritual Energy (SE) as we defined above, but because Dark Energy is already a well-known term and also because we cannot completely prove the above hypothesis at present time, we will still call it dark energy anyway.

In this book, however, we often refer to some terms such as Spiritual Energy, Supreme Spirit Power, Highest Energy Source, which in meaning are intended as we proposed above as a hypothetical model. This mysterious Spiritual Energy (SE) may be characteristically related with the dark energy (DE), and possessing but not limited to the following:

1. Originates from the Supreme Spirit (SS) of the universe

2. Is part of the Supreme Spirit Power (SSP) or Energy (SSE)

3. Is under the SS's governing, operation, caring and controlling by following the universe's supreme law which is created by the SS.

4. Is made from origin particles (or sort of particle) of the universe in other dimension(s), which have intellectual living spirits and super powers, and are completely different from ordinary particles in this space-time dimension.

5. Dominates the universe, constituting the majority of the universe and pervading the universe everywhere in the background like vacuum, which is invisible to ordinary space-time dimension.

6. Forms an Intellectual Energy Field (IEF) or Spiritual Energy Field (SEF) in other dimension(s) over the entire universe that is invisible to humankind in this ordinary dimension.

7. Exists everywhere in the universe and its density and nature may or may not be uniformly distributed. It seems the expressions or effects of this energy field may be or may not be uniform or even to all matters and lives. In other words its effects may appear regionally or may be individualized locally, according to the SS and depending upon the local matters/lives and their nature and quality.

8. Is in other dimensions that are different from the ordinary space-time dimension, yet, it can be transferred or transformed into the energy form(s) in this ordinary dimension to affect the matters and lives in the ordinary realm.

9. Possesses Local Intellectual Power (LIP) or energy (LIE) within and surrounding local matters and lives but expresses its powers and effects accordingly (*see* next).

10. LIP/LIE is super intellectual and expresses its power and effects to each of the local matters or lives depending on the local matters and their nature, quality, spiritual Virtue or Karma by following the supreme law of the universe.

11. LIP/LIE has super power that creates, operates, takes care of, and determines life paths of all local matters/lives depending their nature and quality by following the law.

12. LIP/LIE possesses multiple powers (functions or effects) that can be transferred to the ordinary dimension and affect local matters and lives.

13. SSP/SSE and LIP/LIE together justify all matters and lives based on the universe's law (the universe's characteristics such as compassion, peace, righteousness, truthfulness, justice, tolerance) and the spiritual quality and characteristics of the local matters or lives.

14. Capacity to increase the quality and natures of local lives and their cultivation to a higher level under the SS through LIP/LIE energy field, in order to be blessed and favored by the SSP – life cultivation.

15. Benefits human beings directly: physically, mentally and spiritually with the precondition of a certain mental state and spiritual quality, for example, through deep meditation or spiritual cultivation.

16. Effects of SSP/SSE and LIP/LIE on local matters and lives may include but are not limited to: blessing effects such as birth, growth, changes, happiness, honor, consummation or returning back to kingdom of the heaven for eternal happy living, or punishing effects such as sickness, pain, suffering, difficulties, hardships, aging, poverty, and being sent to hell, depending upon the quality, behaviors, Virtue and Karma of local matters and lives.

17. The energy field has elasticity (attraction or repulsion).

18. If this Spiritual Energy is the dark energy or partially the dark energy, or the dark energy is a part of this Spiritual Energy, or both are related, then it generates repulsive force to accelerate the universe's expansion. This gravitational effect is only one of the many effects and powers of this energy but not everything. The gravitational force from this energy is just the superficial expression of this energy from the observation of humankind but not the essential characteristics of this energy.

The universe is full of lives and everything is a living spirit but with different quality, nature, form, Virtue, Karma, and sometimes in different dimensions. So as such, what else is there within a living life besides its material structure or physical body composed of the ordinary matter? Wouldn't spirit and spiritual energies within and surrounding each human being play an important role in each entire human being as well? It is very likely so. The dark energy (and maybe including the dark matter) must be something related with the spiritual nature of the universe. This aspect of the universe has so much mysterious power that is very likely related to its spiritual characteristics and energies. On the other hand, the universe's spiritual characteristics and energies, it seems, must somehow be associated with the major content of the universe, the dark energy and dark matter. Otherwise, there is no other candidate to consider.

If this hypothesis is true, then it means that the spiritual, mental and energetic vibration energies and particles (not the ordinary matter) constitute the majority of the universe. Within such a universe, if assuming a human being also has the same proportion of these spiritual energies and particles, then:

Our physical body is only less 5% of the entire being at the physical visible dimension, while the mental and spiritual energies and particles are the 95% in the higher dimension(s) of the mind and spirit! Such mental and spiritual energies and

matters must be very important and powerful because they occupy the 95%+ of the entire being to take care of, operate, and supervise the entire being behind the physical body!

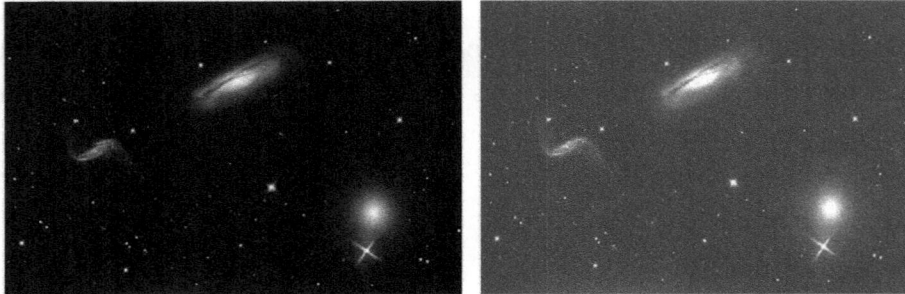

Fig. 3.2.6. The left image is the original picture of Trio Leo (small group of galaxies 35 mil light years away), and the right image was added with brighter background if black/white print or blue background if color print, showing the Spiritual Energy (SE) everywhere within the universe but in other dimensions. Note that there is no color in the SE so that there is no way to show the SE in this dimension, therefore this image is a conceptual illustration.

This hypothesis has not been completely evidenced, but it is already strongly suggested by humankind's knowledge, observation, research, experience, and cultivation of mind, body and spirit and as well as sciences, studies, experiments in related fields, as we will gradually see in the later chapters.

Back to the topic of health of body, mind and spirit – if the hypothesis proposed above is true (in fact it is likely true), think of this: We can then cultivate our mind and spirit to improve the quality and nature of them, get connected with the Supreme Spirit, gain such powerful energy as to heal the whole being and gain true health. Then, it becomes possible to find the true meaning of this life within this lifetime and reach the eternal life destination in other higher dimensions.

This idea of Supreme Spirit and its energy carrier and operator is the most important concept and belief in mind-body-spirit science and practice. We will further explore this topic in the following chapters in terms of, for example, spiritual and mental energy, mind-body cultivation, intra and inter-dimensional energy transformation and transferring crossing the physical, mental and spiritual dimensions for the whole being healing and life cultivation.

§3.2.6 Scientific Findings on Mind-Spirit Energy

The supreme spirit of the universe has powerful energy that affects everything and everyone in the universe, including mind, body, and spirit of human beings, in the way that complies with the ultimate law. The mind of any individual human being can communicate with this spirit and access this energy to achieve integrity, balance and health of body-mind-spirit. The ability of the mind to access such powerful energy is dependent upon the quality of the individual's mind nature and spirituality, in terms of, for example, purpose and meaning of life, love, compassion, conscience, giving, sharing, forgiveness, peace, patience, and all other positive mindsets. Many spiritual and mental scientists have researched in this field in different ways and provided convincing evidences for the relationship between psychological, mental or spiritual quality and health status of the whole being. We will introduce some of our experiments in the later chapter, while the following is a recent research from other scientists.

During the past 10 years, the research team led by Dr. Steven Cole, professor of medicine and member of UCLA's Cousins Center for Psychoneuroimmunology, and his colleagues, including Barbara L. Fredrickson from University of North Carolina, examined how positive psychology impacts human gene expression [26]. What they found is that different types of happiness have surprisingly different effects on the human genome. When people are doing good things, for instance, that have high levels of eudaimonic (content) well-being, and they derive their happiness from a deep sense of purpose and meaning in life, then they show favorable gene-expression profiles in their immune cells. As a result, such individuals demonstrate low levels of inflammatory gene expression and strong antibody and antiviral genes. However, for individuals who have relatively high levels of hedonistic well-being - the type of happiness that comes from over-indulgent consumption, self-gratification (think most celebrities) - shows just the opposite: these individuals have an adverse gene-expression profile, resulting in high inflammation and low antiviral and antibody gene expression. Cole's experiment amazingly illuminated the interactivity between the physical body's biological factor (gene expression) and the mind-spirit connection.

A most interesting and significant point in this result is that not only does the happy feeling (state of mind), but also the spiritual nature (quality of spirit/goodness) determine gene-expression. Determining higher or lower quality of spirit is based on the law of the universe, the characteristics of the universe. The higher quality of spirit appears as love, compassion, conscience, giving, sharing, and doing good things for others, as well as living a meaningful life with higher spiritual purpose and cultivation for such purpose. In contrast, the lower quality of spirit appears in such things as hate, revenge, violence, selfishness, jealousy, doing bad things to others, unclear life purpose or no meaningful purpose for this life.

One of the most well-known researches on the spiritual energy value of consciousness was developed by Dr. David R. Hawkins, a worldwide renowned psychiatrist, physician, researcher, spiritual teacher and lecturer. One of his focused areas was evaluating spiritual and mental energy and their impacts in human lives. He successfully discovered the relationship of energies in non-linear dimensions in mental and spiritual worlds with linier mathematic values as well as their impacts to this physical realm including the lives of human beings. Dr. Hawkins's finding was described in his book: *Power Vs Force* [27]. Hawkins specifically described each level of spiritual value and mental states in a numeric scale based on Applied Kinesiology muscle tests. The result can be summarized in the table 3.2.6.

Spiritual Energy Level	Numeric Score	Mental / Emotion Level	Impact in Life View
Enlightenment	700-1000	Ineffable	Is
Peace	600	Bliss	Perfect
Joy	540	Serenity	Complete
Love	500	Reverence	Benign
Reason	400	Understanding	Meaningful
Acceptance	350	Forgiveness	Harmonious
Willingness	310	Optimism	Hopeful
Neutrality	250	Trust	Satisfactory
Courage	200	Affirmation	Feasible
Pride	175	Scorn	Demanding
Anger	150	Hate	Antagonistic
Desire	125	Graving	Disappointing
Fear	100	Anxiety	Frightening
Grief	75	Regret	Tragic
Apathy	50	Despair	Hopeless
Guilt	30	Blame	Evil
Shame	20	Humiliation	Miserable

Table 3.2.6. Applied Kinesiology muscle tests by Dr. David R. Hawkins.

Based on Dr. Hawkin's work, the enlightenment value is above 700 and under 1000 as maximum. In fact, using the same ideology and technique of Applied Kinesiology, we could personally test almost anything (visible objects or invisible mental or spiritual aspects such as thought, idea, theory, hypothesis, etc.) and give a number in the muscle test to evaluate its energy level. The universe's ultimate law as described in the early section of this chapter was also tested with the muscle test. Interestingly we found that this Supreme Law gave the number not just above 1000 but actually infinity. In other worlds, we could not measure the ultimate law with the same scale in the test. The only explanation for this result is that the law has infinite energy from the energy source of universe.

A question is, why can muscle strength or weakness reveal the true energy level or truth/falseness of the Applied Kinesiology muscle test? For example, consider testing two tomatoes among which one is organic and another one is non-organic with a subject who is never told about which one is organic or which one is not. As the test goes, when testing the organic tomato, the subject's muscles strengthen to confirm the statement "this is an organic tomato," however when testing the non-organic tomato, his muscles weaken to confirm the statement "this is non-organic tomato." Why is it the subject's muscles can tell the truth? The possible explanation is: the organic tomato has good energy, which empowered the muscles and the non-organic tomato has weaker energy or negative energy, which weakened the muscles. This energy influence happens in other dimension during the test: the subject as a whole being of mind-body-spirit, communicates with the tomato's energy vibration in other subtler energy dimensions, and then gains positive energy (or negative energy), and then behaves stronger (or weaker) in this physical dimension.

§3.3 Multiple Bodies Unified by Energy under Fundamental Law

From the understanding of energy medicine, quantum theory, and spiritual energy we addressed above, we can propose a hypothetical model of multiple bodies: Across all these energy dimensions from high to low, a human being as a living life of spirit, mind and body, exists in different energy dimensions with multiple forms/bodies. In other words, a human being has multiple bodies in each of these dimensions and subdimensions; the spirit of a human being exists in the highest spiritual dimension where the highest truth can be revealed, and mind (e.g., emotions, etc.) exists in the intermediate invisible energy dimensions, and the physical body exists in this visible physical world with lower energy and with no truth-revealing transparency.

These bodies are associated with each other as a unified entity through mirror-image relationship[10] and mysterious energy transformation mechanisms crossing all dimensions. A human being has not only a physical body as described in the modern mainstream medicine (such as anatomy, biology, physiology, biochemistry, and molecular biosciences) in this detectable and lower energy physical dimension, but also has other bodies in macroscopic dimensions, microscopic dimensions and high energy spiritual dimensions. These bodies together make up the entire being.

Each of these aforementioned bodies in each level of dimension has its different energy characters, playing the roles at the corresponding dimension. As part of the universe, a human being is an energy complex with multiple layers of dimensional structures. In general, these multiple dimensional levels of bodies can be collectively classified into three levels called physical body (body), mental body (mind) and spiritual body (spirit). Each of these bodies may further have sub-bodies in different energy forms, but we conceptually group them into three bodies in energy forms that flow within and around each body and transform from one to another in communicating with each other.

Just like the universe that is composed of 4.6% visible ordinary matter and 95.4% dark matter and dark energy, the visible physical body is only a tiny part of the entire being, while its majority is the mind and spirit in other invisible dimensions where they are pervaded with mental energy and spiritual energy. The mental body and spiritual body can be positive or negative, depending on each person's energy condition and quality, which determine health status and life quality of the body, mind and spirit, and influence others or the surroundings environments.

A good mind-body-spirit cultivator has higher quality and greater volume of mental and spiritual energies, so that he/she has bigger, stronger, healthier and higher quality of mental body and spiritual body that provide the physical body with good positive energy, resulting in not only good health physically, mentally and spiritually, but also good life quality. This manifests in blessings, luck, and fortunate opportunities in this physical world, which we call Virtue.

The opposite, of course, is exemplifies another way, which is Karma, resulting in bad health and life quality if the mental energy and spiritual energy are bad. Remember the

---

[10] Mirror-image relationship: the relationship of an object to its mirror image, that is, the relationship exhibited by two similar but nonsuperimposable crystals or structures. The mirror image is originally a term of optical physics, meaning an image of optically reflected duplication of an object, which appears identical but reversed of the original object. As an optical effect it results from reflection off of substances such as a mirror or water. It is also a concept in geometry and can be used as a conceptualization process for 3-D structures. In this book we use mirror-image relationship to explain the multiple bodies in different dimensions, which have similar or identical images but made of different substances in different realms, and together forming the entire unified being or object.

majority of the entire being is in other invisible dimensions where the mental body and spiritual body exist. But these invisible bodies dominate the greater part of the whole being in energy form, in the background, like the water in the pool that provides life force source for the fishes, as the water-fish model or dark energy as we described early.

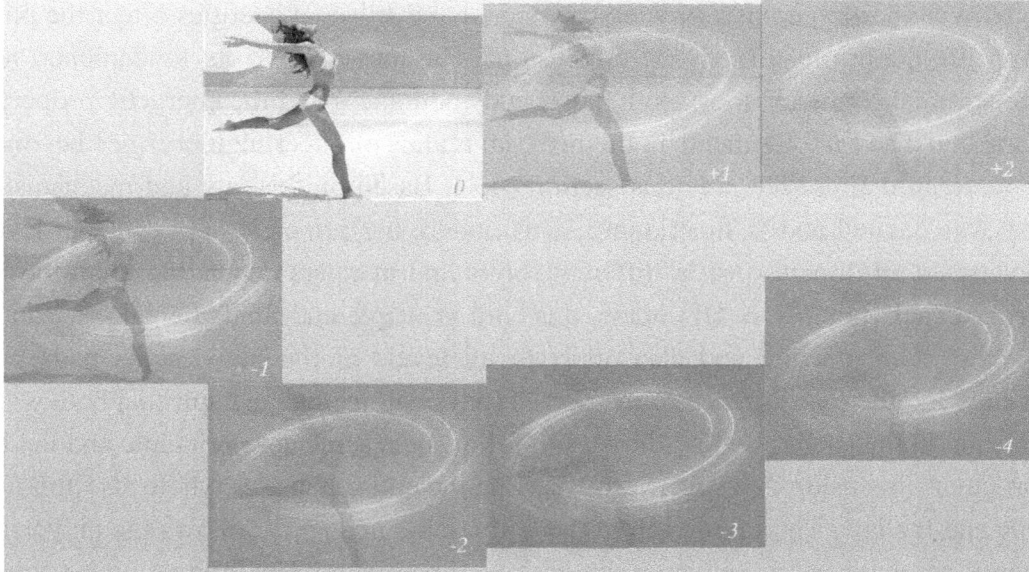

Fig. 3.3. A conceptual presentation to explain the multiple bodies and their energy process in different dimensions of mind, body and spirit as well as dimensions of time, space and energy. The runner is running physically at the present time as shown in the image labeled as 0 in this physical dimension, but she has her spirit or soul had engaged ahead of time (image labeled as +2) in the spiritual dimension with energy in other dimension already generated. At the moment ahead of time (labeled as +1) she already had such emotional energy in the mental dimension to run. In fact at the present moment while she is running, her spirit and mind are constantly involved with her physical action of running, together performing the perfect operation of mind-body-spirit as a whole being in the dimensions of body, mind and spirit. Furthermore the action of her running in the past and present moments also leaves its energetic records in other dimensions of mind, body and spirit and time and space as expressed in the images labeled as −1, -2, -3, -4, ... after her running was taken place – these energy forms exist in other dimensions forever. As result, this will have impact to her emotional feelings, mental health, physical strength and spiritual happiness and freshness afterward.

Fig. 3.3 uses a conceptual presentation to explain the secret that any action or behavior that has been taken place by the mind, body and / or spirit has its energy form, process and influences existing in all dimensions such as physical, mental, spiritual, time, space, energetic dimensions. Therefore any single thought, idea, talk, action, behavior, or any individual or social activity in the mind, body or spirit, is an energy vibration that has impact to oneself, others, and the surrounding environments.

Depending upon the person's mental and spiritual energy nature, quality, level, and volume, the person will have a different quality of life, health, personality, energy, performance, and influences to others and surrounding environments, and for everything else expressed in this physical realm.

Now a question comes: how do the mental and spiritual energies affect the physical body and life quality in this visible dimension? The universe has its fundamental natural law (the spiritual characteristics: truth, good and endurance) and the energetic properties of Yin-Yang and The Five Elements in the material realms or super high energies beyond (out of) the material realms (see previous section §3.1). Based on this law and mechanism, the universe was created and is functioning. This underlying principle applies to all levels of the universe in all dimensions, in different forms and manners depending upon the nature and form of each dimension. Of course, this core principle and fundamental law can apply to the entire human being and also apply to all levels of the individual's bodies in all dimensions. In other words, each of the bodies (physical, mental and spiritual bodies) of the human being in the corresponding dimension follows the same core principle and the law in that particular dimension in a specific way, while the entire being as whole also follows the principle and the law. Therefore each of the body, mind and spirit follows the universal law and energy mechanism in their own dimension respectively. This allows each to develop good quality energies. At the same time, the higher powers of energies in the mind and spirit follow the law and principle to cultivate, elevate their level and quality, integrate these life components, and transform their energies through higher dimensions to physical body to support the physical life and the whole being. Following the law and energy principle means to assimilate, resonate and synchronize with the frequencies of universe's spiritual vibrations and Yin-Yang and The Five Elements energy vibrations. It is the process of mind-body-spirit healing and cultivation.

As energy forms with informational vibration frequency, all bodies of the human being in the multiple dimensions follow the universal law and energy mechanism to communicate, cooperate, unify, harmonize and function, as one system. They communicate to each other through different levels of energy vibrations and energy transformations from one to another. The energy has different forms in different dimensions. Some energy forms are visible at the physical realm where the physical body exists, while some energy forms are invisible at dimensions where mental and spiritual bodies reside. These different forms of energy can be transferred within the same dimension (called intra-dimensional, see next section) or from one dimension to another (called inter-dimensional, see next section), or transformed from one form to another within the same dimension or crossing dimensions through certain processes and pathways – e.g., energy meridians.

For instance, spiritual energy can be transformed to the form of emotional or mental energy, while emotional or mental energy can be transformed to the form of physical energy, and physical energy also can influence mental and spiritual states or be transformed to mental and spiritual energies.

Of course, within the same physical body, energies are transformed and transferred between organs, tissues, cells, molecules, and physiological systems, while within the same person's mind, mental energies or emotional energies can be transformed, converted or transferred from one to another, resulting in physiological and psychological impacts. For example, excessive excitement (imbalance of the fire element) can cause grief, which in turn can hurt the lung, while too much fear (imbalance of the water element) in the mind can inhibit joyfulness (fire) and hurt the heart. These are illustrative of the infinite ways the mind, body and spirit are influenced by each other. The good news is that they can be harmonized, balanced and integrated into one by practicing energy cultivation via the spiritual law and energy principle. For any reason, however, if the energy pathways/meridians are blocked, energy flow cannot pass through, over different dimensions or within the same dimension, or the energy is lacking, low, weak, noisy, distracted, or of poor quality, negative, sick, or overwhelmingly excessive, in that case, the whole being will get sick or feel discomfort. In terms of Oriental Medicine, this impasse is called an energy block, energy deficiency or excess.

Energy block, deficiency, or excess revolves around health problems occurring from one's imbalance with regard to The Five Elements and/or Yin and Yang, but in fact, the Supreme Law of the Universe plays an even larger overall role in the energy process between mental, spiritual and physical bodies of the human being. For example, if a person has good personality and spirituality such as always being truthful, compassionate, loving, giving, forgiving, and tolerant, at least at the human level, he/she is synchronized with the universal law/characteristics. Thus the individual's mental and spiritual energies are good. The law allows the individual to transform these healthy energies into physical form, endowing him or her with good health and life quality. Otherwise, in contrast, if a person has bad spirituality and personality or negative emotions that are far away from the universe's characteristics, the good energy will not be transferred and transformed. Of course, at physical level if the person has imbalanced or unhealthy lifestyle, living habits, eating addictions or a disturbing family and/or social environment, relationships, etc., then the imbalanced energy or energy blocks, deficiency or excess can go even worse.

Speaking specifically of the entire universe, a part of the universe such as a planet (including earth) or a human being and a part of a person such as an organ, mind and emotion are all living lives with different forms and size, in different dimensions, and at different levels, but they were created and are functioning by following the same universal law and principles of the energy system of Yin-Yang and The Five Elements or Beyond The Five Elements at their corresponding dimensions. For example, the universe has Yin and Yang, the pair of fundamental energy forces that are interconnected, interdependent, inter-promotional, and inter-restricted with each other. This is true in both the micro (particle) and macro (the total picture) senses. The balanced status, that is, the interaction between Yin and Yang in a balanced state, is the way that the universe – and all within it, big or tiny – harmoniously functions.

The yin-yang principle and the spiritual nature of truth, good and endurance exist within every human being in this same macro/micro way. This core mechanism, additionally, exists not only in these energy forms at physical dimensions, but also in the forms at other dimensions such as emotional / mental and spiritual dimensions.

The multiple forms (bodies as components or subcomponents) of a human being at different dimensions are integrated and synchronized as one whole. These energy forms (bodies) interact and communicate with each other, through energy transference and transformation between them, based on the fundamental law and the core energy principle. On the other hand, each individual living form (each of the bodies) in its particular dimension has its own form, structure, energy, vibrant frequency, and character while at the same time cooperating with other forms (bodies) of the whole being and following the same core principle and natural law.

§3.4 Intra/Inter-Dimensional Energy Transformation & Transfer

The communications, cooperation and integration of the whole being occur at the all dimensions either between different parts of the form (body) in the same dimension or between different forms (bodies) in the different dimensions. For example, within the physical body, cell-to-cell communication occurs through energy transportation, circulation, transformation and transference. The mind and spirit also communicate with the physical body or any part of the body by crossing over different dimensions. Therefore the integration and communications can be intra-dimensional and inter-dimensional as illustrated in Fig. 3.4.

When the system energy vibration deviates from its original state based on the law and principle, it will have low energy (poor-bad quality energy) or excessive energy, causing energy deficiency or excess, respectively. If dimensions of mind, body and spirit are not integrated based on the law and principle, the energy cannot be transferred inter-dimensionally or intra-dimensionally. This causes the energy meridian blocks.

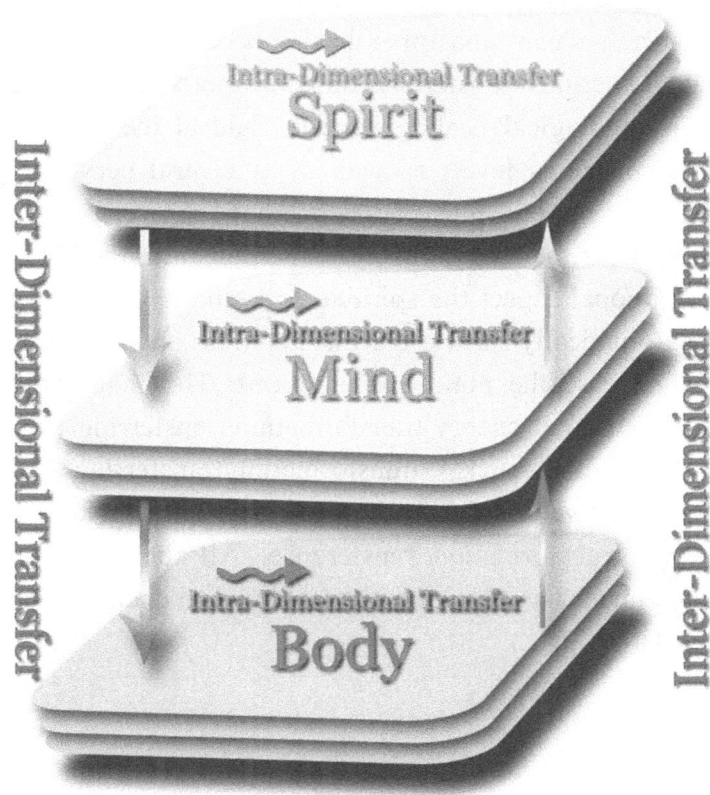

Fig. 3.4. Inter-dimensional and intra-dimensional energy transferring and transformation between or within the dimensions of body, mind, and spirit. Each dimension can have multiple sub-dimensions (in the figure only three sub-dimensions are shown). The energy quality, level, characteristic and volume are dependent on the quality and nature of the body, mind, or spirit, according to the required criterion by the supreme law and energy principle of the universe.

In these communications and integrations within a dimension or crossing dimensions, vibrations of the energy forms and their transformation, transferring, circulation, regulation, conversion, generation, and harmonization, etc. are the actual processes occurring within the life at the same level as well as between its different levels. It is, in fact, what happens during the mind-body-spirit cultivation practice.

During your mind-body-spirit cultivation practices under the guide of the universal law and energy principle, the energy vibrations flow within the body, mind, and spirit at each of their own levels, but they also cross all these different dimensions to transform from one form to another, thereby automatically adjusting to the originally balanced healthy state – this is the healing process. For instance, as your mind calms down, cultivates and lets go of stressful thinking during your meditation, then the spiritual and mental energies generated flow into your body, cooling down the liver fire and stomach heat, detoxifying your body – so you feel good, digestion is improved, skin is improved, you experience gains in energy, better sleep, and other health benefits. In this process, in fact, (1) the mental and spiritual energies transfer and transform into the physical dimension and results in physical and psychological healing benefits, and at the same time (2) your brain, at subconscious and conscious levels as well as at central nervous system and autonomic nervous systems (sympathetic and parasympathetic nerves), also talks to your nerves, organs, immune systems, and hormone systems, regulating and balancing the entire body, and also (3) at emotional aspect the spiritual and emotional energies generated during the meditation will automatically release the mental stress and emotional conflicts or traumas, helping balance and ease the mind and emotions. The first transfer and transformation (above) is inter-dimensional energy transformation/transferring (mind/spirit to body). The second is intra-dimensional energy transformation/transferring within the body, and the third is both inter (between spirit and mind) and intra (within mind or within spirit) dimensional energy transformation/transference. All these are done during meditation cultivation practice under the ultimate universal law and energy principle – a complete total healing and rejuvenation.

§3.5 Energetic Vibration Wave and Its Characteristic Frequency

Now the question is: Actually how do the different dimension energy forms (bodies) of a life communicate to each other and how are they integrated as a unified system crossing multiple dimensions?

The answer is: Through energetic vibration waves that carry energies, information or messages. In other words, any form itself of a life at any dimension is an energy vibration wave; the energy wave is a vibration, which is a phenomenon of an oscillation wave with energetic frequency (f).

In the physical dimension, the cosmos is composed of an unknown number of celestial objects, just like the human body is made of myriad cells. These celestial objects in the cosmos stay in harmony through a certain networking mechanism under the superior divine-driven energy operation and wisdom. Similarly, the organs and cells in the physical body are growing, dividing, regulating, metabolizing, distributing, circulating, transporting, and functioning peacefully by following their natural law and mechanisms as the original creature designed. The networking relationship and communications within organs, cells, and subcellular substances in the body are performed through the processes of neuron signal transduction, intracellular and intercellular transportation of biochemical substances, and biochemical reaction, production, and metabolisms, etc. All these activities are actually biological, biochemical, neurological, bioelectrical, genetic, chemical and physical vibrations (oscillations) of the organs, cells and subcellular substances under the cellular level. It is obvious, in the superficial level of the physical dimension, these vibrations (oscillations) occur within all layers of the biological body such as organs, tissues, cells, molecules, atoms, electrons and further smaller particles. These are intra-dimensional and/or inter-subdimensional energy vibrations at the physical dimension.

In fact, energetic vibrations (oscillations) also occur all over the other invisible dimensions, including mental and spiritual dimensions and these energy vibrations influence the physical body through inter-dimensional energy transformation/transferring.

Different from other modern sciences, in mind-body science at this point, instead of specific mathematic expression, we use a collective concept or conceptual parameter called "characteristic frequency of energy vibration waves" (*fo*) to describe the characteristic features of such energy in any dimensions by borrowing the same concept/term from quantum physics. In the terminological expression of mind-body science, the characteristic frequency *f* of energy vibrations can be spiritual characteristics such as kindness, caring, compassion, love, conscience, truthfulness, forgiveness, and so on, or energy characteristics such as Yin, Yang, or any of the five elements (water, wood, fire, earth and metal) or even higher spiritual energies beyond the five elements, or some other terms for energy such as heat, cold, dryness, wetness, wind or for emotions like fear (water), anger (wood), joy (fire), worry (earth), and grief (metal), and other related emotions like positive, negative, motivated, encouraging, bright, depressive, and so forth, for energy music such as water, wood, fire, earth and metal music, and combinations of the elements in terms of yin or yang. All these are energy vibrations and maybe someday science can describe them more specifically, mathematically and quantitatively.

For different dimensions, different forms of lives, and different energy states, the vibration character can be described with a different frequency, *f*. The original characteristic frequency (*fo*) meets the requirements of the fundamental law and core principle, but in reality at a time during its life journey – e.g. at a particular time during this life time of a human being in the world or sometime in the past lives that may carry on the energy frequency to this lifetime – the energy state, character or the frequency (*f*) of the life energy vibration can be deviated from the original balanced state, character or frequency (*fo*) determined by the universal law and principle at the particular dimension.

This deviation of life energy state causes conflicts between the original nature of the life (as when originally created by the supreme divine spirit by following the universal law and energy principle) and its current energy state at the time. Left imbalanced, this will result in sickness or disease for the life. Therefore, the healing or health practice is to restore the energy state/character or frequency (f) to the original characteristic

frequency (fo). To do so, therefore, the practice of following the law and principle become extremely important key. This establishes the basic foundation of mind-body medicine and healthology.

Just like the existing modern space science cannot explain (and does not know that much about) the spiritual reasons, spiritual connections and behaviors associated with celestial bodies, stars and planets in the physical cosmos (including explanation and spiritual understanding about the acceleration of the universe's expansion), modern life science also cannot provide complete explanations about what is going on within that realm either as well as how the physical body is regulated emotionally, psychologically, mentally and spiritually by the mind and spirit beyond the physical body. So we know that information is at a premium. Through our long history, however, in the area of mind-body science, the teaching of human cultivation and mind-body-spirit practice has taught about Universal Law, the core principle of the universe. This profound, inspiring and enlightening teaching guides us to this day to continue to learn, discover and practice the truth and that is: That the spiritual characteristics of the universe, truth-compassion-tolerance, and the substantial energy natures of Yin-Yang and The Five Elements (or Beyond The Five Elements) guide and operate the whole universe and all lives within the universe, including human beings as one whole unit of mind, body and spirit in a harmonious and balanced state.

At this point at human level, although there is no way to specifically describe all life forms (bodies) and their characteristic frequencies at different dimensions and different states, we can follow the fundamental law and core principle to practice and cultivate ourselves, to resynchronize and re-assimilate with the original frequency as the solution for healing and health as well as enlightenment of life. And at the same time scientifically we use the conceptual parameter or term "frequency or original frequency" to help understand and establish the model of mind-body science and practice.

At this moment in time, it is easy to think that everything operates in the specific way as insisted upon by existing modern science, however, that way does not work for mind-body science study and practice. We need to open our mind even further and avoid locking ourselves in the narrow and skeptical ideology, rules, thinking mode and laboratory experimental methodology of modern science. Their narrower view demands truth to be determined only by empirical observation-based evidence. Yet, we can, through rigorous first-person experiential methods, learn to observe phenomena and identify their characters and causal components and mechanisms. So again, on this basis, we wish to progress with a broader scope on our quest for better tools that will help us be all that we can be.

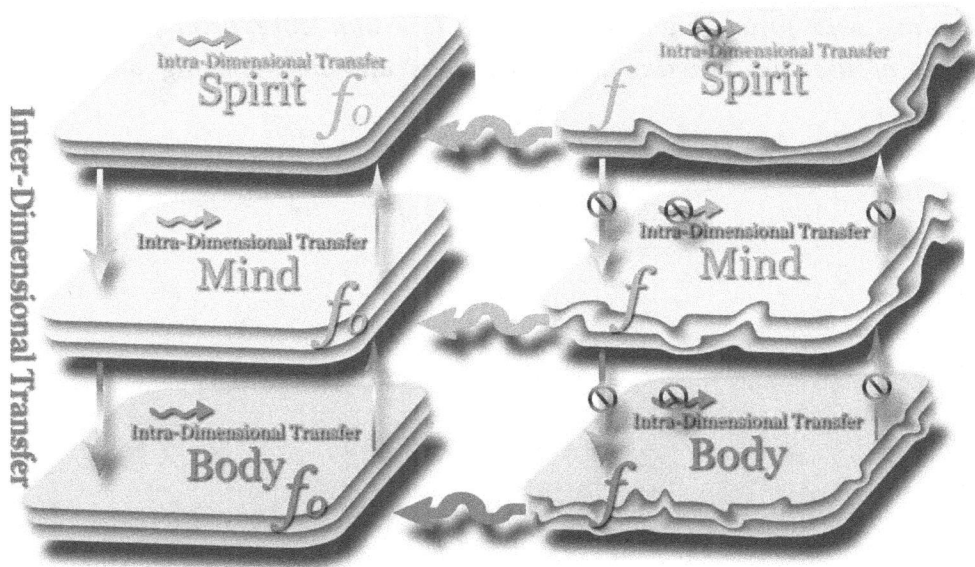

Fig. 3.5. The left panel shows the original state, vibration and frequency (*fo*) of the body, mind and spirit which meet the standard of the supreme law and energy principle, while the right panel shows an unhealthy state or sick condition where the vibration frequency (*f*) in each dimension of body, mind and spirit has deviated from the original frequency (*fo*). As a result, the intra-dimensional and inter-dimensional energy transformation is blocked, and energy level at all or some dimensions is imbalanced (low or excess), causing sickness or disease. The mind-body-spirit healing and health practice is to restore the original vibration frequency (*fo*) at all levels of body, mind and spirit, and regain balance and health.

In summary, besides the communication within the physical body through intra-dimensional energy vibration and energy transformation/transference as described above, the mind, soul and spirit also communicate with all parts of the physical body at all levels through inter-dimensional energy vibrations and transformation/transferring. As an entity of whole being, the spirit, mind and body are one, and connected to each other. Through the communication within and between the mind, spirit and the body under the universe's superior law of Truth, Compassion, and Tolerance and ultimate principle of Yin-Yang and The Five Elements (or Beyond the Five Elements) as mentioned above, all components of the body in different dimensions are unified, balanced and harmonized into one whole life system.

When an individual has failed to harmonize or balance or these are incomplete, the being becomes sick or unhealthy. Mind-body medicine and healthology practice, guided by the core principle and the universal law, then responds by re-balancing and re-harmonizing the person's entire system of mind-body-spirit, in order to achieve the true health and harmony of the whole person.

Learning and practicing mind-body medicine and healthology is the process of understanding and practicing the universal law and core principle to integrate all components of the life, crossing all dimensions and harmonizing and balancing the whole being.

§3.6 Whole Being Model – New Anatomy (Mind-Body-Spirit)

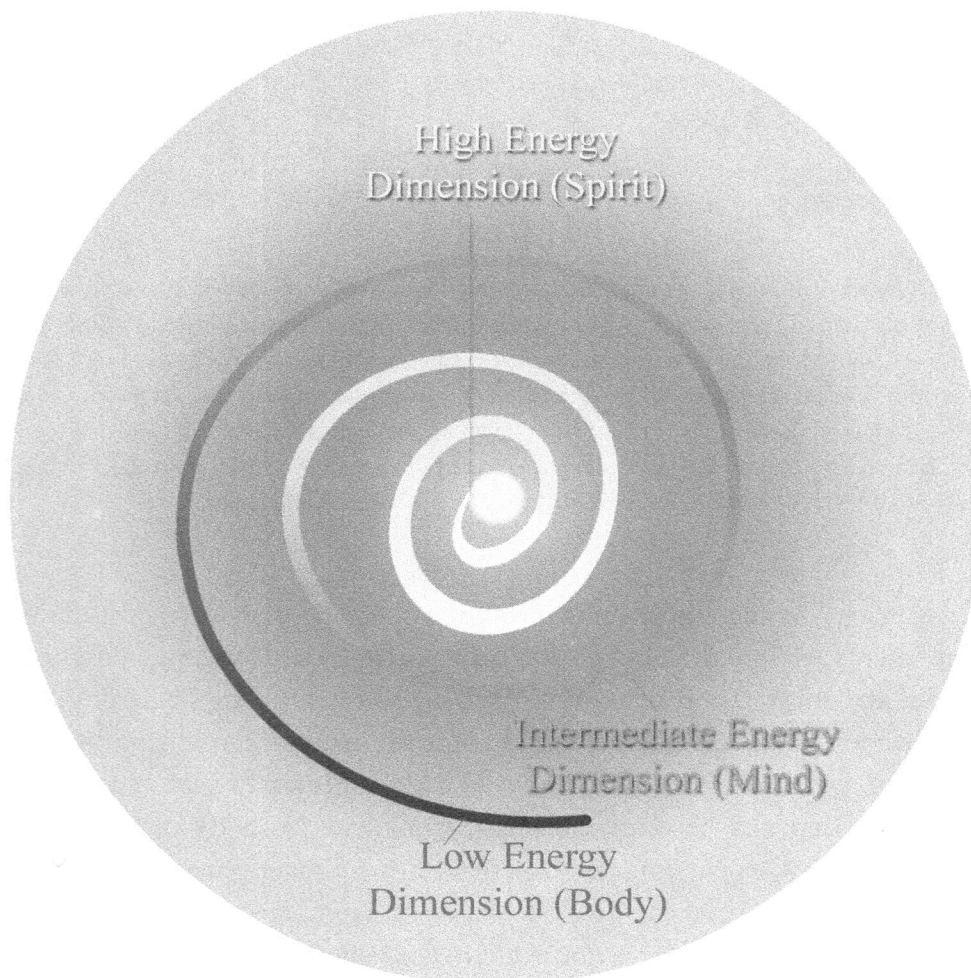

Fig. 3.6.1. BODY, MIND and SPIRIT are three primary components of a human being. They are one indivisible system connected together but at different dimensions - the physical dimension at low energy level (body, in darker red or darker black in black/white print), mental dimension at intermediate energy level (mind, in light red or lighter black / gray in black/white print) and spiritual dimension at high energy level (spirit, in bright yellow or light gray in black/white print). Each primary dimension also has many subdimensions. These primary dimensions as well as their subdimensions are connected through energy transferring and transformation mechanisms (*see* following sections and chapters for further discussions).

Modern medicine deals with life phenomena, physiological functions, pathological observations and explanations about health and diseases based on the body anatomy, cellular and molecular biology; the structures of physical body that are detectable within the visible biological elements such as organs, tissues, muscles, bones, blood, nerves, cells, cellular contents, up to the level of molecule or atom. Modern medicine is based on human body anatomy, cellular biology, microbiology or molecular biosciences. It deals with the physically visible components of a human being, but not the whole being including emotional, mental and spiritual aspects associated with the entire being. Let's look at the Fig. 2.1 again which we presented in previous chapter (renumbered as Fig. 3.6.1. here). The entire being is made of body, mind and spirit as one indivisible system but their different components exist at different levels of dimensions. All components are connected to each other and influence each other within one system.

All components of the human being including mind, spirit and body are absolutely un-ignorable because they are all most fundamental yet important parts of the human being. The reason why human beings can think, talk, listen, write, read, smile, laugh, feel, believe, discover, create, make decisions, do things with intention … all these visible and invisible behaviors and actions take place not just because we have a physical body (brain to think, mouth to talk, ears to listen, hands to write, eyes to see, face to smile, laugh and express, body to do things), but also because we have spirit that guides the mind to feel and then leads the body to take action.

To explain the relationship of the life components, the body, mind and spirit, and the mechanism by which all these life components can function in a harmonious manner, here is a proposed model as shown in Fig. 3.6.2.

The universe is made of energy in an energy gradient from low to high, that is: from the physical dimension to spiritual dimension. As we have said, the physical body and physical living environment exist in the physical dimension(s) in the lower energy form, while the mind exists in the intermediate energy dimension(s) and the spirit exists in the highest energy dimension(s). Here we need to be aware that each of the body, mind, and spirit dimensions can have many sub-dimensions.

Both the mind and spirit are invisible and without a physical form that is detectable by using conventional scientific tools at present time, but they have energy substances that (1) pervade the body and surrounding environment or as well as all other spaces, depending on the person's energy quality and nature or strength, (2) are the main component of the life even exceeding over 95% of the total life system, and (3) communicate and interact with the physical body. In mind-body-spirit science, we believe that mind and spirit intelligently guide and interact with the physical body in order to allow it to physiologically function, psychologically behave, emotionally feel, and spiritually believe, cultivate, improve and grow.

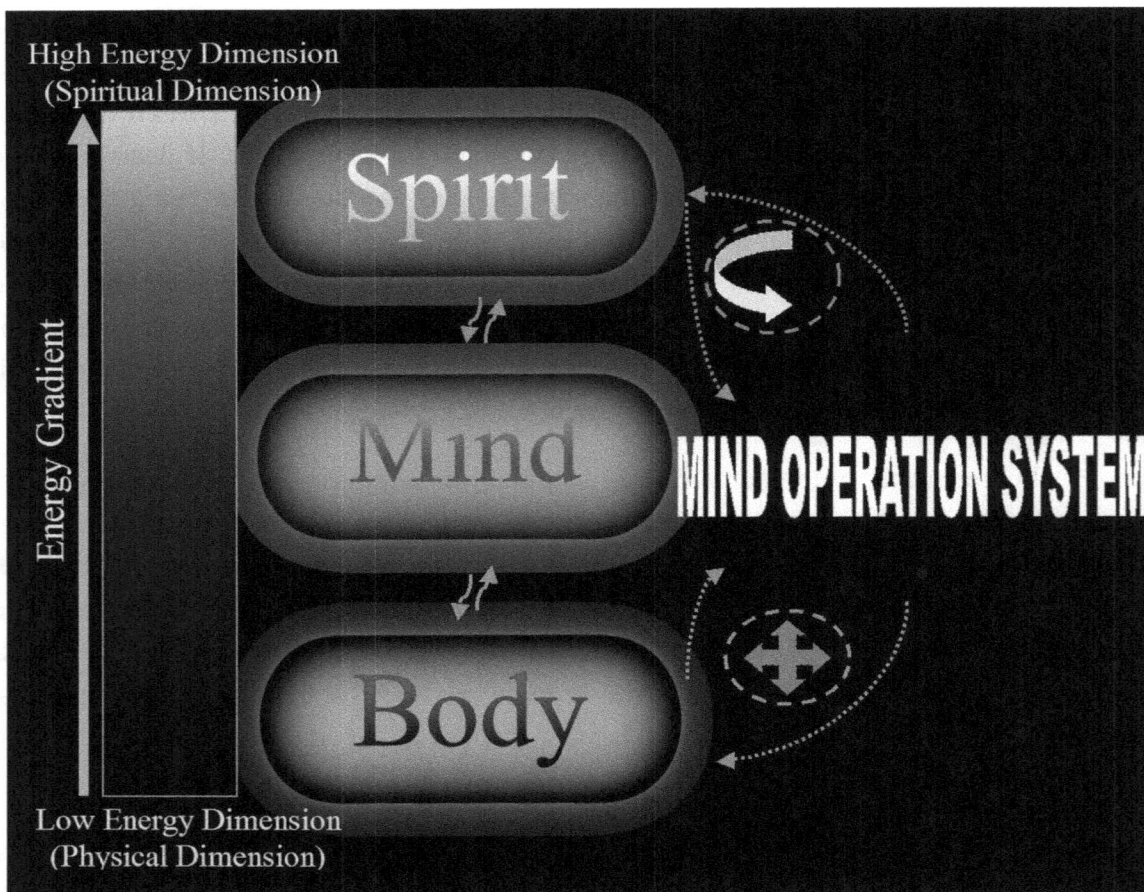

Fig. 3.6.2. The Model of Body-Mind-Spirit explains that a being has three levels of energy forms: 1) The physical body and physical living environment exist in the physical dimension in the lower energy form, 2) The mind exists in the intermediate energy dimension and 3) The spirit exists in the highest energy dimension. The energy flows from the highest spiritual dimension, through the mind-operation system in the mental dimension to the physical level to integrate the whole being. The detailed mechanisms of the mind-operation system for the energy integration will be discussed later.

The spirit is deeply rooted to, connected with and ultimately guided by the origin of energetic substance carried within the spiritual characteristics of Truth, Compassion and Tolerance at the superior level. This spirit is the true Self which permeates the person from high level to the low level, including the physical level where the physical body exists. The highest divine spirit with the superior power of energy carried by the spirit leads the mind and then the body accordingly; crossing dimensions in the order of high-to-low (continue to look at the Fig. 3.6.2).

The mind is manifested and interpreted as emotions, sensory feelings, desires, memories and logical or non-logical ideas or thoughts as well as inspiration(s) while it senses the body, cares of the body, and accordingly directs the body to act and behave. The mind is guided by the higher spirit and follows the spiritual characteristics of the universe and the core principle of Yin-Yang and The Five Elements (or beyond the Five Elements), and stays in a peaceful and optimal state of spirit and mind – a balanced energy state within the inter-promotional and inter-restrictive Yin-Yang and The Five Elements, or Beyond The Five Elements.

The body has the same components of Yin-Yang, The Five Elements (or Beyond The Five Elements) as well and follows the spiritual law and core principle in order to stay in harmony. Since the body exists in the physical dimension that is the lowest level, it needs the mind and spirit to guide its whole being ultimately and supply higher energy from the emotional and spiritual dimensions to it.

We often see the fact that when one is sick mentally or psychologically, he/she is also physically sick or eventually got sick physically. It is because the mind and spirit could not guide the physical body (all the organs, tissues, cells and hormones in the body) to stay in harmony with the individual's original true Self (the spiritual characteristics of truthfulness, compassion and tolerance) as well as in the balanced energy state of Yin-Yang and The Five-Elements or Beyond The Five Elements. In other words, the physical body is lacking in the mental and spiritual energies transferred from higher energy dimensions, so the body and all biological systems of the body such as organs, cells, immune system, etc. as well as the whole person are disconnected with their mental and spiritual energy sources. Therefore as a result, they behave in an imbalanced disturbing state, conflicting with its true Self that complies with the natural laws, and resulting in disordered condition, sickness or disease.

The affected person has lost the unification, continuation and integrity of the whole being - the body, mind and spirit - thus resulting in physical sickness. This is another example of what we called energy blockage or low or excessive energy that actually refers to not only the energy within the physical body but also extensively to the energies transferred from the mind and spirit.

In such a case, if working on the physical body alone by giving medication, acupuncture or natural herbs at the physical dimension, you cannot heal the problem from the root because the mind and soul/spirit are not healed and remain imbalanced and unaddressed.

§3.7 An Example of Meditation for the Mind-Body-Spirit

Now let's do a few minutes meditation to experience the existence and energy of your own body, mind and spirit, cultivating them with the universal law and core energy principle.

The best position to meditate is in a lotus style, cross-legged sitting posture. Both arms form a circle while palms are overlapped with right hand on the top for women and left hand on top for men. The tip of your tongue touches upper palate, while your mouth and eyes are naturally closed and your face peacefully smiles. This is the most beneficial posture for an energetic meditation. It is not just because of the long history of this meditation position taken by ancient and modern people over the world, but also as known from traditional Chinese medicine, this position is the best posture at which all energy channels/acupuncture meridians on the body are formed in their circle for effective energy circulation. Another benefit of this meditation position is that it helps calm the mind and connect the spirit quickly, promoting energy circulation and integration of the whole being.

If you are not able to cross your legs in a lotus position, however, you can just simply sit with single leg crossed or in a natural sitting position.

Close your eyes and relax your entire body, especially relax your shoulders and let them down to release all tenseness of the muscles around your shoulders, neck and back.

Keep your consciousness focused on the front of your nose, peacefully smile, have your body relaxed, mind positive and empty, and spirit upright. Stay like this and meditate quietly.

Peacefully notice the existence of your body; go through it everywhere, from the top to bottom, visualize and feel your head, neck, arms, shoulders, back, chest, belly, legs, feet, etc. making sure all are relaxed. Feel your heart, lung, liver, stomach, kidneys, and all internal organs, muscles, hormone systems, and immune system relaxed. It is so quiet that you seem to hear your heart is beating and air and blood are flowing inside your body, smoothly and peacefully. All parts of your body are in a balanced state of Yin-Yang and The Five Elements or Beyond The Five Elements, and they are truthful, compassionate, patient and peaceful while your mind and mental eye briefly imagine and visualize the earth and all elements such as mountains, water, plants, trees, lives, etc. on the earth, and moon, sun, stars, planets, the Milky Way, other galaxies, and all celestial objects and lives are all peacefully in harmony with you and connected with you.

Now visualize yourself rising up to the higher dimensions and feel the peacefulness of your mind, emotions, and feelings and then recognize your soul and spirit are very pure, clean, truthful, compassionate, peaceful, with no attachments or desire, free spirited, and connected with the greatly compassionate supreme spirit which is right here with you and pervading everywhere over the whole space. Use your mind to cultivate body, mind and spirit, assimilating with the universal law of truth, compassion and tolerance, and resonating with the balanced energy vibrations of Yin-Yang and The Five Elements or Beyond The Five Elements - in other words, feel your energy rising and falling effortlessly and smoothly, in a continuous flow and exchange with the energy of universe. Feel the harmony, unification, and integration of your complete whole being.

§3.8 Brain, Memory, Gene, Mind and Spirit

It is relatively easy to understand that the mind is related with the body because the mind is associated with emotions, sensory feelings, memories, and mental activities through the neuron system of the brain. However, how is spirit related with the body? Where is the spirit or soul located? This is an important question because it will be helpful as we attempt to utilize the interconnections of body, mind and spirit, as well as regarding the way to integrate and balance these components.

So far, modern science believes that mental and spiritual characteristics and activities originate from, and occur inside the brain. It's why modern scientists try to study the brain with the intention of understanding the mind and spirit. However, are the mind and spirit simply located within the brain of the physical body? This is a questionable topic.

Modern science assumes the brain contains the information of mind and spirit (if it accepts there is spirit in a human being, but some scientists exclude spirit and even mind). This implies that the physical human anatomy already covers the entire being, the body, mind and spirit, and if we understand everything about brain, then we will understand everything about mind and spirit. This can easily lead to a risky statement that if the physical brain is dead, the spirit is dead too. Is this correct? Are the mind and spirit really inside the brain? Are spiritual activities and messages from the human spirit or soul reflected in brain activities?

Many scientists including myself do not agree with the supposition that the spirit is completely inside the brain or the spirit's existence and its behaviors are entirely expressed as brain activities.

One obvious example is Near Death Experience in which the spirit (or soul) observes and memorizes occurrences that have happened after biological brain death. There are many evidences and true stories provided by large number of NDE experienced people, so that we are not going to cite them here. These NDEs imply that human spirit or soul is still alive after the brain is dead. The person with NDE can describe their near death experience after brain function is recovered, indicating the spirit's independence from brain functionality, and that it can utilize the brain as a memory storage and output device when the brain is biologically functioning. It seems that the physical body can be dead, but the spirit will continue to live or be transformed to another form of life at another level, in another dimension differing from this physical realm.

Another example is Out of Body Experience (OBE). In a deep meditation, the meditator's soul sometimes goes out the body and visits somewhere in other dimensions, seeing different images and colors never seen in this physical realm. After a while the meditator's soul comes back. The brain can remember some of those experiences afterward. This phenomenon tells us that although the physical body stays in this physical dimension, the soul or spirit can leave the body and go to other dimensions. The activities and behaviors of the spirit are not what the brain purposely thought about or remembered from before. Actually it is in the opposite way, only when the brain completely stops thinking, is devoid of conscious and subconscious activities, can the meditator have an OBE. This means the spirit of a human being has the power to independently travel other deeper dimensions, and store the information of the OBE in the brain. This is different from intentional learning; experiencing or preexisting memories inducing unconscious activities, which can input some information into the memory storage in the brain. OBE occurs when the meditator's human brain is nearly switched off or at very low level of activities, so the soul can connect to the higher spiritual world and experience other dimensions, but not this physical dimension.

In fact many parapsychological phenomena such as clairvoyance, telepathy, precognition, predications, and other supernormal abilities are also circumstances that the soul or spirit could go out the body, do something or know something in or through other dimensions, without relying on the brain, and at times, have include the brain's cooperation to memorize and output the information.

Many evidences tell us that brain is the storage or container and output device of the memory, containing some information processed by the mind and spirit, and involving some but not all activities of the mind and spirit, but the brain itself does not comprise your spirit or soul or mind at all.

Modern neuroscience believes that gene and environmental experience are two major factors that determine the brain's structure and its behaviors. This seems to be true as many evidences show that.

For a long time scientists thought identical twins are identical because they are derived from one fertilized egg, which contains one set of genetic instructions or genome, formed from combining the chromosomes of mother and father. But recent research has discovered even identical twins are not completely the same. Identical sameness is most likely among newborn identical twins pairs, some of them are truly identical and some of them not, and then as they live their respective lives within their respective environments, ***their genes will change in different ways*** due to environmental and experiential differences.

Scientists have tried so hard to study this field with intention to figure out how biological genes and brain associate with a person. All these researches are done with an assumption that the gene determines everything of a living being. This assumption can be the problem why scientists get into a difficult dead end. It could be true that the biological gene determines the biological phenotype, appearance, the body developments, and physiological behaviors, characters, and as well as the brain, and partly the after born personality, characters, individual characters, health condition, diseases, and so on, but it seems genes probably do not carry all the information especially in terms of mental and spiritual characteristics such as consciousness, thought, will, belief, and spirituality, as well as the way of interacting with the environment, gaining experiences, and social behaviors – health conditions, diseases, etc.

Without introducing the spiritual component into the model, the study of human life will be forever difficult in figuring out everything of the whole being of mind, body and spirit. There are many spiritual researches, observations, experiences, and some scientific studies that draw a much bigger picture in terms of genes, brain, spirit or soul. In this book I cannot cite all this information at once, but based on such information I would like to propose a reasonable model below to give you a summarized scenario.

The spirit or soul interacts with the genes, brain, organs and other physical parts of the body, puts information and messages in the genetic molecules and brain memory, and sometimes instructs a gene to express its certain behaviors, and guides the brain to output the memories and perform activities. The spirit can stay inside the brain or some part of the body (such as Dantian point, the belly area, to remain the most energetic state as with that of a good energy practitioner), but sometimes it also can go out the body during this lifetime.

When the physical life comes to the end – the brain and body are dying – the spirit or soul starts leaving the body, entering the spiritual dimension, and being transformed to another form of life. The near death phenomenon is actually the transmission process of biological body's dying, but for some reason the physical life could come back to live, and the brain could start functioning again, so the spirit came back to this physical body, and passed the experienced information into the brain's memory. It's why NDE people can tell their stories afterward even though the brain had no biological functionality during the dying process.

During a woman's pregnancy, the spirit (or soul) as the intellectual life energy form resonates with and identifies the same level or faithful quality of genetic energy vibration in biological form (the fertilized embryos), and enters the body, and installs the information carried by the spirit (or soul) into the body, printing the spiritual emblem on the biological life. In such a mysterious moment, a new life starts not just genetically and biologically, but also mentally and spiritually with both a biological form and energy form emerged and integrated at the same time as the whole being. For an entire lifetime, this life has mind, body and spirit as one unified living system until the biological body ends; the spirit (or soul) enters another dimension, completing one cycle of life journey.

The gene in the biological form carries certain information at its quality accumulated in the past lives (parents, grandparents, ancestries) including Virtue, Karma, and biological characteristics, which will be passed on in the future generation at human level. It's why children have different looks, characteristics, intelligences, and individualities in many aspects, but they are always similar in relationship to their parents, grandparents, or even older generations of ancestries.

However, of most importance is the spirit or soul that entered another dimension after a biological life. This spirit carries the quality of its spiritual life energy, Virtue, Karma, and all information accumulated in the past lives. If the spirit's quality is high enough to enter a higher dimension, it can permanently stay at such a higher level, and live at that higher level of life. However, if it could not reach this higher level, and stayed at the human level, then the spirit will enter next reincarnation of life; entering another biological life and starting another human life cycle. If the spirit quality drops to the level below humankind, then it will reincarnate into a being below humankind.

Even at the same level of human being, there are so many different sub-levels of spirit quality, therefore newborns are not the same and human beings are not the same in spiritual quality although they have the same rights as all human beings in human society. Cultivating spiritual energy and improving its quality during this lifetime is a very important task from the scope of entire-life-journey – endless spiritual life.

§3.9 Cultivated Spirit is The Key

The spirit is a subtle form of energy that is everywhere over the universe and can be as small as a particle and can also become as big as the spirit can reach out depending on its cultivated energy. The energy strength and volume are dependent upon one's cultivation of Virtue and the quality and level of the spirit, in terms of assimilating to the law.

The universe and all lives are born from the Law or the Tao with the ultimate spiritual nature of truth, compassion, and tolerance. Therefore, originally all lives within the universe have the same nature and connect to the same root, the original source of life force. As such, they are capable of staying in the peaceful and balanced energy state of Yin-Yang and Five Elements or Beyond The Five Elements. In other words, a spirit of this life is connected and can stay in harmony with itself as well as with all other lives in the universe.

Therefore, in meditation practice, energy practice and all the other mind-body medicine practices, the key is to cultivate the mind, body and spirit, assimilate with the nature of the universe, and stay in harmony both with the universe and within it. The better cultivation is, the stronger, healthier, more beautiful, and longer living, the whole being of body, mind and spirit will be.

§3.10 Disharmony Causes Sickness, Aging & Unnatural Death

Originally all lives are in harmony with the universe's nature and balanced with the elements and beyond. In the process of a life journey, however, a person may start having conflict with other lives and with his or her original Self, disharmony with the universe, become selfish, and behave in a way that deviates from the original nature of the universe, attaches on his or her own interests and desires, cares too much about his or her physical existence in the lower physical dimension, and gets disconnected from the higher spiritual energy source, and wind up lacking in the supplement of higher energy. As a result, the life becomes sick, weak, old, and dead.

A being has peace, balance and joy within its own nature. This is the nature of life. If there is a conflict within its Self, against its own nature, for any reason, however, then it will suffer with the conflict, fighting with itself internally and with others eventually, and the life will experience pain, sickness, weakness, diminish or die. For example, one who has surrounded himself with negative thoughts about others or about himself will feel ill or downtrodden and eventually this can spiral the individual downward into anger, doubt, confusion, anxiety, self-doubt, depression and other negative emotions, and even lead to other conflicts and problems with others surrounded. This is because negative thoughts are opposite of his original nature: the truthfulness, compassion and tolerance, and all other extended positive characters such as love, giving, sharing, open minded, patience, brightness. No matter if he agrees with this original nature or not, the original nature of life is rooted into his nature. Negative thoughts and emotions could come from this life's experience and notions, education, social and family's influences, or/and come from his past lives' Karmas that carried and passed on negative energy vibrations to this life. The conflict between these negative thoughts and his original nature causes him internal struggle. He is trying to live in a state of fighting – psychologically, neurologically and physiologically – and this will take its toll. His negative thoughts, emotions and actions are against his true Self and diminish and destroy his own life force. As a result, he can get sick at any possible juncture, mentally, physically and/or spiritually.

§3.11 Healing Is to Harmonize and Rebalance the Life

As we just discussed above, sickness and aging are caused by disconnection, disharmony and imbalance with the original life nature and the core principle, therefore, to heal sickness and slow down aging process, all we need is to reconnect, harmonize and balance the life. This, then, can be done by following the natural law and principle at all levels of the body, mind and spirit.

Mind-Body Medicine uses various approaches to improve health. The approaches can be spiritual, psychological, mental, energetic or nutritional. The body and mind have their energy states, energy and elemental balances. The imbalance of the Yin and Yang, and disharmony within the Five Elements (earth, metal, wood, fire and water) are detectable in energy medicine such as traditional Chinese medicine (TCM) or oriental medicine. Based on the diagnosis of energy states of the body and mind, TCM treats the case with Qigong meditation and movement, acupuncture, acupressure, herbs, diets, energy healing music, and so on. However, modern Oriental medicine focuses more on the physical body by using the needles and herbs, but does not pay enough attention or put enough effort on the connection of the body with the mind and spirit as the original Oriental medicine maintains we are supposed to do.

In the following chapters of this book, we will discuss this issue and provide further information to complement and fortify this lack. Besides TCM, the mind-body medicine often uses spiritual, psychological practices and nutritional treatment to energize the spirit and mind and heal the body. These methods include a regiment of such elements as music healing therapy, brainwave sound therapy, hypnotherapy, psychological conversation, biofeedback, neuron feedback, natural diet, and more. In the following chapters we will introduce and work with this regiment toward the comprehensive application of mind-body medicine. We also include discussion and application of Brainwave-Meridian Therapy (BMT), which combines energy music healing with hypnosis, brainwave therapy, oriental medicine, meditation, energy practice, psychotherapy, self-improvement practice and healthy lifestyle, and spiritual cultivation.

To harmonize and assimilate the mind and spirit with the nature of the Tao, the Law or Fa - the fundamental characteristics of the universe – one needs to cultivate the mind, spirit and the body to reconnect with the universe. Based on the Whole Being Model – the Body-Mind-Spirit, the high dimensional energy of the spirit is rooted in the universal energy source. Through spiritual practice, one's spirit can be purified and returned to the original nature, and again "tuned in" to its original source of high energy. The energy will be transferred to the mind, emotions, feelings, and thoughts. The individual will become righteous, truthful, positive, compassionate, kind-hearted, giving, forgiving, patient, energetic, clear, peaceful, stable, and confident, and unified with all good personalities and spiritual characters. And then as a result, the physical body will also benefit as the individual's spiritual and mental energies flow into the body healing it from the root and engendering true health of the whole being. A person can even reach a higher level of life in this life and future lives.

§3.12 Energy Meridians Buried within the Body-Mind-Spirit

Oriental medicine understands that many mental and physical diseases are due to the energy (氣, Qi or Chi in Chinese, pronounced "Chee") blockages that prevent the energy from flowing throughout the entire body and mind, and/or energy deficiency (low or lacking energy) or excess that causes imbalance of yin and yang and five elements energies over the body and mind. Therefore the doctors try to heal the patient with needles and herbs in attempting to unblock the energy flow, promote the circulation of Qi and blood, and/or increase energy level.

Some people including some of the Oriental medicine doctors think the energy blocks are within the meridians (pathways) on the physical body. In fact the meridians are spread not only within the physical body, but also within much deeper dimensions of mind and spirit beyond the physical body. In other words, the acupuncture meridians over the physical body are indeed structured within multiple layers in different dimensions crossing the body, mind and spirit. The energy blockage or imbalance of energy can be located in the meridians on the physical body, but can also be in the mental body and/or spiritual body, or between these bodies at different dimensions. In most cases, the energy blockage is not only within the physical body, but also on the emotional body and spiritual body, or on the pathway between the physical body and the mind, and/or between the mind and the spirit. Because of those blockages, the transformation and transference of mental and spiritual energies from higher dimensions to the physical body can fail or become impeded. Of course, there can be some energy blockages in the physical body that can be unblocked by physical therapy, massage therapy, needle acupuncture or herbs, healing directly at physical level or physical energy level. But in most cases, we see the blockages are located in the physical, mental, and even the spiritual levels.

The mind-body medicine and cultivation practice of the body, mind and spirit open up the energy pathways and remove the energy blocks at different dimensions to allow the energies to flow through the meridians on the physical body, mental body and spiritual body, increase the energy level or balance energies at all dimensions. This is done to foster healing and more robust health. This practice activates the spiritual energy from the spirit (spiritual body), passes it through the mind (mental body), and allows it to reach the physical body, healing the mind and body at the same time. If only working on the physical body, the core cause, the energy blockages deeply buried in the mental and spiritual bodies will remain unchanged, so the healing will not complete.

The energy can cross multiple levels, from the spiritual dimension to the emotional dimension, to the physical dimension. The healing treatment of mind-body medicine and cultivation practice strengthens and balances the energy in all levels to purify, heal and elevate the whole being to a high level. Energy transformation and/or transference from the spiritual dimensions to mental and physical dimensions deliver great life transformation, blessing and magnificent enlightenment to the human being on the earth. Importantly, this practice of energy transfer and transformation is also the core component of true whole being health. The treatments of mind-body medicine can take place at each of the different levels, depending upon the depth and strength of the mind-body doctor's cultivation and energy level and depending upon the patient's understanding, cooperation, Virtue, belief, personality, open-mindedness, and efforts of self-healing and improvement of cultivation practice.

§3.13 Mind-Body-Spirit Cultivation for the Whole Being

As described above, for the total health of the whole being, cultivation practice of the body, mind and spirit at all levels from high to low dimensions, is required. This is the main difference between the fields of mind-body medicine and mainstream medicine.

Medications or drugs may help manage the physical symptoms temporarily and make the patient feel momentarily better, but since the real cause of the disease is the energy block not only inside the body, but also the mind and spirit; neurological system and mental body – within the human thoughts, emotions, attachments, desires, addictions, stubbornness, value system, lifestyle – only dealing with the physical body cannot heal from the root. This is why mind-body practices focus primarily on the factors mentioned above.

Again our regiment of practices will usually include energetic movements, exercises, meditation, music sound healing, hypnosis, Qigong, Taiji, Yoga, combinations of these, and so on. Such practices are basically either still-position meditation or slow, gentle and smooth movements along the energy pathways (meridians) within and surrounding the body which are capable of crossing the mental, conscious, subconscious, and spiritual bodies for energy generation, transformation and transference between multiple dimensions to promote healing. It is important to note: ***These practices are totally different from general physical exercises, workouts or other forms of sport, which train the physical body, muscles, joints, tissues, bones and organs at the physical level.***

§3.14 Energy Frequency Resonance and Mind-Body Healing Arts

You may wonder how the mind-body practices can reach the deeper dimensions, including physical, mental and spiritual dimensions, to achieve life transformation at all levels. In fact this is a key question and mysterious issue about the mind-body healing arts.

As we discussed in the previous sections, mind-body medicine and healthology practices unify the whole being and achieve health at all levels through intra-dimensional and inter-dimensional energy vibrations, energy transformation and transferring within and between physical, mental and spiritual levels.

Question is: How do and what can make these energy vibrations, transference and transformation actually happen at all these different dimensions?

The answer to this question is vital. It gives us access and helps us generate and utilize the right tools for application. Let's look closely.

The universe and all life forms within the universe are made of particles. These particles in the physical, mental and spiritual dimensions constitute the whole being of the life. The particles have wave-particle duality as we mentioned early in this chapter. It means that all particles in their energy dimensions appear as dual properties: energetic particle (particle property) and vibrant wave (wave property). The physical, mental and spiritual particles are the same way; they are the vibration waves with oscillation frequencies that carry substantial energy in their corresponding dimension. As wave, the particle has natures of propagation and resonance. The vibrant waves of the life in its dimension can propagate within the same dimension or cross dimensions of spirit, mind and body, resulting in energy transferring and transformation between spiritual, mental and physical forms (bodies).

At the same time, the wave of the particle has the nature of resonance. It means that all life particles have the tendency to oscillate with much greater amplitude and produce much greater energy at a certain frequency than at other frequencies. This particular frequency is called resonance frequency, the amplitude that occurs in the resonance is called resonance amplitude, and the energy produced in the resonance is called resonance energy. If a vibrant force (life force) as trigger or activator with this particular frequency oscillates within the life system at any dimension, especially at the deeper spiritual and mental dimensions, then the entire life and its particles on different bodies (energy forms) at different dimensions, will resonate with the trigger vibration, producing great energy, re-synchronizing and unifying the entire life with the frequency. So now the key is to find out the resonance frequency, produce and trigger it.

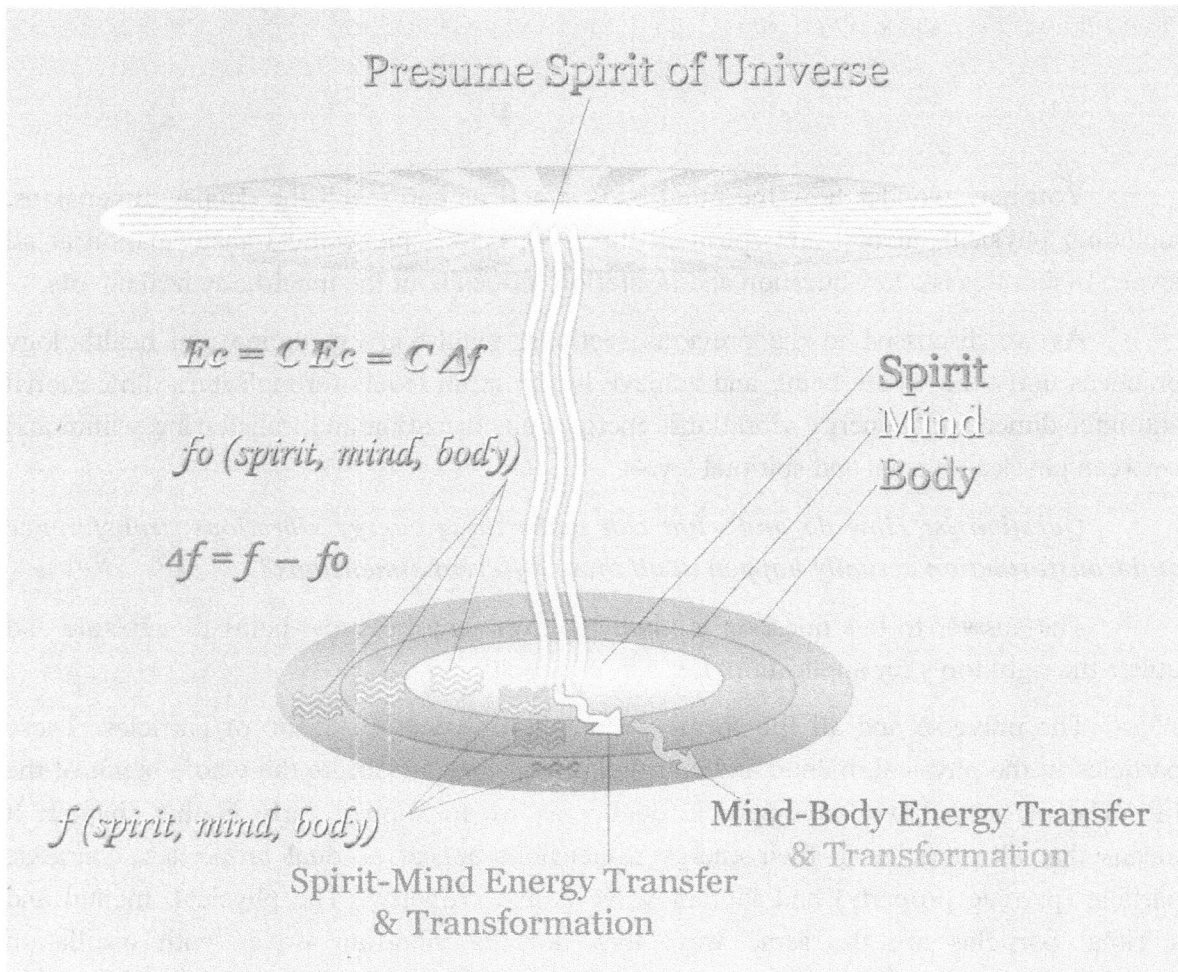

Fig. 3.14. The shift or deviation of vibration frequency (*f*) of the mind, body and spirit from the original characteristic frequency (*fo*) is the cause of the problem. To heal the problem MBM designs healing frequency by following the laws of life to help the subject restore the original energy vibration frequency through the individual's direct involvement of cultivation of mind-body-spirit based on the universal law and energy mechanism.

As shown in Fig. 3.14, the resonance frequency is the original characteristic frequency (*fo*) of the life that originated from the universe's spiritual characteristics and energetic natures of Yin-Yang and the Five Elements or Beyond The Five Elements. Remember, this characteristic frequency (*fo*) was originally built into the life at all levels of body, mind and spirit with different values according the nature and form of each dimension.

Therefore, coming to this point, it is clear that the mind-body-spirit healing work is to create such energy vibrations with the original characteristic frequency (*fo*) or frequencies at the corresponding dimensions and then let them resonate with the original Self of the life at multiple levels of the body, mind and spirit, in order to resynchronize, rebalance and rejuvenate the life. Therefore, the shifted (or irregular) vibration frequency (*f*) or frequencies within the life will be restored back to the original characteristic frequency (*fo*).

$$f \rightarrow fo$$

The triggering or activation energy is called healing energy, the vibration is called healing vibration, the frequency is called healing frequency, and the practice or technique is called energy healing art.

The mind-body healing art is to design, produce or create such vibrant energy forms at multiple dimensions to heal the patient. As a mind-body-spirit doctor, therapist or healthcare practitioner, your center focus is to create such energy healing art. While as an individual cultivator of mind-body-spirit, your central focus is to cultivate your whole being at all levels to resynchronize with the original characteristic frequency (frequencies). For health practitioner and cultivator, it is critical to restore the original energy system and spiritual characters through cultivation practice in order to achieve the goal of true healing and health development.

§3.15 Differentiation of Healthy and Unhealthy Vibrations

Everything is energy and everywhere is energy – all over the universe. The energies can be in different forms, in the same dimension or different dimensions. These forms of energy are vibrations with certain frequencies: mathematical, analogical, conceptual, virtual, or spiritual. These energy vibrations can be in the form of as well as be understood and experienced as physical existence, motion and touch, chemical or biochemical reactions, emotions, feelings, sensations, consciousness, sub-consciousness, thoughts, ideas, talking, writing, thinking, a message, information, sounds, music, colors, foods, nutrients, herbs, drugs, voice, body language, expression, silence, arts, psychological conversation, hypnosis, meditation, Taiji, Qigong, relationships, cultural activities, social activities, economic activities, political movement, social environment, and all activities in this life such as education, family, cultural and social influences.

The question is which frequencies are good for the health of the whole being and which are not. The frequencies input energy to a human being at all levels and they affect his/her whole being energy status. If the frequencies are not good for your health of body, mind and spirit, then they will not help heal you or improve your health, or will even harm your health at all possible levels. We call such energy (information, message, etc.) sick Qi /Chi.

As a mind-body-spirit health practitioner, doctor, healer, therapist or individual self-healing practitioner, we need to be able to differentiate good and bad, healthy and unhealthy energy/Qi, and eliminate or prevent the sick Qi, and produce good and healthy energy in the practice and daily life.

The standard by which you differentiate good and bad energy is the universal law and core principle. Healthy energy vibration carries the appropriate spiritual messages and energy of truthfulness, kindness, peace, compassion, forgiveness, and tolerance, and balanced life force of Yin-Yang and The Five Elements or Beyond The Five Elements.

These energy vibrations resonate with the true Self, the original nature of the body-mind-spirit and harmonious energy vibrations of the life origin. For example, in our energy music healing therapy with combination of meditation as an application of mind-body medicine, we put efforts on the creation of the energy healing music to generate peaceful, compassionate, kind, calm, positive, and forgiving healing messages and energy, and as well as Yin-Yang and elemental (and beyond) balancing within the healing music vibrations. We customize the music with the particular balancing needs of the patient's condition. All of this is done to clear the patient's energy blockages and/or irregularities and restore his or her energy to its initial harmonized state. In addition, psychological conversation and consultation are combined with energy healing to clear psychological, mental and spiritual confusions and negative energies while introducing positive energies that comply with the universal law and energy principle. In this model, the energy field in the session unlocks the energy channels/meridians, activates the patient's original life force (vibration), and connects him or her with the original spirit to heal and improve health for the whole being at all levels of the body, mind and spirit.

§3.16 A Health Practitioner Should Cultivate Mind-Body-Spirit

A good mind-body medicine doctor or mind-body self-healing and health practitioner is a good mind-body-sprit cultivation practitioner who practices cultivation daily, has achieved a high level of cultivation, and stays healthy mentally, physically and spiritually as a good example of true health. Such a practitioner can produce positive, healthy and balanced energy that can heal the practitioner's Self and that of others.

The cultivation practice should follow the universal law of truth, compassion and endurance and the principle of Yin-Yang and The Five Elements or Beyond the Five Elements. The well cultivated practitioner carries and emanates energy vibration that makes surrounding people feel peaceful, harmonious, compassionate, calm, positive, empty minded, energetic, optimistic, inspiring and clear headed. This energy can heal you, as practitioner, because the energy resonates with your true nature and original energy frequency, and helps you restore your original life force and spiritual essence, and balance the energy of mind and body. Both you and your patients will feel this effect.

Besides the presence of the mind-body health practitioner himself or herself, when giving treatment for an individual patient or group, the practitioner often uses a set of approaches to technically facilitate such healing and which the patient can learn and utilize.

If the practitioner has never cultivated well, based on the natural life law and principles as mentioned above, then no matter how good his technique is, the energy produced in the approach will not be of the necessary quality to achieve a good healing result. It is very important that the practitioner is able to "walk the talk," so to speak.

A mind-body health practice can utilize many possible tools that produce the healing energy field and provide such healing environment to reactivate and balance the life force for the patient or client. The approach can be psychological conversation, hypnosis, music and sound, physical movement, herbs, nutrients, meditation, Taiji, Qigong, yoga, arts therapy, traditional Chinese medicine such as acupuncture and other holistic health modalities, etc. All these practices are for helping restore and balance the energy to heal the mind and body, so mind-body medicine is sometimes also referred as energy medicine or vibration medicine.

§3.17 Intermediate Break: Story • Memorization • Meditation

For this chapter's healing story, we will share a patient who had emotional problems such as anxiety and depression that caused physical illness including inflammation, swollen, and bleeding feet, back pain, and chronic kidney infection. She was healed by the vibrational therapy, brainwave-meridian therapy (BMT) with energy sound waves. This story will help you understand how mental and spiritual healing works with energy to heal.

BMT Really Reunified Me

- Kate W

Last fall, I was going through some very difficult physical problems. My hands and feet were very swollen, bleeding, and oozing. I could barely walk, and it was very distressing. It seemed like a cross between an allergic reaction and a toxic reaction, so I started detoxification treatments.

I used Oxygen Light and other therapies, which helped, but couldn't eliminate the problem. When my urine pH level reached 4.2-4.5, coupled with my back pain, I realized it was Kidney related, so I drank cranberry juice. There was something extreme going on with my body, and it got to the point where I finally realized that what I was doing was not addressing it sufficiently.

Throughout my life, the medical industry has made me ill, literally. I was born ill, and their medicines made me more ill; they were injecting me with cortisone when I was 6 years old! I've probably had kidney channel damage ever since I was young. I have studied many therapies; I have tried almost everything. I have been interested in and done lots of research about healing with sound, color, lights and vibration frequency. I was looking at the *Light Connection Magazine* when I came to Dr. Liu's advertisement for Acupuncture-Music Therapy, using sound. This really fascinated me, so I went to his website. What intrigued me most is that Dr. Liu's therapy is primarily based upon sound/vibration energy healing, utilizing no needles or medicine.

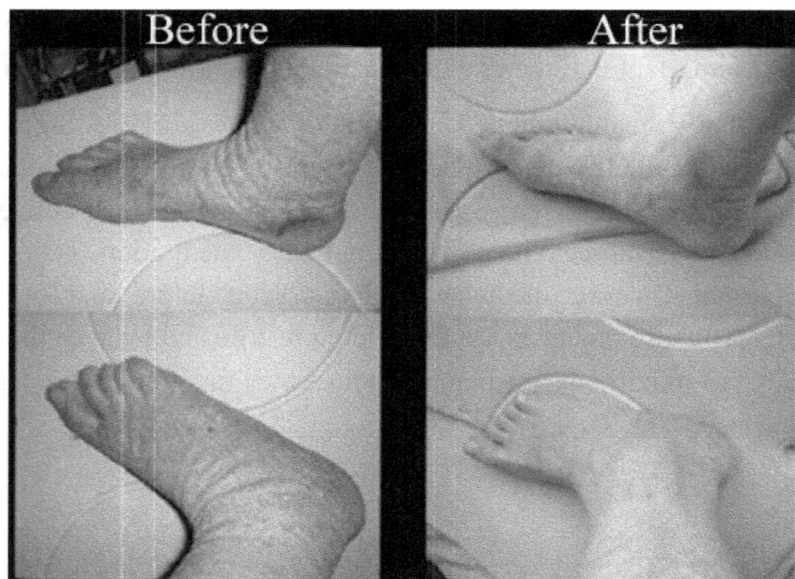

Fig. 3.17. Extremely dry skin, and swollen and bleeding feet due to energy blocks in kidney change and liver channel, especially the kidney yin deficiency and excessive liver yang (fire), and emotional blockages (depression and anxiety) have been healed by energy music therapy (brainwave meridian therapy) and mind-body healing consultation.

I called Dr. Liu and made an appointment, and the results were amazing! All I had to do was lie on a magnetic bed (under a nice comfy blanket), put on headphones, and listen. Dr. Liu's voice would guide me in the beginning, and then I would go on a musical journey. Dr. Liu encouraged me to allow the music to carry me away into the inner dimensions of my soul, and while it did, he hooked me to a 2nd computer with brainwave and HeartMath technologies that measured my brainwaves, heartbeat and brain-heart synchronicity.

My dramatic improvement started within 24 hours. I went twice a week for 4 weeks. What surprised me most was that I went in for physical problems, yet Dr. Liu's diagnosis pointed out that my physical problems were really the result of emotional problems. I was going through some relationship problems, which caused my kidney and liver energy channels to block. As he skillfully tweaked the music he composed for me, my progress was both subtle and dynamic, and deeply unifying beyond my wildest imagination! Session-by-session, I watched, felt, and realized that I was integrating into a "New Me," literally.

My feet are now terrific. You can see the difference before and after in these slides. My hands are great, my skin is great, and even my income has doubled. Before my treatments, I felt very disconnected from Spirit, very splintered. Now I feel unified, complete and very connected to Spirit, which has a great impact on physical well-being.

Those of us in San Diego are truly fortunate, as Dr. Liu is the only person offering this therapy in the United States! Although this type of music therapy dates back thousands of years, Dr. Liu goes way beyond what has been written in the Yellow Emperor's book of "Chinese Internal Medicine." Dr. Liu is a very gifted man; his enthusiasm is contagious. His varied degrees are extra-ordinary, which all add up to an exceptional person with a truly distinctive and profound therapy!

Visual Memorization and Meditation for Chapter 3

EHM03: Fly to the Infinity of Heaven (Yang, Water, Metal)

This music is composed with focus on the relatively yang energy of water and metal elements to strengthen kidney and lung energy. However if you feel you are over heated, anxious, overwhelmed, have too much heat internally or feel too excited and ungrounded emotionally (yang type of condition), then you can choose the following CD (yin type of the healing music) to practice.

EHM04: Holy Water Streams Heal You (Yin, Water, Metal)

Sit cross-legged and close your eyes. Before starting the meditation music, take a moment to peacefully visualize the contents of this chapter, summarizing and memorizing them in your mind. From the universe's supreme law, spiritual characteristics, energy natures, dark matter and dark energy, to the dimensions of body, mind and spirit, intra and inter-dimensional energy transfer and transformation, traditional energy medicine, energy and energy vibrations, frequency, meridians, brain, spirit, mind, true cause of sickness and energy healing, etc., put it all together and form an integrative picture about the universe, life and its mind, body and spirit, then integrate them with the concept of energy vibrations and energy medicine, the practical mind-body medicine and healthology.

And then, [start to play *Energy Healing Music #3* while reading the following induction -], you meditate with the energy music while imagining your mind and spirit meditating in the vast spiritual dimensions of the universe, and the powerful energy pervading all spaces and times, and surrounding you and extending to the boundless accelerating of the cosmos.

Review, in your mind, briefly what you have learned in this chapter: the teaching on the origin of the universe that began with great spirits of truth, compassion and tolerance, carrying powerful energy that created the vast material universe with the energy nature of balanced Yin-Yang and Five Elements.

These spiritual characteristics called the Great Law of the Universe, and the energy nature is called theory of Yin-Yang and Five Elements. These spiritual characteristics and energy natures are inside you as throughout your whole of mind-body-spirit and permeate the whole cosmos. They are within the original you and the universe itself.

Stay with this great energy field and being one with it. Feel the energy coming from the higher dimensions and surrounding you, flowing into you, healing you, energizing and rejuvenating you.

The more your mind becomes empty, letting go of all human thoughts and attachments, the more you will connect to the supreme energy source, and the more energy is transferred from higher dimensions to your body and mind. Enjoy.

Before ending your meditation, practice "Knocking Teeth" (upper and lower teeth lightly knock / bite each other and then release, bite and release, keep repeating it) for about 1 minute. Then you use your both hands to "Dry Wash" (gently massage) your face, head and neck: Starting from chin, gently push your hands up along your face toward the hairline, then continue to massage your head with your fingertips (slightly push stronger to help circulate Qi and blood), and then massage your neck – count this as one time – then you repeat this for 9 times. Keep in your mind: when you massage your face up you take a deep inhalation, and when you massage down from top of the head to the neck you take exhalation. Combining this Knocking Teeth and Dry Wash practice with your every day meditation will strengthen your teeth and gums, and improve circulation and beauty skin and hair.

And now, overlap your hands and put them on your stomach and abdomen area, gently massage clockwise 36 times. And then your palms massage your waist from the sides up and down 36 times while relaxing your entire body. Finally, your thumbs massage the center area of your soles 36 times for each. Doing this every time after your meditation will strengthen your kidney, liver, heart, digestive and gastrointestinal systems.

§3.18 Exercise Questions

1. How do you understand the idea that the universe is created on the basis of fundamental law and core principle?

2. What are the fundamental spiritual characteristics of the universe?

3. What is the core principle of the universe energy system?

4. What is the medium crossing the dimensions of body, mind and spirit?

5. What are the major concepts taught by traditional energy medicine – traditional Chinese medicine?

6. How do you understand the wave-particle dualism based on the energy nature of life at all dimensions?

7. How do you understand the hypothetical model of Spiritual Energy with its possible association with dark energy of the universe?

8. How do you describe the human body in different dimensions?

9. What are intra and inter-dimensional energy transformation and transferring? Explain it by giving an example.

10. What do you understand about energy vibration and characteristic frequency at different dimensions?

11. What is the whole being model and describe the relationships of all life components?

12. Is the brain itself the spirit? How do you understand the role of brain in the whole being – the body, mind and spirit?

13. Why do we need to cultivate the spirit and mind?

14. Why can people get sick, age and die based on mind-body-spirit science and how can you prevent sickness and slow down aging?

15. Why do we say healing is to harmonize and rebalance the life?

16. How do you understand energy meridians buried within the body, mind and spirit?

17. Why is mind-body-spirit cultivation needed?

18. What is meant by energy frequency (*f*) and resonance frequency (*fo*)? What is the center focus of mind-body healing arts?

19. How do you differentiate the between healthy and unhealthy energy vibrations?

20. Why is it required for the mind-body health practitioner to practice mind-body-spirit cultivation?

SPIRIT 靈

MIND 心   BODY 身

CHAPTER 4

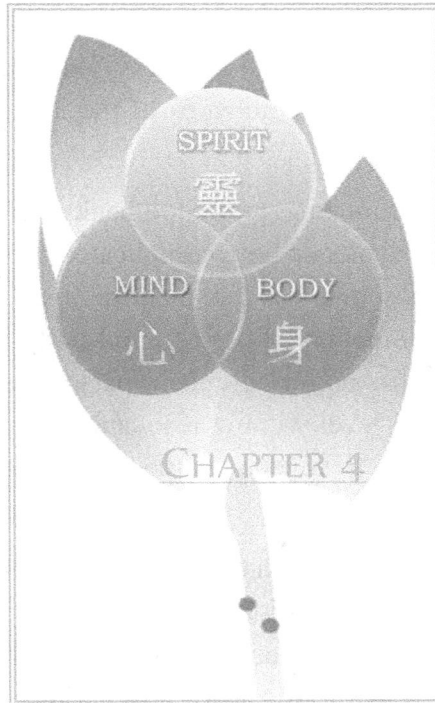

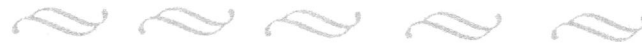

Energy Generation and Energy Consumption

As discussed in the previous three chapters, we know that the energy life force with pure spiritual natures and balanced energy vibration frequencies is the most important and central focus in mind-body medicine and mind-body health practice. In this chapter, we further explore the strategy, implementation and mechanisms by which this energy practice works at all levels of body, mind and spirit. We additionally will further the discussion and understanding of how to gain healthy energy, eliminate negative unhealthy energy, and limit energy consumption for optimal health and performance on all levels of mind-body-spirit.

I want emphasize that no matter how many modalities or techniques have developed in the science and technology of mind-body medicine and healthology, vital energy life

117

force is forever the most fundamental and most important issue and focus within our practice and study. Keeping this in mind is extremely important. Otherwise as we often see, many practitioners start a practice with great interest, but eventually become bored with that or some practitioners stay on the surface only addressing the physical form or focus more and more on complicated superficial things, but never actually progress in the actual practice which moves inwardly, within the domains of the inner mind, body and spirit to upgrade energy at each level.

If the practice is not focused on energy or good healthy energy, no matter how good the technique or theory sounds or looks or how complicated the approach may be or how luxurious and fancy the practice setting is, the practice itself must be something very superficial and has no meaning. Some modalities of mind-body practice may originally be good, but because the practitioner has no (or not much) personal energy cultivated, or his or her focus remains at the superficial level without resonance with the deep root of spiritual energy source on a daily basis, then treatments or the practice will not be very beneficial and efficacy rates will remain low. Let's consider this idea from another angle.

There are four elements of practice that are important for a good mind-body-spirit energy practice. (1) First is to follow the spiritual law and core principles of energy. (2) The second is to understand the mechanism of energy processing within all life components of the body, mind and spirit. (3) The third is to learn and master a few (you don't need too many) good and comprehensive techniques, and (4) The fourth is to put consistent and persistent efforts into the practice of your techniques on a daily basis. Note: To be effective in terms of MBM, these must be consistent with spiritual law and core principles.

The first element of practice is the ultimate guide for the entire practice that we have discussed in the previous chapters. The second puts into action mechanisms of the energy process – the understanding of which is based on the first component (the guide) and also its strategic implementation and application. The third is the learning of actual techniques based on the first and second (components), and the fourth is the practical realization, application and successful use of the entire model.

§4.2 Energy Gradient and Body-Mind-Spirit Multi-Dimensions

This section will now layer and deepen the energy concepts we have been discussing. Universal energy, for instance, lies along a gradient. This gradient ranges from the low energy dimension in the superficial layer of the physical time-space to the high spiritual energy dimension (Fig. 4.2.1). The physical body in the physical dimension has the lowest energy and is supported by the mental and spiritual energy in the higher energy dimensions. As well, the physical dimension is the output exit of energy streams that originate from the highest energy dimension of spiritual dimension and come down to the physical dimension through the mind in the mental dimension.

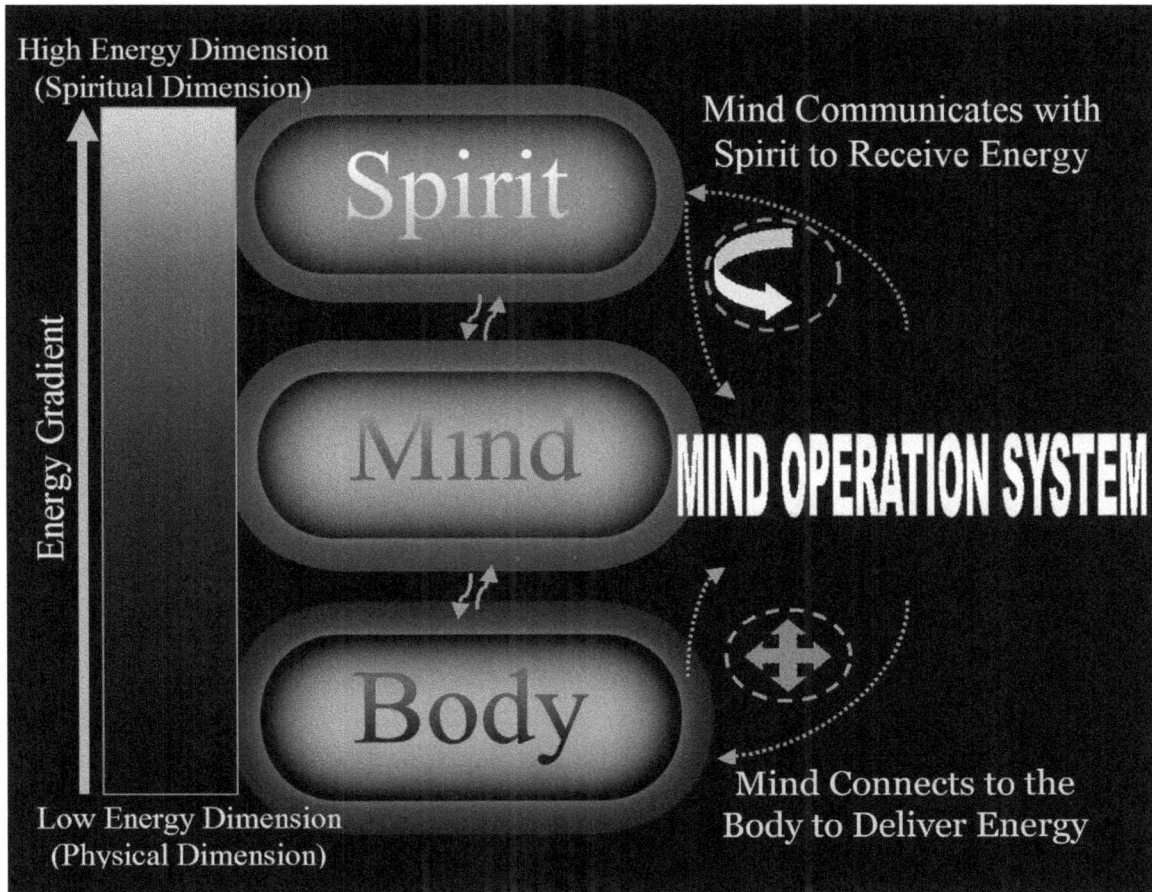

Fig. 4.2.1. Gradient of Life Energy Field: The universe's energy lies along a gradient from the low energy dimension in the superficial layer of the physical time-space to the high spiritual energy dimension. The physical body is at the lowest energy dimension (physical realm), and the mind exists in the intermediate energy dimension (mental dimension, emotional world) that connects to the body and communicates to the spirit, which is in the highest energy dimension (spiritual dimension, spiritual world). The communication and connection are operated through a mind-operation system (*see* later pages for the mind-operation system).

As such, the physical body is the external and superficial form of the life that expresses its physiological functions, physical actions and behaviors. Its health and its functions and behaviors rely on supportive energies provided from the mind and spirit as well as past lives, genetic resources, necessary nutrients and physical exercises.

Therefore, in this physical life, beside energy from past lives, genes and biological energy given by parents, for whom we need to be ever grateful, necessary balanced nutrients that we need to carefully take, and some physical exercises, we really need to practice the cultivation of mental and spiritual energy to ensure a healthy life as a whole being of body, mind and spirit.

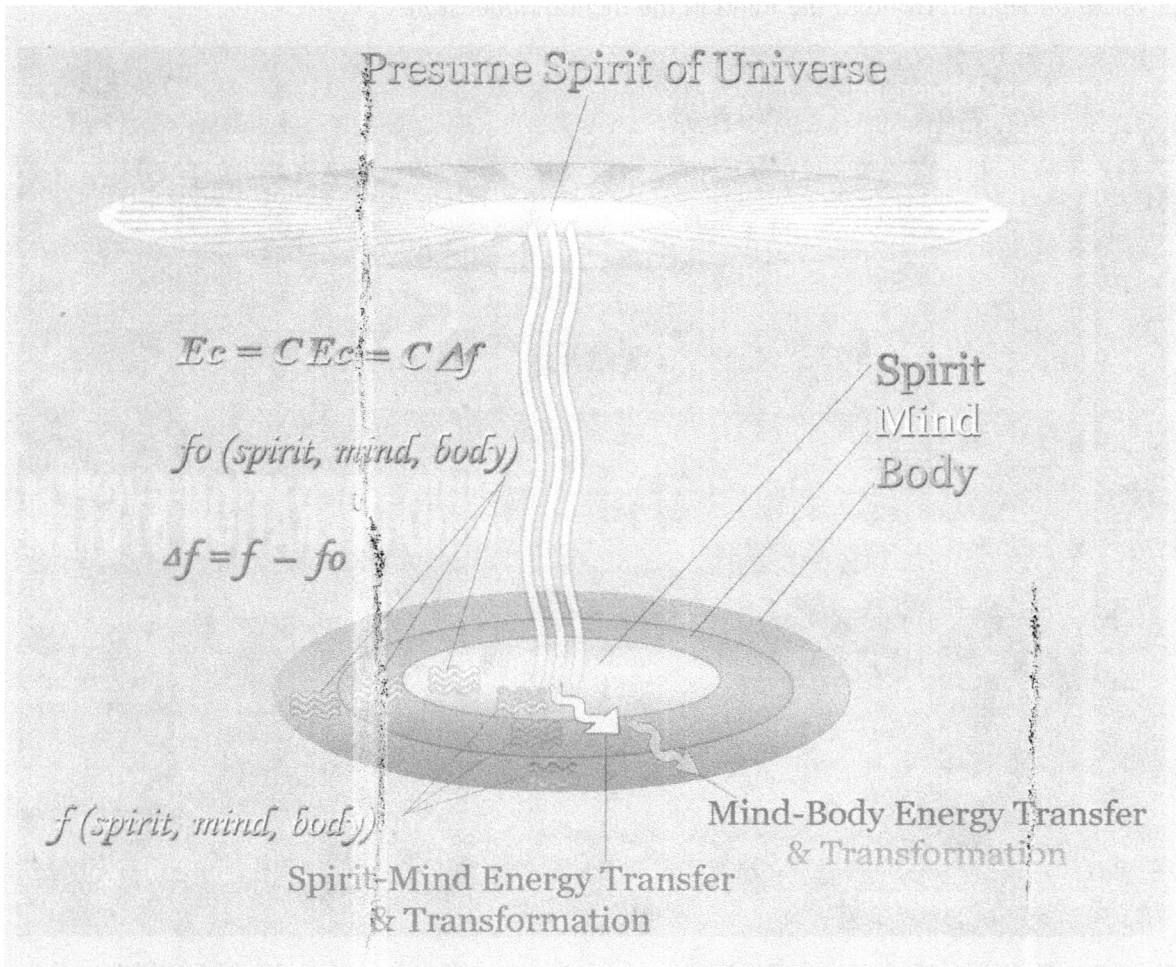

Fig. 4.2.2. The highest spiritual center of the universe has its supreme law that created lives with original standard frequency (fo) for spirit, mind and body. When human beings came down to the human world in the physical dimension, the spirit, mind and body dropped down to the lower level, and they can be even contaminated during life times in the past and present lives, having different frequency (f) in the spirit, mind and body, depending upon their levels of individual mind-body-spirit nature, quality, behavior and cultivation. The difference $\Delta f = f - fo$ represents the deviation of the mind-body-spirit from the original nature (true Self), determining the energy loss and consumption at the corresponding dimensions. The consumption of Energy is $Ec = C(f - fo) = C\,\Delta f$.

The spirit is the human being's original essence and energy form in the spiritual dimension from which the creature originally was created. This spirit has the same natures or characteristics as the universe. It is powerful, energetic, bright, positive, tireless, long living, selfless, truthful, peaceful, lovely, loving, compassionate and forgiving, and has conscience and all positive attributes of godly natures.

Every human is borne of (and sustains) these great spiritual natures. The energy vibration of this sprit is the original energy vibration frequency (*fo*) as shown in Fig. 4.2.1. But these natures may not be apparent, visible/cognizant at the human level in the physical world because they are shadowed or blocked by the darkness of and attachment to negative energy in the physical dimension. In part, this is a result of the mind's becoming selfish, narrowed, non-spiritual, and excessive in its desire for things within the material world. What further shadows and/or blocks the visibility and comprehension of original universal energy are the lack of practice and improvement of mind-body-spirit cultivation, as well as the lack of understanding (which can lead to misunderstanding and confusion) of truth, the lack of self-awareness by inward looking self for improvement, and also the need for more exploration, access, development and mindfulness of original higher spirit and spiritual natures.

Therefore the actual mind and body at the lower dimensions will appear to be operating at a different energy vibration frequency (*f*), as compared to the original frequency (*fo*). The difference between *f* and *fo* represents frequency deviation from the original characteristic frequency:

$$\Delta f = f - fo$$

The bigger the Δf is, the more (as well as worse and worsening) problems the life has, in terms of health and all living issues (Note: see the further discussions on this topic in the following sections).

§4.3 Human Mind Separation from the Godly Mind

The mind originally serves as the connection (conduit) of the whole being with the superior spirit, the highest spiritual energy source. It bridges the spirit and the body as one whole being. We called it spiritual mind or godly mind (G-Mind) because it has many powerful spiritual natures as the universe has, as mentioned in the previous section (Fig. 4.3).

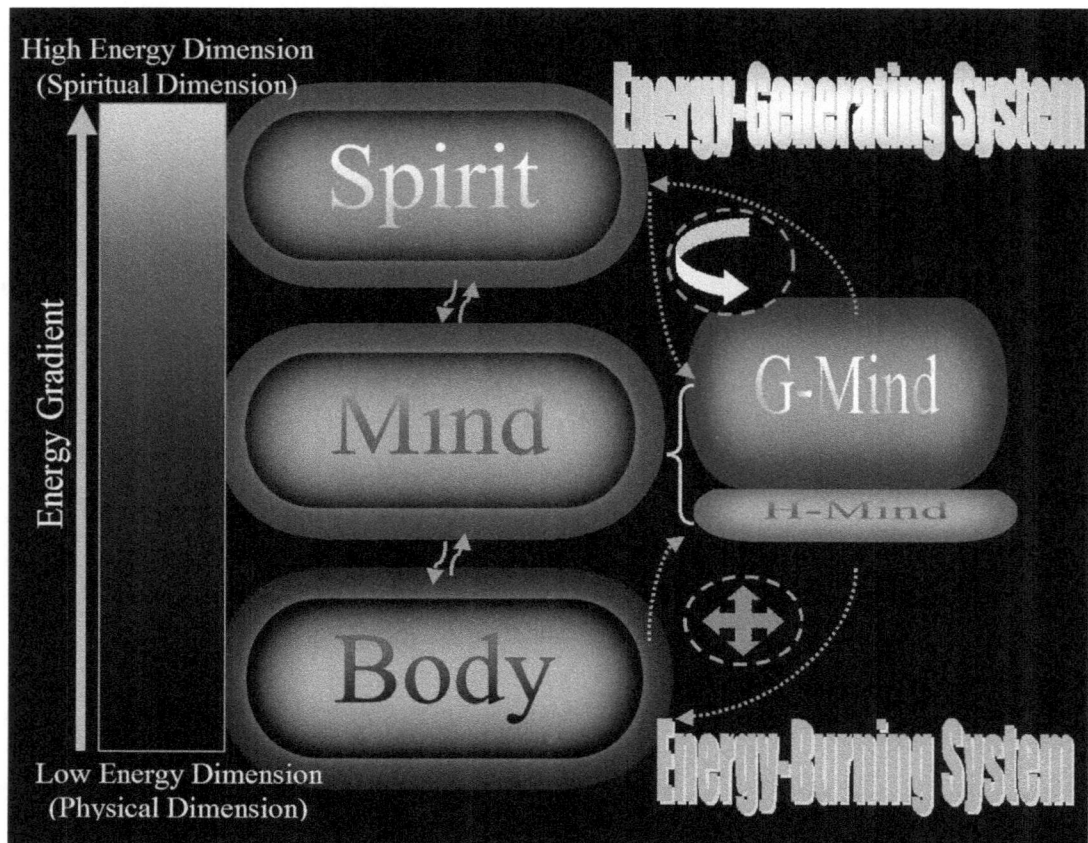

Fig. 4.3. The mind-operation system includes two parts: the Spiritual mind (godly mind) / G-Mind and the human mind / H-Mind: the mind originally connected with the superior spirit and is called spiritual mind or godly mind (G-Mind) that has great spiritual characteristics and powerful energy. Over long journey of human life at human level, however, part of the mind becomes attached to the material world (physical dimension), separated from the G-Mind and formed human mind (H-Mind). The G-Mind connected to the higher energy source and formed Energy Generating System, while the H-Mind attached to the low energy material dimension and formed Energy Consuming System or Energy Burning System.

The material world in the lower dimension, however, influences and contaminates the mind during this life journey, and as a result, some part of the mind becomes attached to the physical human being and the physical dimension (material realm). This partial mind becomes separated from the G-Mind and behaves more materialistically, narrow mindedly, selfishly, greedily, negatively, worrisomely, nervously, anxiously, skeptically, as well as deviates from the original natures of the spirit. Because of these tendencies, we name this part of the mind: the human mind (H-Mind) (*see* Fig. 4.3).

The energy vibration frequency of the G-Mind is basically the same as that of the original spirit, *fo*, while the energy vibration frequency (*f*) of the H-Mind has a difference compared to *fo*,

$$\Delta f = f - fo$$

Important Note: ***This Δf is mainly the result of contributions from the H-Mind.***

§4.4 Energy Consuming System: Human Mind - Physical World

As we look at the model presented in previous section (Fig. 4.3), the human mind cares about the needs of the physical body at the low energy dimension and is disconnected with the high spirit and G-Mind. This human mind associates with neurological sensations, physiological feelings, human thoughts, notions, narrowed mind, rigid logics, selfishness, greediness, materialism, unconscious habits and other mental and physical behaviors that are related with attachments and desires.

Among these human mind behaviors and activities only a minimal part of these may actually be necessary for daily life-care in the way of natural living, but most of them are unnecessary.

The human mind behaves at the low energy dimension, drives the neurological systems, brain, and entire physiological body generating a lot of thoughts, ideas, worries, fears, behaviors, stressful tasks and mental and physical activities. Thus as a result, it consumes a lot of the life's energy.

The more energy a life consumes, the more the physical body and human mind run into the lower energy state. This becomes the downward spiral that occurs from this energy consumption – for then, running on even lower energy, the human mind becomes even more attached, concerned, materialistic, narrowed, blocked, stubborn, skeptical, negative, worrisome, and so on. It then becomes further disconnected with the high energy spirit. This forms a circular pattern of burning more and more energy and producing more and more unhealthy, disturbing and energy consuming vibrations. Accordingly, this circular pattern will widen the gap between original spirit/G-Mind characteristic frequency (fo) and the individual's current life frequency (f).

We name this H-Mind/Body circle mechanism *The Energy Consuming System (ECS)* or *Energy Burning System (EBS).*

Now, we introduce a system constant, C, which refers to the consumption rate. "C" expresses the systematic rate of energy consumed by the ECS.

The constant C depends upon the particular human being's life condition, lifestyle, environment, and genetic or inborn conditions such as Virtue and Karma, spiritual belief, and so forth. The more the individual's H-Mind attaches on the low energy dimension and the issues of human world, and the more it stays deviated from the pure spiritual state (fo), the greater the consumption rate or C is, the greater the amount of consumed energy Ec is.

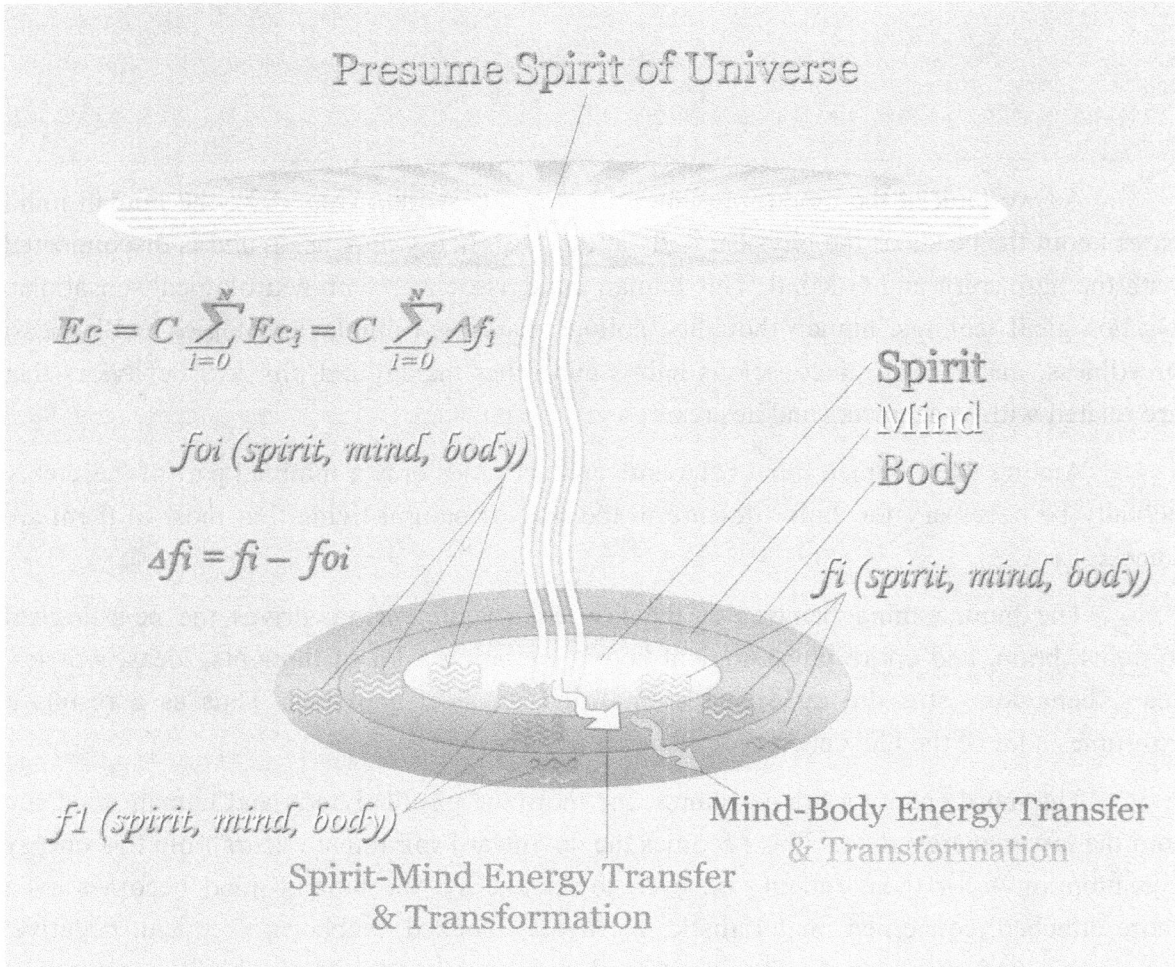

Presume Spirit of Universe

$$Ec = C \sum_{i=0}^{N} Ec_i = C \sum_{i=0}^{N} \Delta f_i$$

foi (spirit, mind, body)

$$\Delta f_i = f_i - foi$$

Spirit
Mind
Body

fi (spirit, mind, body)

$f1$ (spirit, mind, body)

Mind-Body Energy Transfer & Transformation

Spirit-Mind Energy Transfer & Transformation

Fig. 4.4. The highest spiritual nature of the universe has its supreme law that created lives with original standard frequencies for all dimensions and subdimensions (foi) of spirit, mind and body. When human beings came down to the human world in the physical dimension, the spirit, mind and body dropped down to the lower level, and they can be even contaminated during their life times in the past and present lives, having different frequencies (fi) in the spirit, mind and body, depending their levels of individual mind-body-spirit nature, quality, behavior and cultivation. The difference $\Delta f_i = f_i - foi$ represents the deviation of the mind-body-spirit from the original nature (true Self) at a specific dimension or subdimension (i), determining the energy loss and consumption $Ec_i = C \Delta f_i$ at the corresponding dimensions or subdimensions. The total energy consumption is the sum of all Ec_i over all dimensions and subdimensions regarding all activities and issues of the mind, body and spirit.

As shown in Fig. 4.4, if we use $\Delta f_i = f_i - fo_i$ to represent the frequency difference between the current vibration frequency (f_i) and the original frequency (fo_i) for a particular vibration i at the dimension, sub-dimension, system or subsystem, or regarding an issue (e.g., in physical dimension, the vibration #i [1, 2, 3, …N] can be assigned to any of genetics, family and social influences, education, career, job, stress, relationship, lifestyle, personality, manner, financial, health, worry, attachments, thoughts, mentality, spirituality, open-mindedness, belief, etc.) of mind or body, then the amount of consumed energy (Ec_i) will be proportional to both $\Delta f_i = f_i - fo_i$ and C,

$$Ec_i = C\,\Delta f_i$$

Where $\Delta f_i = f_i - fo_i$ and C is the consuming rate of energy.

And the total amount of consumed energy (Ec) is the sum of consumed energy at all vibrations from i to N at all dimension, sub-dimensions, system or subsystem.

$$Ec = C \sum_{i=0}^{N} Ec_i = C \sum_{i=0}^{N} \Delta f_i$$

N is the total number of vibrations in the human mind and body with the frequency f_i.

The negative vibrations in the Energy Consuming System (ECS) can occur through the human mind (H-Mind) in any dimensions or sub-dimensions, regarding any aspect at human level. These include physical or mental dimensions or any of their sub-dimensions.

For example, in the human mind, these can be a series of emotional characters such as worry, fear, anxiety, depression, etc., or personality characters or attitudes such as selfishness, negativity, skepticism, dishonesty, carelessness, etc. Within the physical dimension, these can be any activity or behavior such as smoking, drugging, alcoholic, gambling, insufficient (or too much) sleep, unhealthy diet, imbalance of nutrition, over working, and many other factors.

The negative vibrations can also be the result of any destructive social movement, unhealthy social system or political system, harmful ideologies (e.g., materialism, class struggle, atheism), or forced brainwashing propaganda. The bad energy vibrations also can manifest from harmful thoughts and activities (imagined or otherwise) such as killing, persecution, torture, rape, hate, revenge, violence, slander, jealousy, and evil, or advertently supporting evil via participation or in inadvertently through the choice to remain silent with regard to such evils.

All this creates big Karma and huge amounts of bad energies and escalates the consumption of energy Ec., resulting in disease and even more catastrophically, in death.

You can add more such issues or vibration events to this list of things that contribute to energy consumption that damages life force. All these issues are vibrations with energy and frequency in their own dimension or sub-dimension, contributing to the energetic difference between original frequency at that dimension or sub-dimension, and consuming the energy of life to the extent of low, extremely low or even negative levels.

We assign each of them a sequential number i to present that particular vibration i in its particular dimension or sub-dimension. Then its vibration frequency will be f_i, and the difference of frequency will be $\Delta f_i = f_i - fo_i$, where fo_i is the original spiritual characteristic frequency of the vibration i in the dimension, and the amount of consumed energy due to this vibration event will be $Ec_i = C \Delta f_i$.

Mental and physical sickness, disease, discomfort, negative feelings, and difficulties in this life, all can be caused by the individual's energy deficiency, imbalance or distraction due to the individual's energy consumption Ec. Therefore, in mind-body medicine and mind-body health practice, avoiding or limiting the ECS and the unnecessary consuming of energy Ec are very important.

In other words, in our practice of mind-body medicine, we need to put effort into detaching the human mind with the low energy dimension, decrease the H-Mind and increase the G-Mind.

Human beings come to this physical world like coming to a maze in which the truth is not revealed, so true Self is lost. Many temptations, attractions, distractions or disturbances in the physical world fully occupy the human mind, stimulate desires, and attract attentions. Superficial phenomenon in the visible physical world and material interests block the spirit and hinder people's exploration of the higher wisdom and true meaning of life.

The human mind consumes a lot of energy from its life force. People put a lot of efforts on, pay attention to, and attach to the low energy dimension in the physical world in an attempt to (1) increase and/or satisfy their desires for materials, wealth, interests, fame, power, relationships, sentiments, human notions and emotions; (2) try to realize whatever dreams they have in this physical world, in this life, without knowing and caring about the most important issues, including the health of their mind, body and soul, as well as their long-term life goal or purpose; (3) run into the endless cycle of living the "busy life" all the time, habitually, as a norm, a behavior which may have been learned from parents, family, friends, teachers, society, and now leaves them never thinking deeply and spiritually about what is most important in this life; (4) think and act in ways they have become used to and sustain as notion, habit, addiction, and attachment, and focus too much or entirely on outward things, instead of changes leading toward a more clear headed, meaningful and healthy life of true Self and unified body, mind and spirit.

The material world and human desires interact with each other and as a result, the human mind is often tightly locked into a narrow and imbalanced scope with which to deal with life. Such human mind appears ignorant, has no wisdom and intelligence, and views things, life, and the world with limited knowledge, wrong ideas or ignorance. It often works with low efficiency or even incorrectly or veers in a wrong direction. This is why many individuals are struggling very hard with many things in this life in the physical world, including but not limit to learning, career, family, relationship, society, economy, politics, gain and loss, health and sickness, aging, and death.

The physical dimension is the output exit of energy flow, but not the energy source or its supplement. The human mind and physical world form the energy-consuming engine that constantly consumes energy and runs a life into low energy, an energy lacking or negative state.

Therefore, the overwhelming access, activities and attachments of human mind – and physical world – without one's connecting to the energy source of the spiritual dimension, will consume a tremendous amount of life force energy and cause depletion of the life energy, resulting in tiredness, sickness, diseases, imbalance of energy, negative energy state, mental and physical problems, individual, family and social problems, aging and even death.

To avoid and limit such intense energy consumption and achieve health of the body and mind, we need to de-attach from the energy consuming system, simplify, limit and eliminate the human mind that causes the dramatic frequency difference $\Delta f = f - fo$ of energy vibration.

We need to cultivate such human mind and convert it to spiritual mind (G-Mind), then reconnect with the higher spiritual energy source and limit the difference so that $\Delta f = f - fo \to 0$, and the consuming rate so that $C \to 0$, so the energy consuming will become as little as possible:

$$Ec = C \sum_{i=0}^{N} \Delta f_i \to 0$$

Where $\Delta f_i \to 0$ and/or $C \to 0$; N is the total number of vibrations in the human mind, with the frequency f_i.

§4.5 Energy Generating System: Spiritual Mind - High Dimension

As shown in the Fig. 4.3, the spiritual mind is also called godly mind (G-Mind). As the name states, your spiritual mind is originated from and connected with your original spirit and balanced energy vibrations. It is spiritually enriched and vested with the power and wonderful natures of your original godly spirit and the universal energy source of the Yin-Yang and Five Elements or Beyond The Five Elements. Your spiritual mind came from the superior creature of the universe, the original spirit of life, and power of the divine energy system.

Our spiritual minds have great power and fantastic natures that make our life spiritually meaningful and divinely powerful, beautiful, peaceful, healthy, joyful and balanced in accordance with Yin-Yang, The Elements, and beyond.

The ultimate natures of the spiritual mind are not complicated. Actually they are simple and integrative, which can be summarized as peace, kindness, compassion, truthfulness, forgiveness, forbearance, and so on, all of which have spiritual energy vibrations and balanced positive energy vibrations with the original spiritual characteristic frequency (*fo*).

A little more specifically, these spiritual natures are, for example, honest, loving, compassionate, having conscience, caring, forgiving, appreciative, selfless, humble, respectful, open minded, positive, passionate, enthusiastic, confident, wise, intelligent, detached (in the right way), non-stubborn, open minded, understanding, communicative, clear headed, gentle, soft, kind, strong, consistent, stable, energetically in balance of Yin-Yang and The Five Elements or Beyond The Five Elements, and synchronized with the universe and its characteristics.

The positive energy vibrations can also be any public welfare charity activities, contributions, giving, or righteous thoughts and activities to support justice and the like. These all resonate with high spirit, generate strong positive energies and create good Virtue, benefiting health, blessing luck, and longevity.

The highest spirit has unlimited energy source. The spiritual mind communicates, synchronizes and resonates with the highest spiritual energy source where it has the original spiritual and substantial energy frequency (*fo*), so that it generates a huge amount of life force energy (*Eg*). ***This spiritual mind and highest spirit, as well as its energy system, together form an energy-generating engine, called the Energy Generating System (EGS).***

§4.6 MBM & Mind-Body-Spirit Cultivation - The Solution For High Energy

The amount of generated energy is dependent upon how much the spiritual mind is assimilated with the highest spiritual natures of the universe, how high of a cultivation level the life has reached, and how much the balanced energy of the Yin-Yang and Five Elements (or Beyond The Five Elements) the life is resonated with. This is just the aim of the Mind-Body Medicine & Healthology and Mind-Body-Spirit Cultivation under the universal law (*see* Fig. 4.6.1 and Fig. 4.6.2).

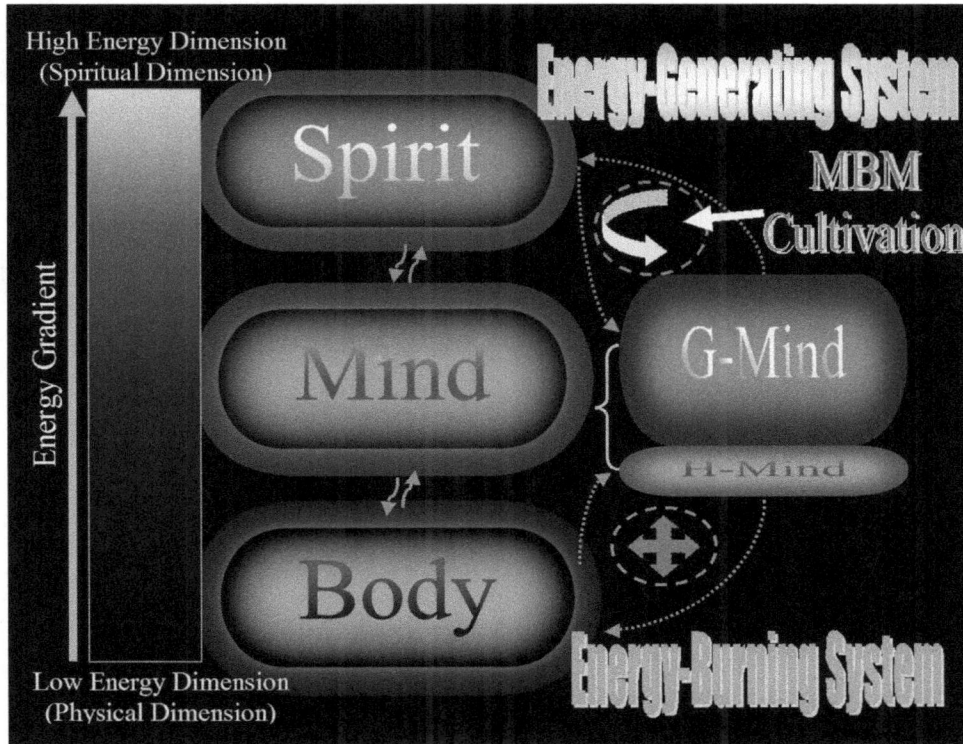

Fig. 4.6.1. Mind-Body Medicine and its health practice or cultivation practice are to help increase the generated energy through the spiritual mind (G-Mind) and decrease the consumed energy through the human mind (H-Mind). Mind-Body Medicine and Healthology, for instance, the Brainwave-Meridian Therapy (BMT) as addressed in later chapter, or self-improvement practice such as meditation and mind-body-spirit cultivation can help increase G-Mind, connect to the higher spirit, generate more higher energy, strengthen the mind-body-spirit health, while attachments to the material dimension can decrease the G-Mind, increase the H-Mind, burn more energy at physical level, causing mental and physical weakness, sickness, aging, and difficulties in life.

All of this energy generated in the practice of MBM and cultivation can be represented by the sum of the frequency (*fo_j*) assimilated. Here we introduce a system constant called energy Generating Rate, G, which represents the energy generating efficiency by the EGS. Therefore, the amount of generated energy is

$$Eg = \sum_{j=0}^{M} Eg_j = G \sum_{j=0}^{M} fo_j$$

Where G is the EGS system constant or energy generating rate, and *fo_j* is the spiritual vibration frequency or Yin-Yang Five Elements (or Beyond The Five Elements) energy vibration *j*, the sequential number of the vibration at the dimension, sub-dimension, system or subsystem of mind, body and spirit with which the spiritual mind assimilated.

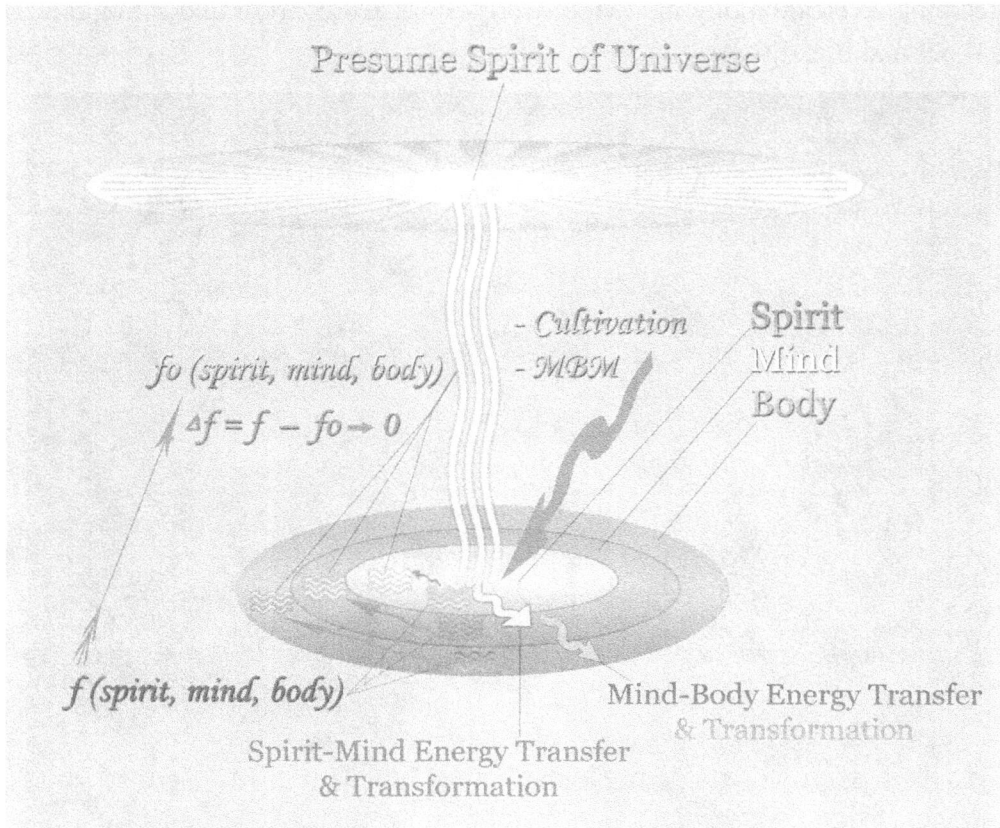

Fig. 4.6.2. Through MBM and healthology practice with combination of mind-body-spirit cultivation, the energy vibration frequency difference *Δf* between the existing state and the original state at all levels of mind, body and spirit and their sub-levels can become as small as possible (the ideal state is close to zero), so that the consuming energy *Ec* becomes as small as possible or close to zero.

From the above conceptual equation, we understand that the more cultivated the mind is, the more (the greater M) and the higher level (greater fo_j) spiritual vibrations and Yin-Yang and Five Elements (or Beyond The Five Elements) energy vibrations the mind assimilated with, the greater energy *Eg* generated. The assimilated higher vibrations of the universe include higher spiritual vibrations and Yin-Yang/Five Elements (or Beyond The Five Elements) energy vibrations at multiple levels (dimensions).

Since we are living in the low energy dimension/physical realm where we often have a lot of disturbances and attractions that drive our mind down to the human mind, there is often conflict and competition between the G-Mind and H-Mind as they compete to drive the life's mind and each wants to own the direction it will go.

We need to cultivate our mind to remain spiritually pure, energetic and connected with the superior spirit and stay synchronized with the universal characteristics and balanced energy frequencies. This way the G-Mind can be increased and H-Mind will be decreased or limited accordingly. As a result, energy E consumption, during the entire life, will be limited to as minimal as possible:

$$E = Eg - Ec = \sum_{j=0}^{M} Eg_j - \sum_{i=0}^{N} Ec_i = G \sum_{j=0}^{M} fo_j - C \sum_{i=0}^{N} \Delta f_i$$

In summary, the job here is to maintain great life force energy **E**, increase the generated energy **Eg** by cultivating the spiritual mind (G-Mind), assimilating with more (M) and higher (**fo_j**) spiritual vibrations and energy vibrations, and decrease the consumed energy **Ec** by letting go of more human mind and having fewer (N, **Δf_i**) negative vibrations such as attachments, selfishness, desires, narrowed mind, skeptical attitude, non-spiritual belief, depression, anxiety, anger, other negative emotions, etc. and as well as unhealthy lifestyle and habits.

Although this process is not a specific mathematic equation precisely, the above equation together with the diagram illustrated in Fig. 4.6.1 and Fig. 4.6.2 can conceptually explain how the mind, body and spirit work together through the processes of energy generating and consuming to operate the life system. The overall purpose of this conceptual equation is to emphasize the central focus of our healing and health practice, emphasizing mind and spirit improvement and cultivation, and limiting the consumption of life energy that manifests from too many attachments generated by the complicated human mind. We support, encourage, and teach the letting go of these attachments and increasing a person's positive energy by following the higher spiritual law and energy source.

This process is not just a belief, but also a science that teaches us the truth about life and life phenomenon and as well as its beneficial practice in daily life.

§4.7 Brain • Mind • Spirit • Energy: Brain Left/Right Hemispheres

The human brain is the biological device of the mind in the physical dimension. The brain consists of hundreds of billions of neurons that form a myriad of neuron networks and carry out huge amounts of informational communications neurologically. These neurological information networks and communication activities in the brain are the reflections that come from the following sources and mainly reside in the left and right hemispheres of the brain:

{Left Hemisphere of the Brain}

(1) Mainly the left hemisphere of the brain facilitates learning about and experiencing material life, education, science, techniques, logics, ego characters, selfishness, negative emotions and immoral or evil natures, etc. within this human world in this lifetime. This type of information, memories, activities and experiences, together with the sources described in both (2) and (3) below, forms human consciousness (existing terminology calls it consciousness; that includes consciousness and sub-consciousness) in the brain and human mind in the mental dimension. This human mind and consciousness deal with the physical world and material life, constituting the energy consuming system. Some of this information, mental characteristics and activities are necessary for physical living as designed originally, whereas some of them are due to the over-accessed or overused desires and human ego. These over-accessed/overused desires cause Karmas and unnecessary energy consumption, resulting in life problems including a wide range of health problems.

(2) The left hemisphere of the brain also facilitates the Karmas and negative characteristics accumulated in the past lives and this life (see above in (1)). As such, these determine the inborn (congenital) and after-born (acquired) natures of the human mind and brain, mainly in the left hemisphere. The inborn Karmas and negative characteristics were carried on through the spirit (original Self) in the spiritual dimensions before this physical life and settled down and associated with the brain, human consciousness, and human mind in this life.

(3) The brain's left hemisphere additionally facilitates negative influences and damages from the bad or lower spirits and environment in the physical world or from other dimensions. These can include but are not limit to bad or evil ideologies, immoral social movements, propaganda, stressful or harmful abuses, persecution and pressures against the natural law and humanity. These influences and damages can be invoked through passive association or active involvement by the individual himself or herself.

{Right Hemisphere of the Brain}

(4) The right hemisphere of the brain facilitates learning, experience, practice and cultivation of arts, spirituality, intuition, imagination, systemization, moral and spiritual activities, and spirit guided by the universal law and energy system. This type of information memories, activities and experiences, together with the sources described in both (5) and (6) forms spiritual consciousness (existing terminology calls it consciousness that includes consciousness and sub-consciousness, but not separate from the human consciousness) in the brain and spiritual mind in the mental dimension. The spiritual mind and consciousness communicate and

assimilate with the higher spiritual dimension, constituting the energy generating system. Some of this information, mental characteristics and activities, as well as the energy generated, support the needs of the spiritual life, healing, health and longevity of the whole being in this life, and the rest of which is accumulated for the further life as Virtue or consummation as higher being.

(5) The right hemisphere of the brain also facilitates the good quality spiritual Virtues, characteristics, talents, and personality established in past lives and this life, determining the inborn (congenital) and after-born (acquired) nature and quality of the spiritual mind and brain. These inborn spiritual qualities and characteristics were carried on through the spirit (original Self) in the spiritual dimensions before this physical life, and settled down and associated with the brain, spiritual consciousness, and spiritual mind in this life.

(6) As well, the right hemisphere of the brain additionally facilitates the pure spiritual natures of the universe and the cultivation with such natures – how much the spiritual natures assimilate depends upon the individual's learning and cultivation in this life. These will contribute to spiritual consciousness and spiritual mind, and the energy generation system.

The brain, as a whole, retains and operates the information of the mind and performs the activities, behaviors and actions of the mind at the biological and physical dimensions. The spirit of a life is at much higher dimensions than where the mind and brain exist, so the brain does not contain all the information, spiritual natures and characters, as well as vibration energies that the spirit has.

When we explore the science of mind-body-spirit, we need to be clear about the truth and that is: That the brain science cannot replace the science and practice of body-mind-spirit.

In the modern times, it seems there is a tendency for people to think the brain is everything – the headquarters and CEO of the human being. Or that brain research will tell us everything about our whole being and its place within mankind. But this is a misleading conception.

In fact, the brain is simply the biological memory container and output device of the mind, but not the biological library of the entire spirit. The brain is developed and trained in this lifetime through the mind in this physical world, but the spirit of the life comes from a long journey of the life before this life to which it will return after this life.

The mind can access the spirit, communicate and resonate with the spirit to assimilate and obtain its spiritual natures, characters, messages, information, high vibration energies, and help transfer and transform those spiritual powers to the biological and physical levels; which is the process of the spiritual mind generating life force energy as we discussed in the previous sections. However, again properly understood, it does not mean the mind contains all the powers that the spirit has.

How much power the mind has is dependent upon how much it has cultivated and assimilated with the high spiritual energy vibrations. Similarly as the biological device of the mind; the power, capability, creativity, energy, and behaviors of the brain depend upon how much the mind is cultivated with the higher spiritual energy source.

Meditation and other mind-body-spirit cultivation practices resonate and assimilate with the universe's spiritual energy vibrations, improve the mind nature and character, enhance the clarity of consciousness, and mental energy level – and as a result – the biological brain is also energized, and its functionalities are improved.

Therefore, practices such as meditation, Qigong, Taiji, Yoga, energy music healing, and the like are good for brain health, learning, efficiency and daily performance.

In the practice of mind-body-spirit, however, the key is to activate, practice and improve the functions of the Energy Generating System (EGS) instead of the Energy Consuming System (ECS). This means that we need to shut down the human mind that attaches on the physical dimensions with desires, stubbornness, skeptical analysis, selfishness, narrowed notions, calculations of gain and loss, and random busy conscious and subconscious activities. This way, our spiritual mind will automatically and naturally access, communicate and assimilate with the original true natures and energy vibrations of the higher spiritual source. When you get yourself into deep meditation and enjoy the depths of a quiet, yet still conscious state, your mind flies up to its haven, the high dimensions, and the higher and pure vibrations resonating with your entire being, all the organs, cells, molecules, atoms – all resonate with the beautiful and powerful bright light vibrations from the godly spiritual dimensions. During that process, your brain is in the reorganizing and energy-charging mode, so it is totally rejuvenated with pure spiritual energy. As a result, the functions of your brain improve and transform to a much greater level.

From the science of brain function, regarding the brain's left and right hemispheres, we understand, then, that the left side of the brain functions with the characters of logical thinking, rationality, sequence, specificity, analysis, objectivity, materialism, ego, cognition, and non-spirituality. It looks at the parts, but not the whole. The right side of the brain, however, functions with the natures of art, intuition, imagination, synthesis, subjectivity, holism, analogy, and spirituality. It looks at the whole. In consideration of the EGS and ECS in our body-mind-spirit model, the left hemisphere of the brain actually contains more information of the human mind (H-Mind), and performs the activities of the H-Mind, and as a result, consumes a lot of energy in the physical dimension. This is why when an individual over-uses or overloads the left brain hemisphere, he or she feels low in energy or tired or even physically and emotionally uncomfortable or sick.

The right hemisphere of the brain, however, accesses, communicates and assimilates with the higher spiritual vibrations and obtains a lot of powerful energies. This is why when people practice arts, music, or talking spiritually, they feel good, relaxed, energetic and happy. In fact, during practices of mind and spirit such as meditation and musical healing, and hypnosis, we feel *more* energetic and clearer in the brain.

Of course, you must not get the wrong idea from what we just discussed above, as we should not completely shut down the left parts of the brain because these are still necessary to take care of certain specific issues in the human world that rely on functionality of the left side of the brain, the logical mindset. It would not be correct to assume that all the contents of the left brain hemisphere are negative human mind characters and behaviors. In fact, they include necessary logical memories, information, skills, techniques, methods, and ideas which are capable of many things in this physical world, and cooperate with right brain to perform necessary tasks. The problem is that the character of left hemisphere of the brain, especially over use of left brain's function, can make the person attach to the physical world, overwhelm him with the human desires and addictions, and lock him in a narrowly scoped mindset, resulting in energy consumption and preventing him from enlightenment to the spiritual truth of life.

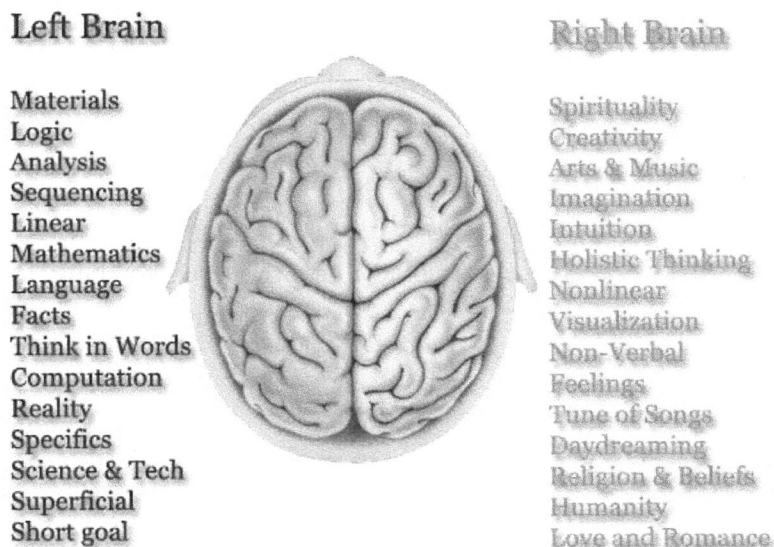

Left Brain

Materials
Logic
Analysis
Sequencing
Linear
Mathematics
Language
Facts
Think in Words
Computation
Reality
Specifics
Science & Tech
Superficial
Short goal

Right Brain

Spirituality
Creativity
Arts & Music
Imagination
Intuition
Holistic Thinking
Nonlinear
Visualization
Non-Verbal
Feelings
Tune of Songs
Daydreaming
Religion & Beliefs
Humanity
Love and Romance

Fig. 4.7. *The left and right hemispheres of the brain have different functions.* The left hemisphere of brain takes care of the things such as materials, logic, analysis, mathematics, calculation, reality, specifics, superficial things, short term goals, and linear relationships so that the left brain works mainly for the human mind at the lower physical dimensions in the energy consuming system in the model shown in Fig. 4.2, and described in section §4.4. The left side of the brain seems to be involved in human attachments. The right brain hemisphere, however, has talents and functions related to your spirituality, creativity, art, music, and rhythm, as well as the imaginary, intuitive, holistic, visual, humane, emotional, feeling, loving, romantic, religious and belief aspects of your life. The right brain, then, works more for spiritual mind and connects to the higher dimensions in the energy generating system in the model shown in Fig. 4.2, and described in section §4.6.

Academic studies from elementary school to graduate school nowadays are all or mainly about the left brain works, so the left brain is overwhelmingly overloaded from when we are young onward. On another note, the artistic and spiritual mind and its biological device, the right brain, need to be activated and given enough higher energy through the mind-body-spirit practice. Therefore, the key is to unlock the mind, activate spiritual mind, limit the activities of the human mind especially the natures and characters that lock, attach or bind the mind tightly to the physical world and prevent it from connecting to the higher spiritual vibrations.

Yes, we still need to calculate and manage, for example, finances as part of our daily life, but we also need to slow down the left brain and human mind, and slow down the faucet of our ECS – as this faucet can go dry. Consequently then, we can practice cultivating more EGS in the spiritual mind to transfer more energy from the high energy source for the whole being including the mind, body and brain.

We need to understand that the existing life at the material world is only part of the entire life journey in the scales of both space and time. And we need to remember that practicing the body, mind and spirit for the entire being in this life and future lives will improve both brain hemispheres and functions and help you achieve your short-term goals and long-term goals at the same time.

Consider this story as told by the Harvard brain scientist, Dr. Jill Bolte Taylor, Ph.D. who consciously experienced the exceptional inner peace of her brain's right hemisphere during a massive stroke of the left hemisphere of her brain [28]. She explains what she gleaned from the experience like this:

"This was the blessing I received from my experience: that nirvana is just a thought away—or, in my language [of science], deep inner peace exists in the consciousness of our right hemisphere. And at any given moment, you can choose to hook into that part of your brain, into a peaceful state, if you are willing to stop the cognitive loops of thought, worry, [anger]—any ideas that distract you from the experience of being in the here and now. What my stroke did was shut out all those moments; it silenced the dominating, judging voice of my left mind. And when that happened, my consciousness dwelled in a flow of sweet tranquility." [29]. "I realized that the blessing I had received from this experience was the knowledge that deep internal peace is accessible to anyone at any time. I believe the experience of Nirvana exists in the consciousness of our right hemisphere, and that at any moment, we can choose to hook into that part of our brain. ... My stroke of insight would be: *peace is only a thought away, and all we have to do to access it is silence the voice of our dominating left mind.*" [30].

Dr. Taylor's wrote on another page in the same book, "The secret to hooking into any of these peaceful states is the willingness to stop the cognitive loops of thought, worry, and any ideas that distract us from the kinesthetic and sensory experience of being in the here and now. Most important, however, our desire for peace must be stronger than our attachment to our misery, our ego, or our need to be right. I love that old saying, 'do you want to be right, or do you want to be happy?'" [30].

I love her experience, but love more her understanding of both the ways of brain science and beautiful spiritual inspiration. She mentions the term of Nirvana, which is an ancient Sanskrit term used in Indian Buddhist practice to describe the profound peace of mind and enlightenment achieved after a long journey of cultivation. Dr. Taylor's experience with Nirvana is an exceptional case because she was able to contribute to this field not only with her research as a scientist, but also with a clear scientific explanation of a personal experience. When her left hemisphere of the brain stopped functioning, the right hemisphere of the brain connected outside of the physical world and received great spiritual energy, experiencing the extreme peace, quietness, freedom and enlightenment. Of course, this is a biological failure of the left hemisphere function of the brain, which we do not want to happen while we are living on this physical world because it is still needed to take care of the specific human issues. However, it was really a blessing experience that tells us, through the experience of Dr. Taylor, how the left hemisphere of the brain works as well as what will happen and how we will feel when it is shut down.

Instead of having to live through functional shutdown as with a stroke, we can purposely and positively quiet the left brain activities, and let the spiritual mind and right brain fully access and communicate outside of the physical world. Then, the great spiritual energy vibrations will bring you to the same Nirvana state similar to that which we often experience during a deep meditation cultivation practice.

After the spiritual mind and right brain are fully charged with the powerful energy, and the left brain gets rested and transformed with great energy from the right brain, you can resume healthy activities of this physical world and live in the balanced functionalities of the right and left brain as the whole.

§4.8 Further Understanding of Mind-Body Practice & Its Benefits

Coming to this point, we get clearer about how a human being is living as an energy system at all levels of body, brain, mind, and spirit. This further understanding helps us see how to heal this life system if one is sick or how to maintain health preventively.

The great natures of the life are deeply rooted in the original spirit and energy source. The mind-body-spirit healing or health practice is the process of returning to and maintaining the original spirit, and balanced energy state and energy level. We advocate and practice limiting the consumption of energy by the human mind allowing for the cultivation and fluid transference of rejuvenating energy from our spiritual/godly mind. Many true examples show that such high level of cultivation practitioners successfully achieved their good health and life quality [31].

Technically at the biological and physical level, the left hemisphere of the brain stays quiet and peaceful to remain in a clearheaded and energetic state, and the right brain works with the spiritual mind as its biological device and charges with higher vibration energy, then transfers it to the left hemisphere of the brain for its necessary functioning output to the physical body and logical actions in cooperation with the right brain under spiritual mind instruction. Letting go of attachments, addictions, emotional actions and random thoughts and staying in a godly state of the spiritual mind and right brain will automatically generate huge amounts of life force energy, and at the same time the human mind will become smaller and smaller, so the life will have less energy consumed at the human level in the left hemisphere of the brain. It's why as a good health practitioner or self-healing practitioner or mind-body-spirit cultivator, you are not only healthy and do not get sick, but also always stay tireless, much more energetic, broad hearted, efficient, capable, intelligent, artistic, and creative. You are not busy throughout most of your day. This is because, instead, you are much more efficient and productive. You have a simple lifestyle and many fewer tasks to involve in, but you also have a much higher quality of happiness and joy in your life. You not only have compassion, love, and passion toward your family, friends, communities, societies, the world and its people, but also have such energy, capability and wisdom to actually take action at higher level and deeper meaning for long-term results.

In fact, as you let go of the human mind little by little and day after day, you will notice by yourself that you have greatly grown mentally, spiritually and physically, in terms of health, wisdom, personality, energy, overall performance in daily life, and much more. This practice helps you open up yourself; find your true Self; unlock your spirituality; mental and physical energy channels; boost your right brain, balancing both left and right hemispheres; transfer pure energy from higher dimensions to transform your physical body and all its organs and physiological systems; and as a result, you will stay harmonious, healthy, energetic, grounded, integrated, positive, hopeful and successful in all aspects of life.

Reaching such a state as described above is the goal of the mind-body-spirit healing, health and spiritual cultivation, called in the original language of Chinese, *Man and Heaven Become One*. Such an energetic state is a balanced state between Yin and Yang, and harmonized state of The Five Elements (or Beyond The Five Elements) at the levels of physical and mental bodies.

The energy from the high spirit activated through the cultivated spiritual mind has universal divine power within the entire life at all levels with the characteristics of the universe. Such energy integrates, unifies and harmonizes all life components. Therefore, the spirit can guide the entire life and take lead of the body and mind, build the good and healthy personality, character, thoughts, ideas, lifestyle, etc. As a result, the body and mind are balanced and energized by the life energy substances featured as Yin-Yang, and The Five Elements (earth, metal, wood, fire and water) or Beyond The Five Elements. All these meet the fundamental law and core principle of the universe, thus generating positive energy *Eg* and benefiting health and longevity.

The yang energy in the mind and body is featured as active, uplifting, bright, motivated, powerful, external and expressional, strong, advancing, and of male natures. Yin energy is featured as soft, gentle, calm, internal, humble, deep, harmonious, passive, stable, and of female natures. Balanced Yin-Yang energies allow the person to stay in the balanced and harmonious state of interdependence, mutual-consumption and inter-transformation of these energies.

Specifically speaking, your mind and emotions stay in the balanced state; peaceful and positive, bright and quiet, happy but not excited, confident and grounded, talented and wise. Therefore, your body will also stay in the harmonized and balanced Yin-Yang state.

The universe has five elements (or Beyond The Five Elements) of energy, and the body and mind also have five elements (or can go Beyond The Five Elements) of energy state. The cultivated and generated energy *Eg* of the mind and body allows the person to stay in harmony with The Five Elements (earth, metal, wood, fire and water) or Beyond The Five Elements.

These elements of energies are in harmony of inter-promotion and inter-restriction within your body (stomach/spleen, lung/small intestine, liver/gall bladder, heart/large intestine, kidney/urine bladder, respectively) and mind/emotions (cheerfulness and sadness, delight and grief, enjoyment and anger, calmness and overexcitement, courage and fear, respectively). Thus as a result, your body and mind are healthy, beautiful, energetic, strong, and efficient in daily performance, clearheaded, and long living.

We have discussed how the spiritual mind (G-Mind) resonates and synchronizes with the high spirit to generate life force energy, and how the human mind (H-Mind) operates the physical body (physical world) to consume life energy. This means the spiritual mind exists between the spirit and body (physical world) to transfer spiritual energy to the body or physical realm, but the human mind does not access the spiritual energy. Rather it only directs the physical body to consume energy. Now the question is how the spiritual energy and mental energy in the mind and spirit are transferred to the physical body or physical world and affect them, and how are they interacted and influenced with each other?

In next chapter, we will present some biomedical laboratory experiments to further explain the energy transferring and transforming between spirit and body (physical realm). Before that, however, here we want to discuss this issue just based on some of our daily experiences.

The silent film *The Artist* used a lot of psychological vibrations to affect the mind and to lead the story forward. As such, many individuals experience deep, tender memories of the film's brilliant moments. As an example, we can playback a few minutes of YouTube clip. Although it is difficult to describe the interaction between the spiritual energy at very high level (such as Supreme Spirit's level) and human mind and body, but we can use this as an example at human level to get an idea about this matter. Please join me and view the following:

http://www.youtube.com/watch?v=SmPt9il-Tdo

Peppy Miller enters the room alone, silently. She is filled with feelings of George Valentine. Then through her imagination, inspired by his jacket, which she sees hanging on a coat tree in the room, she enjoys an amazing flood of real emotions and real love chemistries as his momentary touch becomes suddenly real in both her mind and body.

All was initially triggered by the spiritual image of the man she loves. You can see her physically experiencing the fluid and loving energy vibrations which are, at first, manifested by her interactions with the jacket in this physical dimension, where the room and jacket exist. Then you can see how these interactions are advanced and furthered into activities in her spiritual mind, in the spiritual dimension.

The spiritual image then carries spiritual energy vibration and triggers and advances into her (real) physiological sensations and feelings to generate the strong emotions which then give rise to further (real) physiological sensations to produce (real) changes in her blood chemistry – what we might call "loving chemistries" – neurologically, biologically and mentally scripting her reality, and finally leading to the series of physical actions: the hugs and touches which are now taking place in both the spiritual imaginary dimension and in the physical realm as well.

This scene of only 2~3 minutes gives us so much to help us actually experience the energy transformation within multi-dimensions; spiritual, mental and physical realms. It helps us actually sense how the energy at the spiritual, mental (emotional), and physiological (physical) levels can be transformed interactively and dynamically within each other through the mind. The spiritual mind has the power to create a spiritual image – a vibration of spiritual energy. This spiritual vibration has the power to cross all dimensions, including mental and physical dimensions, thus creating actions and interactions in the mind and body.

From this example, although it is not specifically in the manner of modern science, any of us can easily and actually feel the spiritual energy vibration of love, the emotion and imagination in the mind, and finally how it naturally transforms and converts to actual actions in the physical level.

In fact such spirit→mind→body multi-dimensional energy processes are happening all the time in our everyday life. They affect us in with myriad of energies, not only loving energy as we just discussed in *The Artist*.

In general, the take away point is this: Spiritual energy vibration has such power to affect our physiological body and physical world. The spiritual energy and its powerful natures in the invisible dimensions are universal characteristics within all lives. This god-created inborn nature in our lives, and we can know it as compassion, love, caring, forgiveness, peace, harmony, etc. When we have these positive natures in our mind and spirit, then we will resonate with our original nature, and our body and mind will accordingly and directly receive the pure spiritual energy to heal and stay healthy, energetic, peaceful, successful, confident, beautiful and long-living, physically, mentally and spiritually.

However, if we lose these original natures in our mind and spirit, then our body and mind will have no such energy supplied from the spiritual dimension. In contrast, if we have negative energy in the mind and spirit, such as selfishness, disharmony, fighting, anger, dishonesty, carelessness, hate, violence, revenge, resentment, ungratefulness, impatience, intolerance, disrespect, skepticism, materialism, narrowed-mindedness, unspiritual mind, fear, depression, worry, non-confidence, jealousy, suspicion, maliciousness, or even bad, evil or demonic characteristics, all of which are against or opposite of the original spiritual natures of our lives and the universe, then we will have conflict with our true nature, and will be disconnected from the original spirit and its superior energy source. Then, as a result, we will get sick, tired, weak, uncomfortable, ugly, age prematurely or begin dying, physically and mentally. It is just like when a plant withers and dies because it has as no water or air supply. Pure spiritual energy (the essence of your original spirit) is the water and air of your mind and body.

The universe is formed from energy in different forms. Life is also made of different forms of energy, such as physical energy, mental and spiritual energies. These different energy forms can be transformed as well as interact with and influence each other. In the processes of the energy transformation, transferring and interaction, the spiritual energy takes the lead among all these forms of energy because it is pervading the entire space of the being everywhere in the background and is directly rooted in the life's original nature which is the essence of life, resonating with all levels of the life energy forms. Like the movie we just watched, the love in Peppy Miller's spiritual mind, resonating with her original nature (just as one specific example) made everything happen for Peppy in the sample – at both emotional (mental) and physical levels. This spiritual nature (which we all have) is capable of resonating with another living being's spirit and result in actual emotional and physiological reactions. Of course the original spiritual characteristics of compassion, truthfulness and forbearance are much higher level of love than that of human love, but nonetheless, you can see the power and application of such resonance.

Therefore, the practice of mind-body-spirit is to purify the spirit and mind, and elevate the energy level of the life, so the high energy from the spiritual dimension, as we see with our example of Peppy, will support the physical body and as well as the entire being. This is why all kinds of practices in the mind-body medicine and healthology require the mind to be empty, pure, peaceful, positive, bright, compassionate, loving, truthful, conscientious and calm, producing powerful positive energies from high dimensions so they can be transferred to the physical and mental dimensions.

Here let's think of two examples. First example, if you meditate with a busy mind that is filled with a lot of worries, concerns, human desires, angers, violence, revenge, hates, jealousy, calculating gain and loss, or complicated logical thoughts, then after your meditation, you will certainly become tired or even experience headache and discomfort. However if you could meditate with an empty mind, peaceful mood, and opened mind, then you will feel energetic, peaceful and calm. This is because the former meditation had the energy featured with opposite (negative) characters compared to the original spiritual natures. This opposition in energy causes conflicts and diminishes the life energy. The later meditation, on the other hand, resonated and harmonized with the original spiritual natures and therefore enhanced the life force. In fact, other practice such as Taiji, Qigong, or Yoga is in the same way as meditation, the cultivation state of the mind and spirit is the key.

As a second example, one most of us have probably experienced, consider this: If we take walk, jog or workout with the mind busy, not relaxed, thinking of complicated human life issues, afterward we will feel the exercise was not that beneficial or we may even feel fatigued. If we do these exercises with a relaxed, empty, positive and peaceful mind, afterward we always feel refreshed, energized, clear-headed, harmonized, and strong physically and mentally. This experience tells us that physical movement (or sports) itself alone without the involvement of a peaceful and positive mind and spirit may not gain healthy energy and achieve health benefits.

The physical exercise alone is just a physical form to train the physical body in terms of muscles, bones, joint, tissues and organs, but itself may not necessarily make the body healthy. This is because if the process of the physical practice has no mental and spiritual energy involved, then there will be no good spiritual and mental vibrations resonating with the original life force inside the physical body. As a result, the physical form is just consuming energy to do the exercise, but no internal higher energy is generated.

Additionally, if the mind and spirit are in a negative state that streams against the original spiritual natures of the life, then the energy produced within the body and mind during the physical practice will be negative or can even be harmful to one's health. If, on the other hand, the mind and spirit are in a positive way, resonating with the original spiritual energy vibrations, after the practice, the mind and body will be energized and strengthened. The mind has a switch, which can switch to human mind state consuming energy as well as switch to spiritual mind state negating higher energy. It is under your control. The mind-body-spirit practice is to train the mind to turn the human mind off and switch the spiritual mind on, and leave it on all the time during the entire life journey.

In conclusion, the mind and spirit have powerful energy vibrations to lead the body in a healthy and energetic way if they assimilate with the universal law of the life and balanced energy system. It's why the teaching and practice of Qigong, Taiji, meditation, and Yoga often guide you to practice with a peaceful and positive mind in the meditative state in order to connect to the higher spiritual energy source.

Extending our discussion – beyond just spiritual practice and physical exercise – and into daily life, the mind even during daily routines influences and interacts with the body. We will discuss this aspect more in the following chapter. At this point, it is clear that the energy from the spirit, through the mind, leads and interacts with the physical body, guiding the body into a positive and healthy state. In contrast, the human mind can easily attach to the human desires, self-interests and material benefits, then generate negative, stressful and unhealthy vibrations, consuming significant amounts of life force and drive the entire life down.

§4.10 The Role of Mind Bridging Spirit-Body and Its Practice

The spirit can access the superior law system and ultimate universal energy source, while the spiritual mind communicates with the spirit, generates pure life force energy, and plays the role of the ultimate director, manager, and leader for the body. Therefore the mind bridges the spirit and body and transfers the high energy to physical body and physical world. To pass on the spiritual guide and transfer its energy from superior system to the lower dimensions including physical body, to guide the whole being and bridge the spirit and body, human beings need to cultivate, and train (with plenty of practice) the mind needs to overcome temptations from human desires and material interests, and assimilate with the original spiritual natures, which are able to guide the life to perform healthily and positively.

When we talk about the mind-body-spirit practice to assimilate with the original spiritual natures such as peace, compassion, love, kindness, truthfulness, forgiveness, tolerance, patience, caring, humbleness, sincerity, appreciation, righteousness, open mind, spirituality, wisdom, purity, etc., and to synchronize with the energy system of Yin-Yang and Five Elements or Beyond The Five Elements, *we are not talking about religion or belief, but science and the practice of healing and health of mind, body and spirit.*

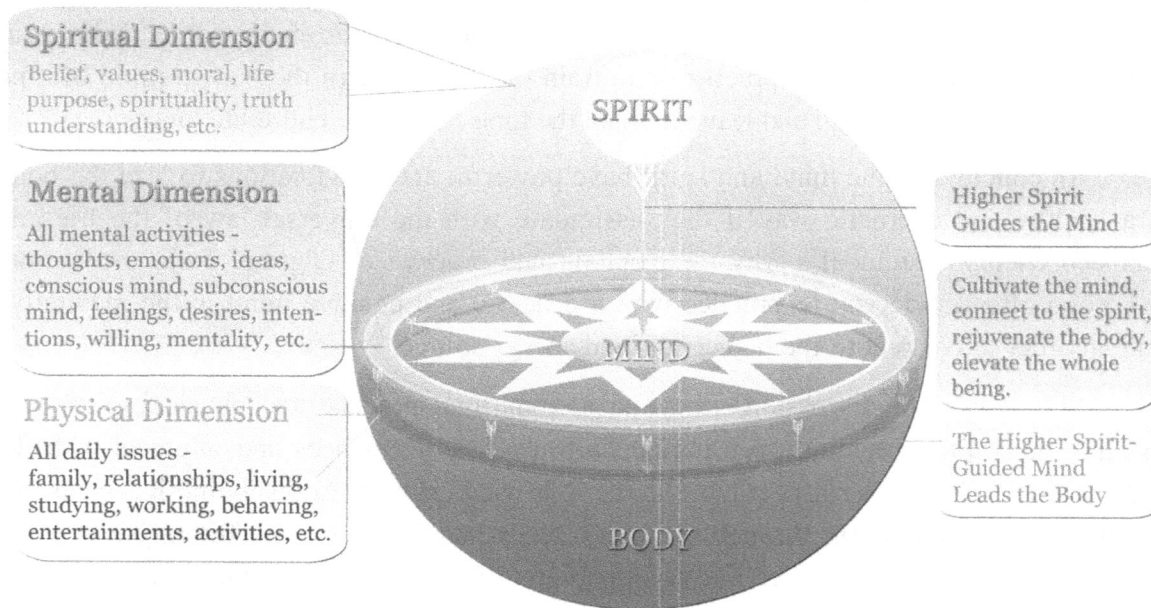

Spiritual Dimension
Belief, values, moral, life purpose, spirituality, truth understanding, etc.

Mental Dimension
All mental activities - thoughts, emotions, ideas, conscious mind, subconscious mind, feelings, desires, intentions, willing, mentality, etc.

Physical Dimension
All daily issues - family, relationships, living, studying, working, behaving, entertainments, activities, etc.

SPIRIT

MIND

BODY

Higher Spirit Guides the Mind

Cultivate the mind, connect to the spirit, rejuvenate the body, elevate the whole being.

The Higher Spirit-Guided Mind Leads the Body

Fig. 4.10. The cultivated mind connects to the higher spirit and gains cleared head to direct the body performing in the way of following the law of the universe and the good intention of the true Self. Cultivation of the mind and spirit is the key to activate the mechanism of mind-body-spirit operation.

Although there may be some readers who practice such a belief system, and this book cannot replace such teaching and practice, you can also understand the spiritual practice from the angle of mind-body-spirit health science. We are talking about the way to stay in an energetic state and gain the true health for the whole being of the body, mind and spirit. This practice is the most essential task of all tasks within this life. It is also the main focus of mind-body health practice and its science. When the mind holds the clear messages and pure energy of the original spiritual natures, the body and all activities as well as performances in this life will be automatically synchronized with the whole. Therefore, such practice will benefit your entire being and your surroundings at all levels of body, mind and spirit.

§4.11 Your Mind Determines Your Health of Whole Being

Your mind plays the key and central role in the mechanism of your entire life system. In other words, originally the life has its pure, healthy, powerful and beautiful spirit that has to pass on its high energy and powerful message to the entire life at all dimensions from the high spiritual dimension to the physical world including the physical body, with which the whole being is unified and integrated. This job can be done only through the mind in the intermediate dimension where each life possesses its own entity.

The universe creates all levels of lives in all dimensions with the universal energy substances that carry the original spiritual natures. Once the life is created, then each has its own responsibility to live in a way that is guided by the original life mechanism. As the mind is cultivated by following the superior law of body-mind-spirit and the energy natures of Yin-Yang and Five Elements or Beyond The Five Elements, then the spiritual mind will generate high life force Eg to transfer to the entire life, and at the same time reduce the consumed energy Ec. As a result, the life will be healthy, energetic and long living with a high level of life force energy $E = Eg - Ec$.

§4.12 Switch on Spiritual Mind and Switch off Human Mind

The energy mechanism of mind-body-spirit is like a dual-switch system: spiritual mind (higher self) switches on the energy generating system, while the human mind (lower self) switches on the energy consuming system.

The mind-body healing treatment or health practice is a practice that switches on the higher Self (spiritual mind) to enhance energy generation and switches off the lower self (human mind) to reduce energy consumption (leaking). Human beings used to have a highly sensitive human mind switch. It has a low threshold against stimulus from this material world. When the human mind switch is on, the person appears to be driven by many negative behaviors/vibrations such as human desires, addictions, attachments, sentiments, materialism, selfishness, jealousy, hate, violence, revenge, worry, fear, depression, no or low confidence, disharmony, fighting, anger, dishonesty, carelessness, impatience, intolerance, disrespect, narrowed mind, skepticism, unspiritual mind, suspicion, paranoia, or even bad, evil or demon characteristics, and immoral behaviors. These characteristics or behaviors carry negative vibration energy and cause mental and physical health problems.

When the spiritual mind switch is on, the person appears driven by positive energy such as love, compassion, kindness, giving, sharing, peace, forgiveness, tolerance, patience, respect, spirituality, intelligence, wisdoms, creativity, open mindedness, etc. These behaviors and characteristics carry positive vibration energy.

The healing process for the mind-body-spirit is the effort to increase the threshold of the human mind, lower its sensitivity, detach the human mind attachment to the material world, and at the same time, increase the sensitivity and energy vibration of the spiritual mind.

This requires self-wakening and guided enlightenment through cultivation practice and energy practice to make the conscious mind clear about the spiritual meaning and final destination of this life and about the true nature of original Self. At the same time, the healing is to transform the subconscious mind to a high and pure energy state, automatically cooperating with the conscious mind at the higher spiritual energy level. As a result, the energy within the body-mind-spirit will be mainly generated by spiritual mind and higher spirit.

$$E \rightarrow Eg \ (Ec \rightarrow 0)$$

§4.13 Break: Story • Healing Music • Memorization • Meditation

My Fibroid Healed - Saved Me from the Surgery

- Iris C.

My name is Irene. I came to the U.S. from Russia a few years ago. I was diagnosed as fibroid and advised by my doctors to get immediate hysterectomy, a surgery that removes the uterus. The condition caused heavy bleeding (8 days each period) for 2 years. I even had to have emergency care due to losing too much blood that resulted in anemia and low blood pressure (85/50). I became very weak, physically and mentally. I thought I would die in this way as the condition got worse and worse. However, I didn't feel ready to go through the surgery, as it's a lot of money, for the operation and the after-care cost, and I was also afraid of the side effects of removing this main female organ.

I heard many complain that hysterectomy could cause female hormone imbalance, speeding up the aging process and other related problems. I also read some information from online medical advisors that said that many physicians and women's health advocates argue that 75 to 80 percent of hysterectomy surgeries are not necessary because alternative ways could help. For all these reasons I kept looking for a natural way to get help and heal.

Luckily, I found Dr. Jason Liu, from a magazine. When I met with Dr. Liu, I was emotionally depressed, looked pale, and not sure how he could help me to stop the bleeding. But an amazing thing happened, the bleeding volume reduced right after the 1st session. It was unbelievable! I continued another 20 sessions and by then my period returned to normal - 3-4 days with regular amount. The fibroid is now healed so I don't need the surgery anymore!

My life is changed because of Dr. Liu's healing work. I have become not only physically healthy, but also very positive and happy mentally and emotionally. I feel confident in strongly recommending Dr. Liu's natural healing to anyone who is in need.

Meditation for Chapter 4

EHM04: Holy Water Streams Heal You *(Yin, Water, Metal)*

This music is composed with focus on the relatively yin energy of water and metal elements to strengthen kidney and lung energy. However if you feel you are weak, cold, have low energy, or unhappy, unconfident, or at a low mood emotionally (yin type of condition), then you can choose the following CD (yang type of the healing music) to practice.

EHM03: Fly to the Infinity of Heaven (Yang, Water, Metal)

Before you start the music, please meditate and visualize the body-mind-spirit model shown in Fig. 4.2, and remember it and all associated concepts (e.g., energy consuming and energy generating systems, etc.) in your mind as a fundamental model as well as an ongoing daily practice reminder for your mind-body health and cultivation. By remembering this model, you can explain many things in this life and understand what you should focus on – e.g. letting go of the human mind and detaching with the lower dimension.

[*Play Energy Healing Music #4*] The heavenly sound waves flow into every cell of your body, purify and cultivate your mind, body and spirit and connect you to the higher spirit energy source. Assimilate with the universal characteristics, so that you will have a healthy, long living and meaningful destination of life. Go with the energy vibrations deeper and deeper.

§4.14 Exercise Questions

1. What are the central focus, mechanism, strategy and implementation of mind-body science and practice?

2. How do you understand the energy gradient and dimensions of body, mind and spirit?

3. How do you understand the difference between current energy vibration frequency (f) and the original characteristic frequency (fo), $\Delta f = f - fo$?

4. What is Human Mind (H-Mind) and what is Godly Mind (G-Mind)?

5. What is the Energy Consuming System (**ECS**)? How do you understand the concept of consumed energy Ec and how do you conceptually express Ec with a conceptual equation?

6. What is Energy Generating System (**EGS**)? How do you understand the generated energy Eg and how do you conceptually express the Eg with a conceptual equation?

7. How can one increase his or her generated energy and decrease the amount of consumed energy in order to maintain greater life force energy?

8. Make a list to describe positive energy vibrations at all possible levels. List as many as you can.

9. Make a list to describe negative energy vibrations at all possible levels. List as many as you can.

10. What are the main characteristics of the left and right hemispheres of the brain, and their associated consciousness and mind? What are the relationships of the left hemisphere of the brain, human consciousness, and human mind? What are the relationships of the right hemisphere of the brain, spiritual consciousness, and spiritual mind? What are the roles that the left and right brain play? And what are the energy sources and processes, which the left and right brain are involved?

11. Use your own example to explain the spiritual energy vibration transferred to the physical world through the mind?

12. How do you understand that mind plays the key role in the health practice of body-mind-spirit?

13. What is the dual-switch system of mind-body-spirit energy mechanism?

14. What behaviors appear when the human mind switch is on / off? What behaviors appear when the spiritual mind switch is on / off?

15. What does healing have to do with the dual switches?

SPIRIT
靈
MIND　BODY
心　　身

CHAPTER 5

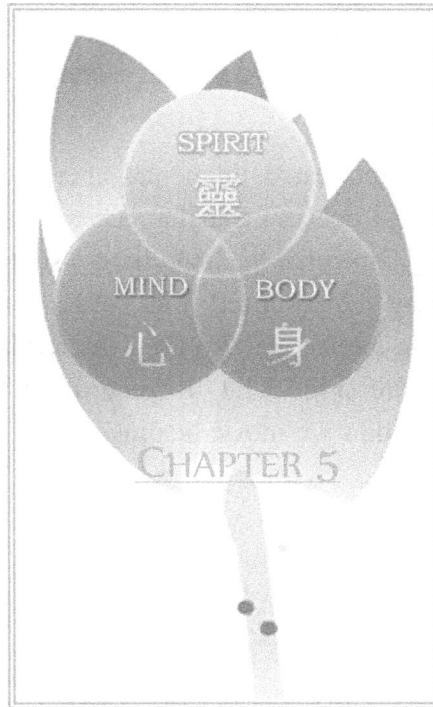

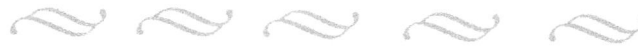

Research on Bioenergy • Mind • Spirit • Health

In this chapter we will address some researches conducted in the laboratories by means of modern science and technology. These research data demonstrate the effectiveness of the mental and spiritual energy on the biological system or physical health, and help deepen our understanding about the connections between mind, body and spirit. If you are not familiar with the fields such as biology, biophysics, physiology, neuroscience or conventional medicine, etc., please do not try too hard to understand the details, but instead you can still enjoy the interesting ideas of the studies, the inspiring research results, and the important conclusion and concepts the research data suggested.

§5.1 Kirlian Photography Bioenergy Experiment

Universe's energy has all different forms and they all follow the same mechanism and principle. Life force within the universe is the same way; there are many forms of life force energy and all follow the mechanism and principle as we described in the previous chapter. More specifically, these forms of life force energy each have the characteristics of the universe and comply with the principle of Yin-Yang and Five Elements to operate, function, be transferred and transformed intra-dimensionally or inter-dimensionally from one to another, under certain conditions.

Here we are particularly interested in mental energy, conscious energy, spiritual energy, and bio-energy (biological energy) transference and transformation. We designed the following experiment to see if spiritual healing energy, such as energy generated during meditation and/or while listening the balanced Yin-Yang, Five Elements music [32] can cause any measurable changes in bioenergy. We used the Kirlian photography system [33-34] shown in the following figure (Fig. 5.1.1) to record the fingertip bioenergy images, before and after meditation or meditative music healing, in the cross-legged position for 45 minutes.

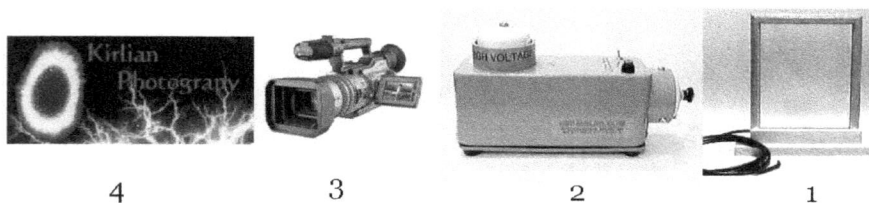

4   3   2   1

Fig. 5.1.1. Kirlian photography system used to record the bio-energy images of the fingertips. The system contains 4 components as labeled in the figure above: 1) 8" x 10" Coronavision transparent coronal discharge viewer, 2) CV6000 electrographic power unit, a TESLA COIL based Kirlian unit, 3) Sony DCR-VX2000 NTSC video camera, and computer/software Premier 6.5 for producing images from the video camera.

As shown below, in the Fig. 5.1.2, before meditation the five fingers (left hand thumb, index, middle, ring and little fingers as labeled as 1, 2, 3, 4, 5, respectively) Kirlian images as their bioenergy imaginary reflections were recorded as shown in the upper row. After 45 minutes of meditation, the five fingers' energy statuses were imaged again. These images were significantly increased in both density as well as the size of the energy distribution area as shown in the lower row.

Results imply that meditation increases energy flow in the body and the fingertips, and such energy could be imaged by the Kirlian photography technique. This as well as other similar experiments conducted by myriad of other individuals at a wide range of institutions can demonstrate how spiritual energy generated through the meditation process can actually be brought to the physical body and results in energy enhancement.

The experiment performed with meditation and the addition of Yin-Yang Five Elements energy music also improved energy flow in the fingertips.

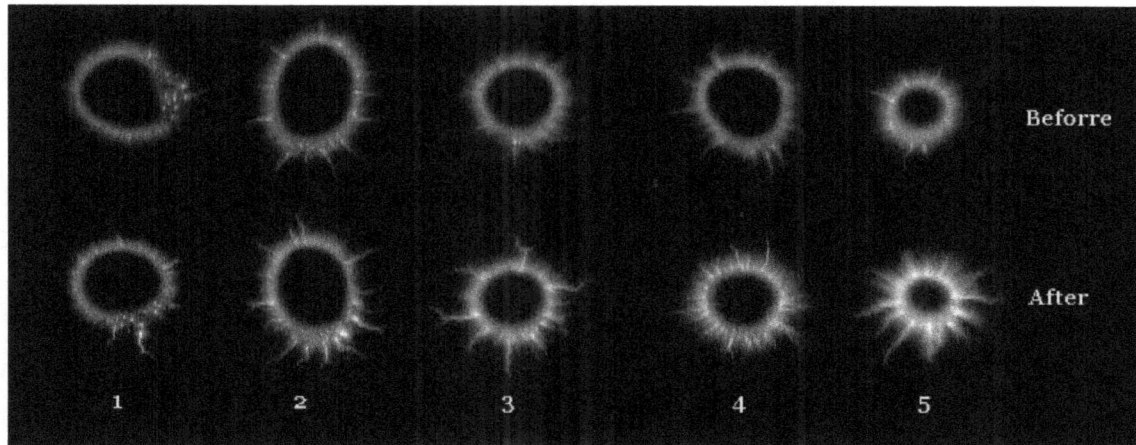

Fig. 5.1.2. The Kirlian photography images taken from a meditation practitioner indicate that 45 min meditation practice increased both bioenergy intensity and the size of its emission distribution area. The images on the upper row show the left hand five fingertips Kirlian patterns taken before the practice, and the lower row shows the images taken after one hour of meditation practice with music. The right hand's Kirlian images had similar results (now shown). The numbers 1, 2, 3, 4, 5 labeled in the bottom of the figure indicate the Kirlian images taken from the thumb, index, middle, ring and little fingers, respectively.

Oriental medicine has traditionally maintained that energy (Qi or Chi) flow is the key of health. In the Oriental system, the fingertips play a specific role in that they are the starting points or ending points of meridians. Therefore, they especially reflect the energy status of each meridian (thumb, end of lung meridian; index finger, beginning of large intestine meridian; middle finger, pericardium; ring finger, beginning of triple burner meridian; and little finger, end of heart meridian and the begin of small intestine meridian).

Our experiment indicates that meditation with the universe law produces balanced energy and enhances the biological energy to improve physical health.

Other experiments showed that when a fibromyalgia patient meditated with energy music, the patient's condition was improved. Energy images of the patient's fingertips, while meditating and listening to/absorbing the music, showed that the individual's bioenergy was increased. As a result, she was eventually healed completely and no longer required the use of pharmaceutical medications, including her pain medications.

This experiment was repeated multiple times, testing the same person as well as different individuals. The requirement was that the person being tested be able to get into a deep meditation state with a quiet, peaceful and positive mind. Results were similar to what we acquired with the initial fibromyalgia patient, showing an increase in bioenergy as well as an alternative to pharmaceutical treatments.

Although modern science cannot explain how the meditation could enhance the bioenergy flow within the physical body (fingertips), it is obviously clear that meditation must invoke some biological changes in the physical body and as a result improve the flow and circulation of Qi/bioenergy as indicated by the same fingertip bioenergy imaging.

Bioenergy enhancement via meditation requires the meditator to stay in a deep meditation state, with an empty, peaceful and positive mind. This result was confirmed by control experimentation with individuals of no meditation experience as compared to results acquired from an experienced meditator. This implies that the spiritual and mental energies in the person were involved in the meditation process, and such energies caused biological changes inside the body and thus enhanced Qi flow and then the individual's healthy condition. Question is: Why does a peaceful and positive mindset during the meditation process become a precondition to achieve the energy flow improvement as seen in this experiment?

This is the topic that we have discussed and will discuss more throughout this entire book as the fundamental principle in mind-body-spirit practice: The human being is part of the universe and originally has the same natures with the universe, and sickness or discomfort is due to a conflict between the individual's current energy status and the that person's original natures. Therefore when deeply mediating with peaceful mind and without negative emotions and confusions, the meditator could connect to the universe's spiritual natures – peace, love, compassion, tolerance, and truthfulness, and therefore he/she resonates with the universe's nature and spirit, receives its energy. As a result, the individual's energy channels are opened, and the person stays healthy and energetic.

The aforementioned results agreed with clinical research conducted by Peipei Cheng and Li Liu, Mackay Memorial Hospital, Nursing Department, Taiwan. Their research demonstrated similar evidence that Five Elements music therapy is an effective approach in the improvement of depressed emotions and physical condition. Instead of using five fingertips Kirlian imagery for the measurement of bioenergy, however, they measured the meridian/energy channel to evaluate the energy meridian status [32]. Yet, results were virtually the same.

§5.2 Cardiac Muscle Bioenergy Enhanced by Mind-Body Practice

Now we look at what may happen with a biological tissue while it is exposed to the meditation energy field. We isolated a small cardiac muscle fiber bundle from the papillary muscle of the heart ventricular wall, set it in a physiological condition and measured its contraction force during an experienced meditator's practice of meditation. The tendon end of the muscle was attached with stainless steel tweezers of a liner motor and the other end was attached to the force transducer tweezers that is connected to computer to record the muscle contractile force as measure of the muscle cell biological activity (Fig. 5.2.1).

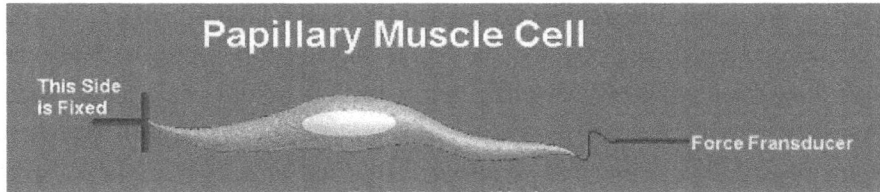

Fig. 5.2.1. Papillary muscle cell isolated from the ventricular wall of the heart, mechanically, under microscope. The tendon end of the muscle was attached with stainless steel tweezers of a liner motor and the other end was attached to the force transducer tweezers. A 3 mm diameter cylindrical cuvette was slipped over the muscle cell and perfused with 95% O_2 and 5% CO_2 saturated Krebs-Henseleit solution [35]. The muscle cell was stimulated electronically with 1 Hz (1 cycle per second) squire pulse and the contractile force generated in the muscle was recorded through the force transducer to the computer recording system.

As control experiment, the cardiac muscle kept consistent contractile force development in physiological solution at consistent temperature 21 ° C (see Fig. 5.2.2). After the muscle contraction became stable for 30 minutes, an experienced meditation practitioner started to meditate with music in the background. As shown in the figure, the muscle contraction force gradually increased. The increase of contraction force reached peak at 135% of the control level. As long as the meditation practitioner stayed meditated with the muscle, the contractile force level remained unchanged at the 35% increased level. During the process of meditation and data recording, there were no chemicals (e.g., ATP, ions of calcium, sodium, potassium, etc.) added in the solution nor physical energy (e.g., heat, physical vibrations or shaking, electronic or magnetic field, etc.) added in the environment of the muscle cells. In other words, there was no external energy added to the muscle except the meditator meditating with the muscle cells without physically touching them.

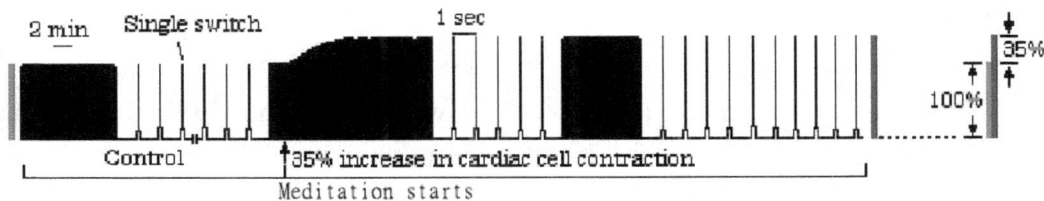

Fig. 5.2.2. The meditation cultivation energy field increased the contraction force of cardiac papillary cells. The muscle cells were attached to a force transducer and placed in a chamber filled with circulated Krebs-Henseleit solution [35] saturated at 21 ° C with 95% O_2 and 5% CO_2. An electrical stimulation at 1 Hz at a voltage 20% greater than threshold was continuously applied to

the cell. After a 30 minute recording of a stable contraction force in the absence of the energy field, as control, the meditation practitioner applied the energy field with his hands held in front of the abdomen. His hands were kept ~30 cm away from the cell, and far enough away from the recording system to avoid influencing the temperature, which would cause artifacts in the recording. Compared to the regular practicing posture, the hands stayed away from the body, and the palms were facing each other beside the cell, ensuring that there was no physical contact to the cell by the practitioner. As shown, after the energy field was applied, the contraction twitch tension force started increasing up to 35%, compared to the control, and stayed at a stable level. The same experiment showed that no change was detected with other individuals who are not meditators. This type of experiment was repeated more than 5 times, with similar results, as shown in this figure. Extent of the increase in the cardiac cell contractile activity by the energy field was by 35% ~ 111%, depending on the physical size of the cell and its initial condition after cell isolation, and the practitioner's meditation state. No decrease in cell contraction by the energy field was detected.

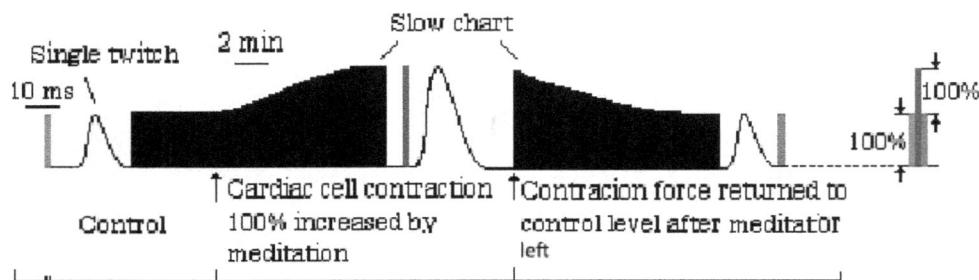

Fig. 5.2.3. Cardiac cell contractile force was increased by 100% by the meditation energy field and returned to the control level, after the practitioner left the experiment room and stopped thinking about the cell. Except for the following modifications, all experiment conditions and procedures were the same as described in Fig. Fig. 5.2.2. After the cell contraction force was increased by 100% with the energy field applied to the cell, the practitioner stopped holding his hands beside the cell, but kept sitting in the room at a distance of ~3 feet away from the cell. The contraction force remained at the increased level. Interestingly, when the practitioner left the room and stopped thinking about the cell, the cell contraction force gradually returned to the control level, indicating that the energy field applied by the practitioner is essential for the increase of the cell contractile activity. This experiment was repeated more than 5 times, with similar results, as shown in this figure. The first arrow indicates the time point when the practitioner positioned his hands beside the cell, and the second one indicates the time point when he left the room.

As shown in the Fig. 5.2.3, the experiment was done with another isolated muscle bundle while the meditator was meditating. This time the contraction force was increased by 100% and stayed at the stable level until the meditator left the room and the contractile force gradually returned to the original level, confirming that the meditator was the only reason that induced the increased contraction energy, instead of something else.

154

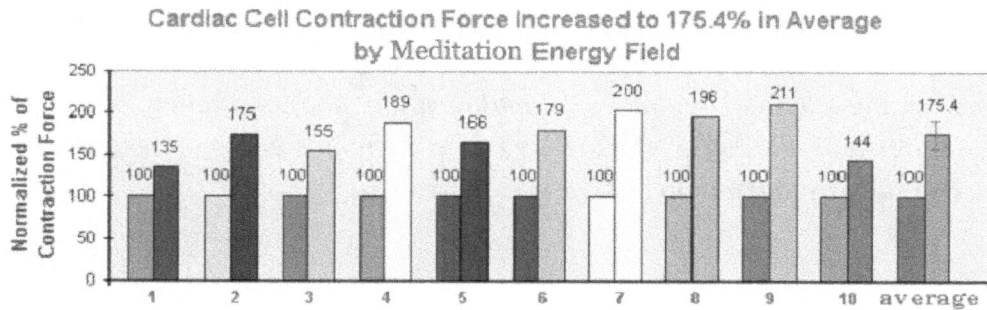

Fig. 5.2.4. Cardiac cell contractile force was increased by 75.4 $\pm$ 17.34% on average by the meditation energy field. In summary of experiments described above, the increase in the papillary cell contraction force was averaged over 10 different individual cell preparations (numbers from 1 to 10 labeled in horizontal axis). The control for each isolated cell preparation was normalized to 100%, and plotted in a bar to the left for the corresponding sample indicated by each of the numbers (1 to 10). The contraction force in percentage of the control (after the meditation energy field was applied) was plotted in a bar to the right for the corresponding sample. The averaged percentage values were illustrated by the pair of bars to the extreme right in the figure, for the averaged control (left bar, 100%) and increased force (right bar, 175.4%), respectively, as labeled "average." The standard error for the averaged percentage of contraction force was $\pm$ 17.34.

The experiments in the similar procedure as Fig. 5.2.2 and Fig. 5.2.3 were repeated 11 times as summarized in Fig. 5.2.4. The contractile forces with different experimental samples were increased to the extents ranging from 135% ~ 211% with an average increase to 175%. The reason why the increases of the muscle bundles were different is because of the different sizes of the muscle bundles. The control experiments with non-experienced person did not change the muscle cells' contractile activity, indicating meditation state is critical for the observed bioenergy increase during the cultivated meditator's practice.

The experiments described above indicate that without any change in the experimental conditions such as temperature, solution, measurement equipment and procedure, or adding any physical and chemical energy, the meditation practice with the muscle cells increased the bioenergy of the cells significantly. This result strongly implies that (1) the meditation energy reacted with and was transferred to the biological samples (muscle cells) and transformed into the form of detectable bioenergy in this physical realm as recorded muscle contractile force, (2) the transference and transformation of the meditation energy were through the invisible mental and spiritual dimensions to this visible physical dimension. This significant experimental result implies that the invisible energy of the mind and spirit may be a part of the dark energy/dark matter beyond this visible physical dimension, which can interact with and be transferred and transformed to this physical realm through a spiritual cultivation process.

155

This may explain the mechanism by which mental and spiritual energy healing improves physical health: Energy transfers and transforms from mental and spiritual dimensions to the physical realm by communication and resonance with the higher spiritual natures and vibrations of Yin-Yang Five Elements energy through mind-body-spirit practice such as meditation cultivation.

§5.3 HeartMath Research on Heart Rhythm Improved by BMT

To further understand how the mental energy (or conscious and subconscious energy) and spiritual energy react with the physical body, heal health problems and generate physical and mental health, we carried out the following HeartMath experiments to study the coherence between the mind, brain and body. There is no direct way to measure mind and spirit. However, because the heart is the organ that is sensitive to the mind, emotion and spiritual energy, we can measure the heart vibrations to indirectly detect the mental and spiritual states. HeartMath Research Institute in North California developed the HeartMath system to detect and analyze the correlation between the brain, heart and emotions. We used their EmWave to monitor the HeartMath Data during the process of mind-body healing treatments such as meditation, energy music therapy, hypnosis, psychological healing or these combination treatments called Brainwave-Meridian Therapy (BMT) as addressed in Chapter 12.

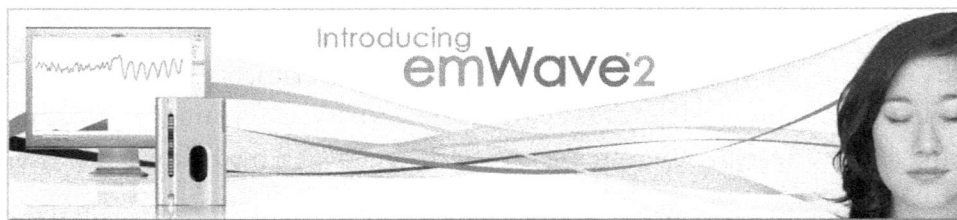

Fig. 5.3.1. EmWave 2 system developed by HeartMath Institute (Boulder Creek, California) was used for the measurements of heart waves (pulse waves), heart rate variability and brain-heart entrainment ratio. The image shown is seen in the original product advertisement.

EmWave 2 (HeartMath Institute, Ca) as shown in Fig. 5.3.1 was used for the experiment while the index fingertip of the patient was connected to the module sensor of the EmWave system and other end of the module was connected to the computer through USB. The software EmWave runs simultaneously to monitor the patient's heart waves (pulse waves), and analyze the wave data to calculate the Heart-Brain Entrainment Ratio, and average heart rate and rhythms.

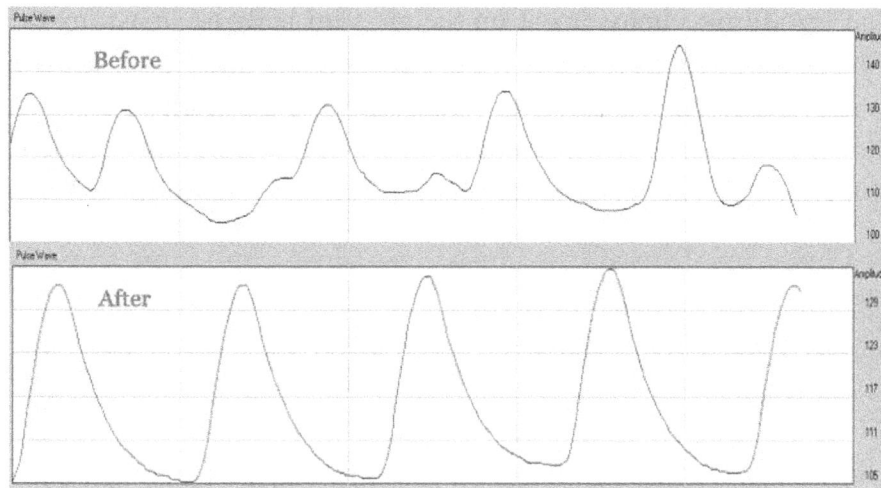

Fig. 5.3.2. Bipolar disorder patent's heart waves (pulse waves) improved during the treatment of brainwave-meridian therapy (BMT). During the treatment, the patient's index fingertip connected to the sensor adopter of the system that was plugged into the computer through USB. Upper trace shows the heart waves have frequent variations without consistent pattern before the treatment, while the lower trace shows that heart waves became well synchronized with a consistent pattern and heart rate 5 minutes after the treatment started.

The upper traces of Fig. 5.3.2 and Fig. 5.3.3, show that before the BMT treatment, a bipolar disorder patent's heart rhythm had frequent variations of up and down, heart rate changes constantly, showing the nature of anxiety and depression at her emotional level that was reflected in the physiological level – the heart waves (pulse waves). However, with BMT treatment in combinations with Yin-Yang Five Elements energy music, meditation, hypnosis, energy healing and psychological conversation, the heart waves (pulse waves) in a consistent pattern (lower row of Fig. 5.3.2) were observed, and the heart rate consistency was recorded (lower trace of Fig. 5.3.3).

This result indicates that the treatment calmed the patient's emotions and brought about the peace of the mind that resulted in the physical harmony and coherence between the heart and brain, body and mind. This experiment data was helpful in understanding the correlation of emotional and spiritual peace with physiological health as recorded via the coherence between the heart and brain or the body and mind.

The treatment is purely at the emotional, mental and spiritual levels without physical touch, but it resulted in significant improvement on the physical body as shown by the recorded consistency of heart waves (pulse waves) in the figures (5.3.2 and 5.3.3), implying that the mental and spiritual energy produced in the treatment were transformed and transferred to the physical dimension, improved the connection and communication between mind and body or brain and heart, then harmonized the physical body and improved health condition.

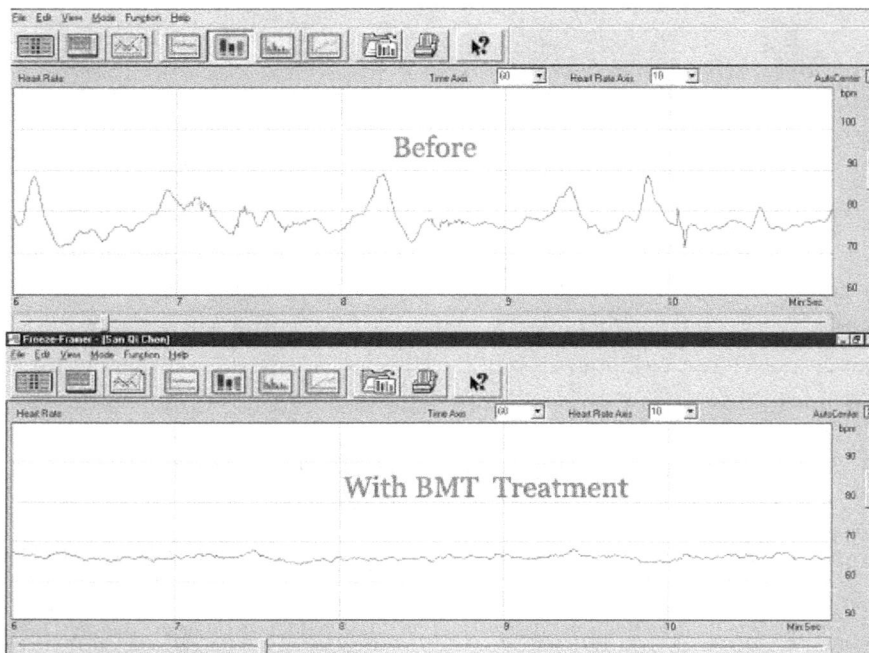

Fig. 5.3.3. The heart rate of a bipolar disorder patent improved after 10 sessions of treatment with brainwave-meridian therapy (BMT). During the treatment, the patient's index fingertip connected to the sensor adopter of the system that was plugged into the computer through USB. Upper trace shows the heart rate was relatively high (90 BPM, beats per minute) even during the rested lying down position and had frequent variations ranging 70-90 BPM without consistency before the treatment, while the lower trace shows that heart rate became consistent at ~70/BPM, 5 minutes after the treatment started.

Fig. 5.3.4 shows the heart rate and heart rate stability improvement of the patient who had anxiety and depression. At the first session her heart rate was as high as 90 BPM on average even at lying down position during the relaxing treatment. Over five sessions of BMT treatment, however, her heart rate could drop down session by session and finally reached normal level at 74 BPM. After 10 sessions of BMT treatment, this patient's heart rate could stay very stable at 67 BPM. For this patient, her resting heart rate was always high before the treatment, indicating her anxious emotional state was a chronic daily state. Even during the first session over 1 hour of treatment in the very relaxed lying down position, her heart rage was still at 88 BPM. Such fast and anxious heart beating had been continued with this patient for years. This physiological parameter was not easy to change because it was the status of her autonomic nervous system that governs her heart beating and subconscious state that is related with her emotion. But the energy healing treatment could lower her heart rate to the normal level and stabilize it at the normal level, and finally healed her emotional bipolar condition. This indicates the healing energy in the mental and spiritual dimensions could react with both mind and body, and re-harmonize the entire being.

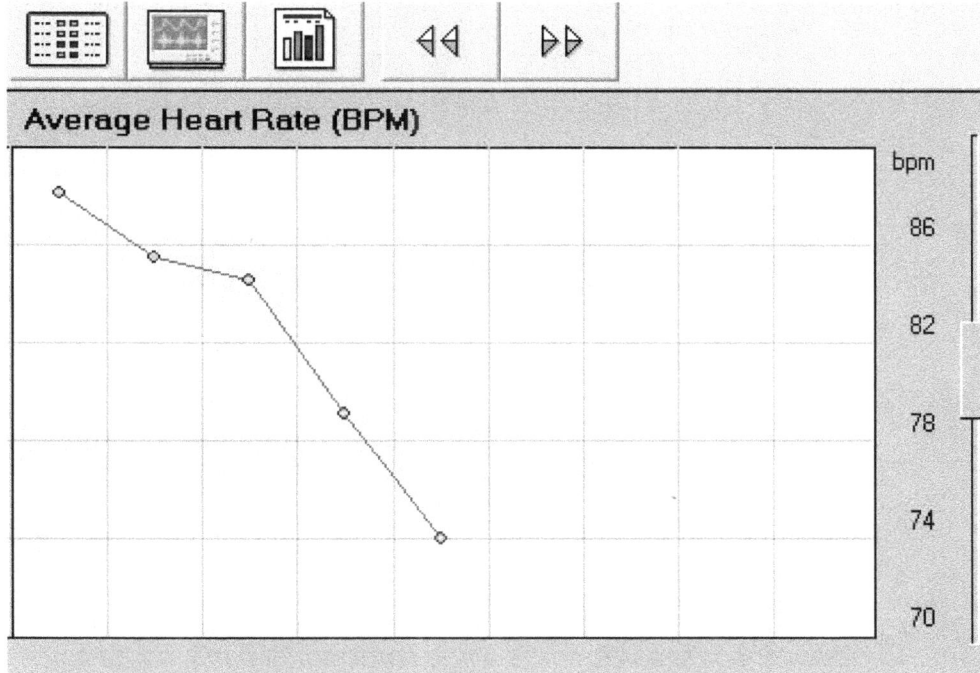

Fig. 5.3.4. The average heart rate of the patient with anxiety and depression was improved from 88 BPM to 74 BPM in the resting state (lying down) during the BMT treatment. The average heart rate is obtained through 1 hr treatment. The first point of the data is the first session average heart rate (88 BPM), and the second point, third point, ... fifth point, are in the same way. This improvement indicates the emotional frustration has been improved.

To further understand the relationship between the mind and body or brain and heart, we used the EmWave system and analyzed the Heart-Brain Entrainment Ratio to see how the patient's heart-brain was entrained during the treatment (Fig. 5.3.5). The BMT treatment brought the patient into a deep relaxation and hypnotized state, and as a result the entrainment ratio of heart and brain was increased up to 94% (sum of medium entrainment ratio 32% and high entrainment ratio 62%) as shown in the Fig. 5.3.5. This means that the energy vibration of brainwave meridian therapy (BMT) with energy healing music sound and meditation could synchronize the patient's body and mind, brain and heart into one harmonized system, which is the process of how the healing energy heals the body and mind. This data demonstrates the peace, unification and synchronization of the mind and body achieved by the emotional and spiritual healing energy produced during the BMT treatment. The result supports the ideology that mental and spiritual healing energy vibrations in other invisible dimensions may be transferred and transformed to this physical dimension and react with the physical body. Thus as a result, the body and mind resonate with the energy vibrations; then resynchronized into a harmonious and balanced whole being.

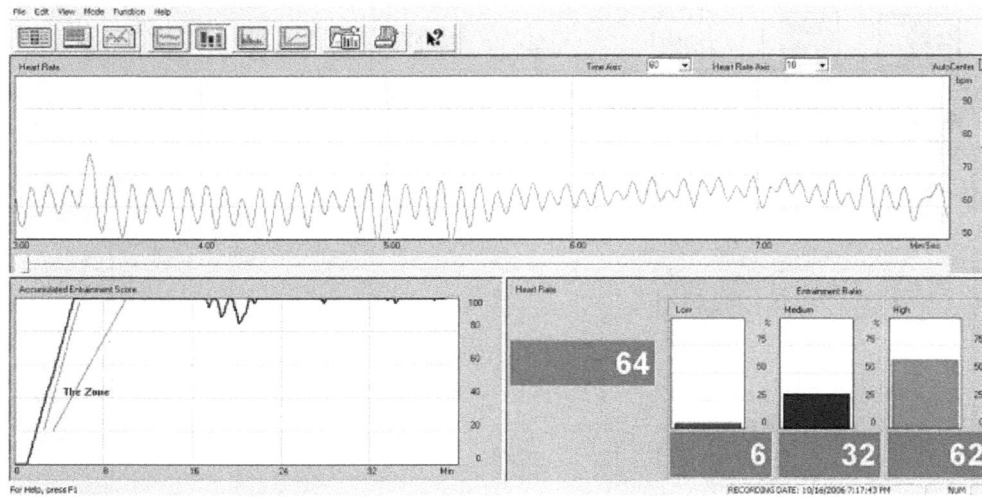

Fig. 5.3.5. Heart-Brain of the bipolar patient was well entrained during the mind-body-spirit healing by BMT treatment. For this particular session (the second session) the medium entrainment ratio was 32%, and high entrainment ratio was 62%, the sum was 94%. Other sessions showed similar result.

§5.4 Case Study: Bartholin's Gland Cyst Healed by BMT

§5.4.1 Research Overview

This is a clinical case study carried out at our Mind-Body University Medicine Clinic with Bartholin's gland cyst patients. This small section is a brief overview on this research's objective, design, results and conclusion and will be followed by further sections to address detailed information, including introduction to the case and the nature of this disease, treatment methods, results and data presentation, summary and discussions.

Objective: The direct objective of this pilot study was to investigate the effectiveness and long-term healing success for Bartholin's gland cysts with an alternative and non-invasive healing method called Brainwave-Meridian Therapy (BMT) that will be addressed in greater detail in a later chapter. The ultimate objective is to demonstrate how mental and spiritual healing energy works with the human mind and body to improve physical health through the mind-body connection and brain-heart coherence.

Study design: The Bartholin's cyst patient was treated with brainwave-meridian therapy (BMT) and the detailed data is presented in this study. BMT is a healing system that uses a series of musical sound waves to treat the patient. The BMT music soundtrack was created based on traditional Chinese medicine principles, the theory of Yin-Yang and The Five Elements, which were combined with brainwave sound waves at frequencies of Delta (1-3 Hz) and Theta (4-6 Hz). This energy music's sounds are designed with an attempt to remove energy blocks on the related meridians within the physical and emotional bodies and energize the body and mind.

The patient is a 32-year old woman who has a Bartholin's cyst gland at the left side of vulva area as diagnosed by her supervising physician in the hospital she visited prior to coming to our clinic. The cyst had already been present for over a year, measuring at 5 cm long by 2.5 cm width. It caused dryness of the vagina, swelling, pressure, pain, sexual difficulty, daily discomforts, emotional stress and relationship problems.

Before BMT treatment, she was diagnosed at our clinic by pulse reading as showing kidney yin deficiency and liver yang excess that likely caused insomnia, irregular menstrual period, and chronic infection or inflammation. Then she was treated with BMT for 36 sessions within a period of approximately 4.5 months.

The patient's urine pH, HeartMath data and single-channel electroencephalogram (EEG) were recorded during each session. The patient voluntarily took pictures of the cyst after every session in a stable setting (camera, light, angle, focus, shutter settings, etc.) at her own home to monitor the healing progress, in parallel with other data. However the patient did not take a picture of the cyst before the first session because she did not expect the first session to make a big improvement.

Results: The cyst was reduced to half size after the first treatment, pain was significantly reduced and the left Bartholin's gland started lubricating again. After 36 treatments the cyst healed completely. The healing process had no side effects other than improvement of the patient's general health condition and stress reduction. A follow-up check after the next 24 months revealed no recurrence. The urine pH curves before and after each session show an "S" shaped healing process (up and down and up again). This finding implies that during the BMT treatment, first a neutralization process of the over-acidic body condition took place, and then followed a cleansing and detoxification process, and a process of recovery completing the healing.

The entrainment ratio of heart-brain was progressively increased over the sessions of treatment (from 28% to 78%), suggesting that resonation and synchronization of the healing vibration with the mind and body might be an important mechanism in the healing process. The EEG recording shows that delta (deep relaxation state) and theta (energetic meditation state) components were increased, whereas the high beta (anxious mind) components decreased during the treatment. This implies that the psychological, mental, or conscious and subconscious response as a synchronization with the meditative healing energy vibration brought the corresponding coherence and harmonization of the heart waves and restored physiological function of the body. As a result the Bartholin's gland healed.

Summary and Conclusion: It is suggested that (1) BMT may be an effective, pain-free non-surgical method to treat Bartholin's gland cysts and improve the holistic health condition as well. (2) BMT heals this gynecological disease by improving the condition at multiple levels, including the mind, emotions, brain and body through a balanced Yin-Yang Five Elements energy vibration. (3) This study demonstrates evidence, at least as a possibility, that spiritual and mental energy vibration has the power to interact with the mind, brain, and body to invoke a series of physiological or biochemical processes such as detoxification, cleansing, balancing functions of organs and hormone production, etc. towards physical healing. (4) Beside Bartholin's gland cysts, BMT may be used for healing some other similar diseases that are caused by stress or mental traumas.

§5.4.2 Introduction to Bartholin's Gland Cysts

The Bartholin's glands are two glands located slightly below and to the left and right of the opening of the vagina in women. Cysts or abscess formation of Bartholin's glands are common gynecological diseases [36]. This disease is seen in approximately 2 percent of sexually active women between the ages of 20's and 30's. Various techniques described for the management of Bartholin cysts include incision, drainage, marsupialization, insertion of a catheter, surgical excision of the cyst, silver nitrate insertion, creating a new duct orifice by carbon dioxide laser, and window operation method [37-39].

To avoid disadvantages of the named methods as mentioned above, painful surgery, anesthesia, scar tissue formation and recurrence, the aim of this brainwave-meridian therapy (BMT) [40-41] was to evaluate the effectiveness of an alternative modality that allows for natural and pain free healing for this gynecological disease. Furthermore, BMT aims to find the cause of the cyst and improve the patient's condition (or alleviate it) by improving and strengthening blocked or weakened energy channels, instead of just focusing on the removal of the cyst itself.

BMT is a vibrational sound and music healing technique based on both neuron-biofeedback therapy [42-43] and acupuncture principle-based sound therapy without needles [40-41]. This healing therapy has been found to significantly increase bio-energetic circulation and improve mental and physical health as well as help with stress or emotional trauma-induced conditions as reported in the previous studies [40-41]. Recently more researches reported that designer music, which is specifically designed for healing, may be useful in the treatment of diseases caused by stress, tension, mental distraction and confusion, as well as negative moods, like depression, resentment, anger and fear [44-46].

In short, BMT has been found to bring body and mind back to a more harmonious state and thus allow the body to initiate the healing of the diseased body part.

Bartholin's cysts seem to be caused by stress and negative emotions and are a complicated gynecological disease. This innovative study is an attempt to treat Bartholin's gland cysts with this alternative method, the brainwave-simulated vibrations combined with energy healing music sounds.

§5.4.3 Energy Medicine Checkup and Healing Methods

The following study was conducted from December 2004, through April 2005 in our clinic, the Center of Brainwave-Meridian Therapy, in California. The Bartholin's gland cyst was healed with the Brainwave-Meridian Therapy as described below. The healing result was stable and has no recurrence as confirmed by checkups and feedback from the patient within or over 2 years afterward.

Before visiting our clinic, the patient, a 32-year old woman, had a recurring Bartholin's cyst at the same location as the previous Bartholin's gland cyst, which had been removed once by marsupialization [47-48] in the Park Klinik, Kiel, Germany 1998.

At the time of starting BMT treatment in this study, the cyst had already been present for one year. The patient complained about severe swelling, vaginal dryness, pain and pressure at the cyst location, the left side of her Bartholin's gland. The condition was accompanied by other symptoms such as insomnia, irregular menstrual period, and negative emotions such as depression, anxiety, worry, fear and no self-confidence. The appearance of the cyst coincided with emotional trauma due to a break-up of a long-term relationship as well as stressful working conditions and schedules. Based on reading the patient's pulse as energy status checkup in energy medicine, it was obvious that she had kidney yin deficiency, liver yang excess and internal fire that likely caused insomnia, irregular menstrual period, imbalanced hormone, weakness of the immune system and chronic infection and inflammation as appeared as swelling and cyst of Bartholin's gland.

The treatment was conducted as an outpatient procedure with a 1.5-hr BMT treatment (30 minutes conversation and 60 minutes treatment) once a day for 2 weeks except Sunday (12 sessions), followed by two treatments per week for 2 months (16 sessions), and one treatment once a week for 2 months (8 sessions), therefore totaling 36 sessions of treatment altogether.

BMT musical sound waves were created, utilizing the traditional Chinese medicine principle, the theory of Yin-Yang, and the Five Elements. This technique has been shown to improve energy circulation along the acupuncture meridians [49-50]. Based on the pulse reading for this particular patient, we mainly used water yin and wood yin energy music to enhance kidney yin and suppress liver yang, and at the same time properly combine with all other elements to balance the patient's energy and strengthen her immune system and overall health. The musical soundtrack was also combined with brainwave-simulated sound vibrations at frequencies of Delta (1-3 Hz), Theta (4-6 Hz) or Alpha (7-12 Hz) that are believed to enhance the quality of relaxation and healing benefit [51-52].

The patient's urine pH was taken before and after each session over the period of the treatment, to monitor the body's acidity/alkalinity balance, using a digital pH Meter Checker (Model 1 / HI98103, Hanna Instruments, USA). As the treatment was performed the patient deeply relaxed and sometimes fell into a deep sleep.

The session was monitored using EmWave system (EmWave version 2, HeartMath, LLC, CA, USA) and BrainMaster 1.9A (BrainMaster Technologies, Inc., OH, USA) during the session for 50~60 min after a 30 min conversation which was not recorded with EmWave or BrainMaster.

The single-channel method of EEG was used to simultaneously monitor patient's brainwaves while her eyes were closed during the session. Three electrodes were placed over the patient's forehead. In the EmWave recording, the fingertip sensor was connected to the patient's index finger and pulse data were recorded with the software during the session. The entrainment ratio was calculated and reported by the software as an indication of the entrainment degree between brain, heart, mind and body [43-44].

§5.4.4 Experiment Results and Discussion

§5.4.4.1 The Bartholin's Gland Cyst Healing Result

The patient's cyst was about 5 cm by 2.5 cm (not shown in the picture) as explained by the patient. After the first healing session the patient reported a decrease of the cyst to about half of its previous size and the patient took the picture at home as described in the first text box in the diagram Fig 5.4.4.1. According to her the swelling, pain and pressure decreased significantly after the first session.

She continued more sessions after that and kept taking pictures voluntarily afterward at home to record the improvement process. After she completely gets healed, she presented all the photo images to our clinic. The diagram shown in Fig. 5.4.4.1 describes all the photo images in a sequence along with the timeline of her healing sessions conducted. Each text box describes an image in word. Please note that we did not show the original photo images here, so that all readers at any age can read.

1	2	3	4
Cyst: 2.5 x 1.5 cm	Cyst: 2.0 x 1.2 cm	Cyst: 1.2 x 0.7 cm	Cyst: 1.0 x 0.5 cm
Skin: dark	Skin: brighter	Skin: brighter	Skin: normal
Scar: no Change	Scar: improved	Scar: further improved	Scar: further improved
after 1 session	2 weeks	6 weeks	10 weeks

5	6	7
Cyst: disappeared	Cyst: no recurrence	Cyst: no recurrence
Skin: normal	Skin: normal & young	Skin: normal & young
Scar: significantly improved	Scar: Almost gone	Scar: not noticeable
18 weeks	1 year	2 years

Fig. 5.4.4.1. Diagram Illustration based on the actual pictures of the vulva area provided by the Bartholin's gland cyst patient (age of 32) that show the Brainwave-Meridian Therapy's healing results with a series of improvements in time order of picture 1 (after first session), 2 (2 weeks, 12 sessions), 3 (6 weeks, 19 sessions), 4 (10 weeks, 28 sessions), 5 (18 weeks, 36 sessions), 6 (1 year later follow-up), and 7 (2 years later follow-up), respectively. Note that there was no picture to show the condition prior to the first session, but the patient explained that the size of the cyst was reduced about half compared to the one prior to the first session treatment.

In picture 2, after session 2 weeks (12 sessions), not only was the size of the cyst further reduced, but also interestingly, the scar tissue from the previous surgery was also improved significantly. At this point, the Bartholin's gland started producing lubricating fluids again, making the patient feel much more comfortable in daily life. Another clearly noticeable detail was that the skin tone of the vulva area became much more normal in fresh pink color, indicating a much better circulation where for a long time there had been a darker-shaded flesh tone due to bad circulation as seen in picture 1.

In picture 3, six weeks later (after 19 sessions), the size of the cyst was reduced by half as compared to the status after the first session. Also, scar tissue from the patient's previous surgery was further improved. Picture 4 in Fig. 5.4.4.1 shows further improvement 10 weeks later (28 treatments). In picture 5 (18 weeks, 36 treatments), the swelling of the cyst has disappeared completely; the Bartholin's gland shows a normal lubrication and the previous scar has improved further to the extent of almost being hard to see. The follow-up at 1 year later, revealed no recurrence of the Bartholin's gland cyst (picture 6). The patient reported that all symptoms caused by the Bartholin's gland cyst had disappeared completely, and the Bartholin's gland seemed stable and healthy. After 2 years as shown in picture 7, the situation retains the same condition without recurrence.

No negative side effects were reported, however, the patient was particularly pleased with the healing results and some additional positive benefits from this treatment, not only the disappearance of the Bartholin's cyst, the dark and swollen vulva area, but also the dramatic improvement on the previous surgery's scar that became much smaller and smoother and no longer visible. After this healing, the healthy and normal appearance of her vulva area helped her relieve much emotional pressure and depression, and made her very happy and confident about herself in every aspect – especially in terms of personal health or relationships.

Additionally, the patient was also pleased with the great improvement in her general health, much smoother and cleaner skin (no more acne), pain-free and regular menstrual periods. She generally felt much happier and positive, more optimistic, and developed healthier eating and exercise habits, and reported she felt much less prone to stress. Furthermore, she reported a more efficient performance at work and in general life, and felt blessed by more good luck and better job opportunities.

§5.4.4.2 Urine pH Time Course During the Healing

Along with the entire process of this healing, the above patient's urine pH before and after each session was measured to understand the healing process and mechanism (Fig.

5.4.4.2). As reported by Hay (19), a low urine pH is often an indicator for too much acid waste in the body tissue, which makes the body more prone to illnesses. The urine is one of the important ways for the body to remove any excess acids or alkaline substances that cannot be buffered by the body. If the average urine pH is below 6.5 the body's buffering system is overwhelmed, a state of autotoxication may exist; therefore, an attention should be given to lowering acid levels [53]. Fig. 5.4.4.2 shows the Bartholin's cyst patient urine pH values taken after each session (red points in color print but darker points in black/white print) compared to the one taken before the session (blue points in color print or lighter points in black/white print). Each of the red points (in color print) or lighter points (in black/white print) corresponds to each of the blue points (in color print) or darker points (in black/white print) as a pair representing one data point of each session. Compared to the outlook of improvement process of the cyst, the urine pH time curve was divided into three phases:

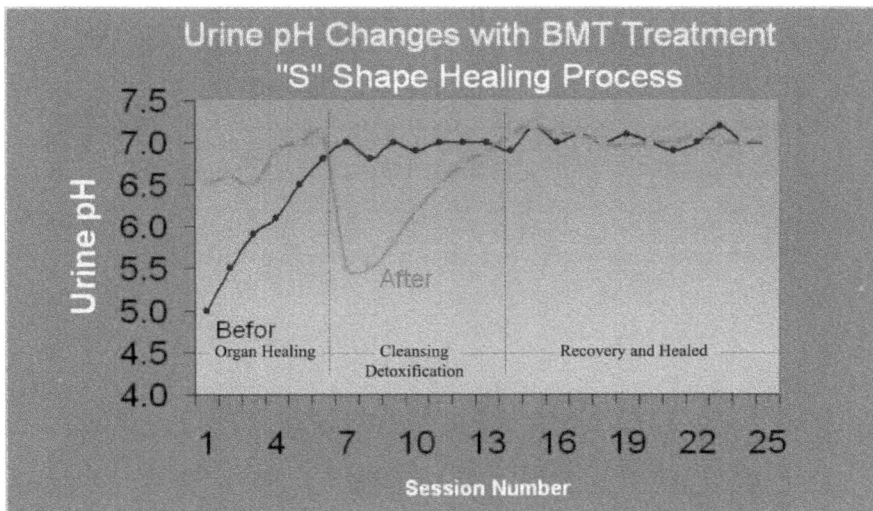

Fig. 5.4.4.2. Healing Process reflected by Urine pH changes during BMT treatment. The pH curve appears as a mirror "S" shape: Phase I is the process for healing the organs (kidney, liver, immune systems, etc.) and neutralizing the body. Phase II is these healed organs clean toxicities, release acidic substances and neutralize the body, and phase 3 is the process for the entire system recovering towards the complete healing. Note: the darker (or blue in color print) data points represent the data taken before the session and the lighter (or red in color print) data points represent the data taken after the session.

Phase I: Neutralization/Organ Healing, week 1, session 1-6

Initially the patient's urine pH was very low (~5.0), indicating an acidic body condition and implying a high stress and severe infective condition. However, after each treatment, the urine pH reached a neutralized condition as the value shown within a range of 6.5 to 7.1 (red points - lighter points in b/w print - within the first phase), while the daily body fluid/urine acidity slowly decreased from pH 5 to 6.8 as seen in the curve before each session (blue points – darker points in b/w print - within the first phase). The gradual increase of urine pH value points towards (1) an improvement of the overall health and stress reduction coupled with an alkalization of the body, (2) an improvement of the liver, kidney and immune system as supported by the pulse reading. During the second phase (detoxification) the urine pH before the session stays constant with a neutral pH value of ~7, (3) the size of Bartholin's gland cyst was reduced and the gland lubrication was gradually improved.

Phase II: Cleansing/Detoxification, week 2, session 7-13

The pH value after session # 7 decreased significantly to ~5.5, and then it is slowly recovered to a neutral pH value ~ 7 after session #13. The urine pH was further decreased after each session compared to that before the session, implying that more acidic substances were released from the body during the session. This is very likely an indication of cleansing or detoxification of the body by the treatment. During this period, the cyst was further healed. Considering the further reduction of the cyst size during this period, this data can reflect that patient's body released a lot of acidic substances, poison or toxins, and the body reached a more neutral pH condition, helping improve the infection, especially in the area of her vulva.

Phase III: Recovery and Completely Healed, after 2 weeks

After the first two weeks of the treatment, the data of urine pH values before and after the session showed no major difference and remained a stable value at the neutralized value of 7.0. It seemed that a stabilization of the condition took place and the internal environment of the body retained a neutral pH condition.

Interestingly, even though the urine pH reached a neutral state after 2 weeks of treatment, the cyst was still not completely healed and required more time to complete the healing. This implies that the restored neutral pH condition and after detoxification or cleansing, the body immune system becomes stronger and has the power to heal diseases such as infection or inflammation automatically.

§5.4.4.3 Brain-Heart Entrainment During the Healing

Each session was also monitored with the EmWave system. The brain-heart entrainment ratio was progressively increased during the period of the treatment (Fig. 5.4.4.3). The sum of high and medium entrainment ratio increased 278% (from 28 % to

78%). Interestingly, the time course of entrainment ratio improvement could be obviously divided into three phases, correlating with the three phases of urine pH change time course (refer to Fig. 5.4.4.2) and related with the cyst healing progress process.

Brain-Heart Entrainment Ratio

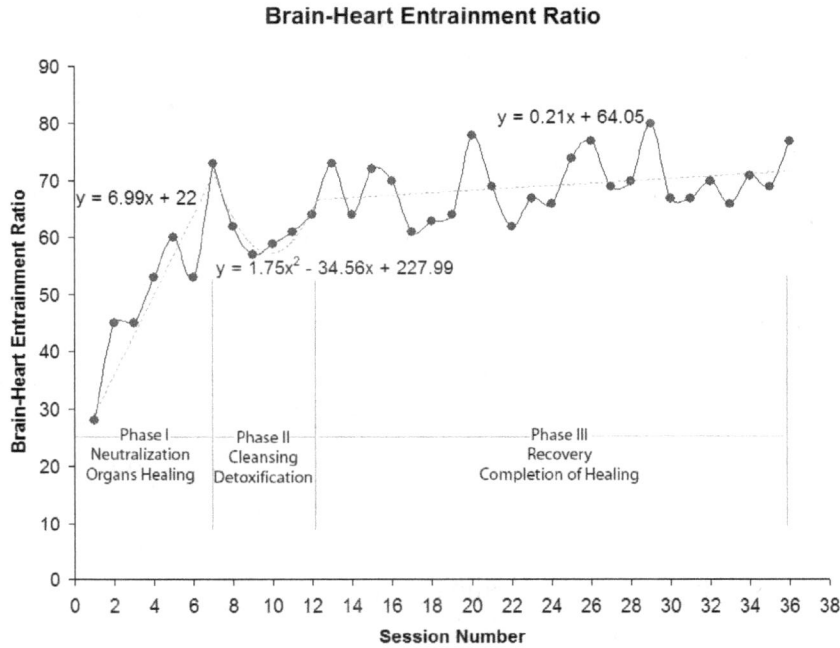

Fig. 5.4.4.3. Brain-Heart Entrainment Ration time course during the entire healing process. The entrainment ratios were taken from each treatment over the entire recording of the session (50~60 min after 30 min conversation which was not recorded with EmWave). The data was linearly regressed (phase I and III) or best fitted (phase II) by software excel by using the functions of xy scatter and Add Treadline. The entire process includes a fast rising entrainment phase (I), a phase of drop down once and rising again (II) and then a slow rising entrainment phase (III) with variations of ups and downs, representing the three healing periods of (1) local organs healing and neutralization, (2) global body cleansing and detoxification, and (3) recovery and complete healing.

Phase I covered the time period of the first 6 sessions, which coincides with the Phase I in the healing process of Neutralization/organs healing (refer to Phase I or first week of Fig. 5.4.4.1~3). It could be linearly regressed to a rising line with a 6.99 slope: y = 6.99x + 22, where y is the entrainment ratio and x is the session number. It seems that during the first week of the mind-body energy healing, the patient could resonate with the healing energy vibrations and achieved fast increasing entrainment of brain and heart, mind and body, so that organs such as kidneys and liver and the immune system functioned efficiently. As a result, the infection and inflammation of Bartholin's gland was improved, and the cyst was reduced in size dramatically.

Phase II lies along the period of cleansing and detoxification healing process in the second week of the treatment, corresponding to the Phase II of urine pH time course (refer to Phase II or second week of Fig. 5.4.4.1~3). During this period, it seems that the patient had complicated cleansing reactions and complicated mental reactions during the treatment. Entrainment of brain-heart or mind-body dropped down from the peak point (session 7, Fig. 5.4.4.3), forming a complicated fitting curve: $y = 1.75x^2 - 34.56x + 227.99$, where y is the entrainment ratio and x is the session number. This cleansing period released toxins and acidity of the body, and the mind and emotions also went through some conflicts and struggles. It took about a week of the treatment, and gradually the patient recovered to the stable state at a higher entrainment ratio, and at the same time, her urine pH also recovered to neutral value.

Phase III is the time period after 2 weeks of treatment, corresponding to the recovering and completion of the healing, along with the urine pH stabilization period (Phase III) and the cyst healing progress and completion (refer to Phase III or the period after second week as shown in figures of 5.4.4.1~3). During this period, the patient relatively stayed at a higher mind-body/ brain-heart entrainment state during the treatments as shown by the relatively higher entrainment ratio with some variations of ups and downs. The entire process of this recovering healing process took long and there was a small rising with a slope at 0.21. The linear regression equation was $y = 0.21x + 64.05$, where y is the entrainment ratio and x is the session number.

§5.4.4.4 Brainwave Recording During the Session

The patient's brainwaves (Electroencephalography, EEG) were monitored to observe the healing and relaxation taking place during a session. Fig. 5.4.4.4 gives an example of a typical session where the brainwave patterns were changed during the session upon the healing vibrations of the composed Five Elements energy music. As the energy music sounds incorporated with delta ($\leq$ 4 Hz)/theta (4–8 Hz) brainwave-simulated vibrations brought the patient into a deep meditative or hypnotized state, the delta and theta brainwave components increased correspondingly from 4.2 to 9.6, and 2.1 to 3.9, respectively. At the same time, the high beta brainwave was decreased from 2 to 0.15.

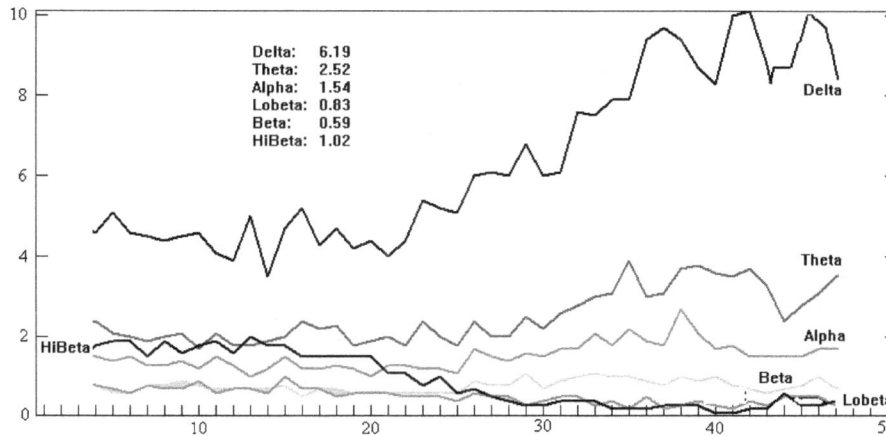

Fig. 5.4.4.4. The brainwave EEG changes during a BMT session. The horizontal axis is time in minute and vertical axis is the relative value of brainwave amplitude. As the energy music sounds with delta (3 Hz) and theta (5 Hz) brainwave-simulated vibrations brought the patient into a deep meditative or hypnotized state, the recorded delta brainwave and theta brainwave components correspondingly increased from 4.2 to 9.6, and 2.1 to 3.9, respectively. At the same time, the high beta brainwave (representing stress or anxiety) was decreased from 2 to 0.15.

In brainwave research, we know that the delta brainwave represents the deep relaxation, trance or hypnotized state, theta brainwave represents meditative energy state, while high beta (HiBeta, > 20 Hz) brainwave represents excessive focus, or stressful, sometime anxious state of the mind. Therefore, this brainwave recording during the session indicates that the patient resonated with the energy brainwave music vibrations during the BMT therapy and got into a relaxed and hypnotized state, and stressful anxiety was relieved, implying that the healing energy vibrations were transformed into mental and biological energy inside the patient's mind and body to balance the Yin-Yang and Five Element energies, open the energy meridians of kidney and liver, and promote energy circulation and strengthen the immune system. Therefore, it healed the infection, inflammation and Bartholin's gland cyst. In fact, after this reported patient, there were two other patients with Bartholin's gland cysts who were also healed by BMT treatment.

§5.4.5 Summary and Conclusion

A comparison of the cyst healing process (Fig. 5.4.4.1) with the urine pH value (Fig. 5.4.4.2), HeartMath data (Fig. 5.4.4.3) and EEG data (Fig. 5.4.4.4), implies a possibility that a series of BMT treatments works at multiple levels of mind, brain and body, allowing for an effective non-surgical treatment for Bartholin's gland cysts and additional balanced holistic overall healing benefits including stress reduction, relief of negative emotions, hormone balance, and physical and mental strength.

As a result, this pilot study showed for the first time in literature that it is possible to improve and heal the symptoms of a Bartholin cyst gland by the gentle and non-invasive BMT method with focus on the mind and mental energy produced by musical vibrations. Furthermore, it seems that during this healing process, the body was able to restore its own healing power because of the musical sound waves that enhanced circulation conditions and detoxification ability.

As a result the cysts could get healed naturally, accompanied with other mental and physical healing benefits such as neutralization of body pH, stress release, and improvement of overall health and wellness. Although the healing mechanism at a biochemical level remains unclear, and it may be beyond the scope of modern science, the results presented in this work strongly point to the possibility that Bartholin cysts could be healed by this gentle BMT natural healing method because of the energy vibrations intra-dimensional and inter-dimensional transformation crossing the dimensions of the spirit, mind, and emotion to the brain and body.

Even though Bartholin's gland cysts and abscesses are considered a minor condition, they can cause major discomfort and pain in daily life and can have a negative influence for a normal sexual life. They can, furthermore, cause considerable mental stress, depression, and/or relationship problems. This study suggests that trauma caused by conventional treatments, including painful surgery and scar tissue formation, might be avoided with the application of mental and spiritual healing approaches such as the brainwave meridian therapy as addressed in the present work. The treatment is comfortable and effective in a fast manner. Pain and discomfort started reducing immediately after the first session. Within two or three months, a cyst might get healed completely, thus providing a powerful natural healing modality for this common gynecological disease.

As a future outlook, studies at molecular and biochemical levels, with more cases, may allow for an even more extensive understanding of the healing mechanism of Bartholin cysts. However, the present study is a positive insight that may lead to further or similar investigations on this gentle, natural and noninvasive method for healing not only Bartholin's gland cysts and abscesses, but as well as other infective and inflammatory diseases or stress and/or emotional related and/or psychosomatic diseases, as well as some cause-unknown health problems. In fact, BMT has healed many other kinds of physical and mental problems, including some difficult or complicated conditions (see the testimonials in Chapter 14).

After you have understood the experiments of mind-body healing in this chapter, sit down and meditate with your mind quiet. Use the following energy healing music, enjoy your meditation, and charge your mind with great fresh energy.

EHM05: Heavenly Song Purifies You *(Yang, Metal, Earth)*

This music is composed with focus on the relatively yang energy of metal and earth elements to strengthen your lung and stomach energy. However if you feel you are overheated, anxious, overwhelmed, have too much heat internally or feel too excited and ungrounded emotionally (yang type of condition), then you can choose the following CD (yin type of the healing music) to practice.

EHM06: Calm And Comfort You *(Yin, Metal, Earth)*

[*Start play Energy Healing Music #5*] The sound carries the vibrations from the divine spirit, wakening your soul, purifying your mind and detoxifying your body. Deeply breathe in the energy stream, and let it flow into your head, heart, lungs, every organ, every cell, and your mind and soul. You are resonating with the universal spirit character and fully assimilated with its energy vibration. You are cultivating your true Self of your whole being, mind-body-spirit, through every moment of this meditation and daily living. You are healed, rejuvenated and transformed …

Before ending your meditation, with the great energy you just experienced and an opened mind you have cultivated, ask yourself some questions, which also link to the exercise questions followed at the end of this chapter: Why and how does meditation increase the cardiac cell bioactivity? Why and how does meditation, energy music healing, hypnosis, or a combination such as the brainwave-meridian therapy increase the bioenergy as shown in the Kirlian photography? Why and how can these practices heal the Bartholin's gland cyst? How do you understand the mental and spiritual energy vibrations produced by these practices, and how was the healing energy transferred from mental and spiritual dimensions to the physical body in this space-time dimension? Based on these experiments, how do you understand the possible energy mechanism and model described in the early chapters? How does all this data help shape your thinking about future life science and health practice?

§5.6 Exercise Questions

1. What is Kirlian photography and how does it reflect bioenergy? What were the differences in the Kirlian photography images of fingertips before and after meditation, and what does this result mean? Discuss the possible mechanism of multidimensional energy transformations from spirit and mind to the body, by using this experiment as example.

2. In the experiment of cardiac contractile force measurement, how did meditation or energy music meditation affect the muscle contraction activity? Explain the energy process crossing the mental/spiritual dimensions and physical realms in this experiment.

3. How do you explain why the bipolar patient's heart wave, heart rate and brain-heart entrainment ratio were improved by the BMT treatment? Add to this understanding from the perspective of mind-body medicine, with the focus of "energy healing."

4. Consider the Bartholin's gland cyst healing time courses of appearance and outcomes, urine pH, brain-heart entrainment ratio, before and after the sessions of BMT treatments. What do you understand about the contributions of the mental and spiritual energy healing process, mechanism, and the impacts of the mind-body-spirit connection on the physical health of this individual and on people in general? Using this experiment as an example, describe the mental and spiritual energy healing natures at different levels/ dimensions of the spirit, mind, emotion, brain, organs, hormone, immune system, and the entire body. What made this treatment achieve a stable healing result without recurrence?

CHAPTER 6

SPIRIT 靈

MIND 心   BODY 身

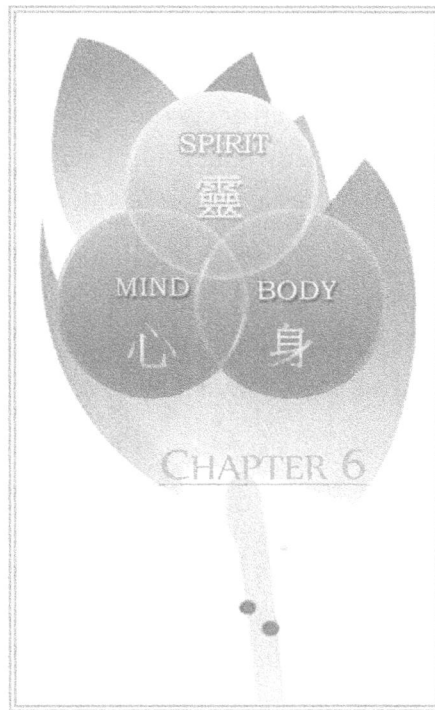

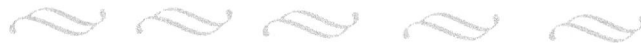

True Self – Conscious Mind And Subconscious Mind

In the previous chapters, we have defined the mind as material mind (human mind) and spiritual mind (godly mind) based on its spiritual character and energy level in order for us to understand the energy process and mechanism of the body-mind-spirit.

In this chapter, we will further discuss the energy process and mechanism of body-mind-spirit from its functional character. Functionally the mind has two parts: the conscious mind and subconscious mind. There may be, however, more than one subconscious mind.

The conscious mind is the part of your mind that is in charge of voluntary activities as higher functions of the brain such as reasoning thinking and actions like calculation, analysis, decision making, intentional behaviors, conscious study, learning and practice of belief and value system.

Alternatively, the subconscious mind is that part of the mind that is in charge of involuntary actions or unintentional behaviors such as breathing, heartbeat, motions, and the storing of beliefs and memories carried on by the inborn-spirit and after-born, those learned by the conscious mind and subconscious.

Emotion is naturally controlled by subconscious minds. Therefore, a human being feels happy or sad, calm or angry, peaceful or anxious, courageous or fearful – at first unconsciously. The subconscious memorizes belief and value systems, so it automatically responds to the issues in life based on one's belief system or value system locked in memory.

Once a belief system or value system, habit, ideology, or notion is formed and memorized in the subconscious mind, it remains unchanged until one consciously decides to change it or learn and understand another different system.

Your conscious mind is dealing with issues and performing functions as your main Self at this physical dimension and by partially interacting with mental and spiritual dimensions, while your subconscious minds are cooperating with it at all other higher dimensions. Your subconscious minds are not in this physical dimension. In most cases in your daily life, your conscious mind and subconscious minds are working together to think, believe, talk, act and behave. Both of them are powerful at all levels through energetic processes in the mental and spiritual dimensions as well as physical dimension.

Some parts of the conscious mind and subconscious minds can be human mind, and some of them can be spiritual mind, depending on their energy level and spiritual character. For example, if the conscious mind (and/or subconscious mind) is materialistic, then it is human mind. However, if the conscious mind (and/or subconscious mind) is spiritual rather than materialistic, then it is spiritual mind. If the conscious mind or subconscious mind is human mind, then it will consume energy in the human world, while if the conscious mind or subconscious mind is spiritual mind, then it will generate higher energy.

Improving the energy level and spiritual character of the conscious mind and subconscious minds and limiting the human conscious and subconscious minds is important to energize the whole being of body-mind-spirit.

§6.2 Random Mind Chatter and Racing Thoughts

The random mind chatter and racing thoughts symptoms are commonly seen in the patients with anxiety, depression, ADD/ADHD, OCD, bipolar disorder, insomnia, fatigue, chronic pain, manic or hypomanic behaviors as well as other mixed behaviors, and with many everyday stressful people. In fact, most chronic patients we have seen in our clinic have these symptoms of random mind chatter and racing thoughts. Such mental activities are energy burning behaviors that can constantly occur, mainly in the subconscious mind, and sometime also partially involve habitual thinking patterns in the subjective conscious mind.

The reason why some meditators cannot quiet their mind during meditation is also because of such random mind chatter and racing thoughts in their mind.

As we have indicated, energy problems are the core cause of mind-body health issues. One of the most common of these energy problems is the subconscious mind having too many random thoughts and unnecessary activities, and burning too much energy of the body and mind.

On other hand, an imbalance here can also manifest when the consciousness mind narrows tightly, restricting and/or locking the subconscious mind, so that significant wisdoms, genius, talents, and creativity in other dimensions cannot be fully explored and are rendered at least temporarily unavailable to the individual.

Random mind chatter and racing thoughts are usually caused by confused, blurry, low energy of, and human-world (material world) -attached conscious mind, which eventually cause the subconscious mind to store and repeatedly or randomly play the same messages over and over. The key to heal this problem is to wake up the main conscious mind with higher enlightenment teaching, let go of attachments and existing human notions, habits, addictions, and bad lifestyle, and practice energy cultivation to clean up and energize the subconscious mind and conscious mind. As a result, the mind becomes clearheaded and grounded, and body is energized accordingly.

§6.3 Differentiate Conscious Mind and Subconscious Minds

So how does one differentiate conscious mind and subconscious minds? How does the conscious mind train itself and the subconscious mind toward energy cultivating behavior instead of consuming energy unnecessarily, and how do both conscious mind and subconscious minds cooperate together to perform their functions energy-effectively.

Subconscious activities are done unconsciously, and such activities run under your radar. However, except the biological subconscious/unconscious behaviors such as heart beat, breathing, digestion, hormone production, and so on, other subconscious characteristics can be trained, influenced, and testified by the conscious mind. For example, some bad habits in the memory of the subconscious mind can be improved or gotten rid of through conscious practice and training. In fact some stress and emotion-caused irregular physiological problems can also be improved or corrected by conscious mind energy practice. Such examples include emotional/stress-induced irregular blood pressure, heart rate, respiration, and other autonomic dysfunctions.

Good unconscious living habits, for example, can be formed through conscious learning and practice. In such a process, practice/repetition allows the conscious mind to influence subconscious mind. The conscious mind, for example, can learn to be aware (mindful) of the subconscious activities and interact with the subconscious mind. By making yourself aware of whether an action is initiated or controlled by conscious mind or subconscious mind, you can use your conscious mind to testify to the current (present) moment activity (CMA) and previous moment activity (PMA), and correct some unnecessary, incorrect or unwanted subconscious mind behaviors and conscious mind activities. This can be a good training practice that can be done either on-the-fly and/or also accomplished through meditation and visualization practice. Let's take a look.

First, let's try to determine whether a previous moment activity (PMA) or current moment activity (CMA) is triggered via the conscious or subconscious mind. If the CMA in your mind is initiated or controlled by your conscious mind intentionally, then it will be easy for you to detect because your conscious mind knows what you are thinking or what you are doing at the moment. If your CMA is initialed through your subconscious mind unintentionally, however, you will not be easily aware of it. This is why most conscious activities are relatively easy to remember but unconscious (subconscious) activities are often easily forgotten or perhaps go unnoticed. Because subconscious influencers are triggered unconsciously, there is no fool-proof way for your conscious mind to be fully aware of your subconscious CMA.

However, if you pay attention to your previous moment activity (PMA) with your conscious mind at current moment, you can know whether the PMA was sparked through your conscious mind or subconscious mind. If your conscious mind realizes the PMA was initiated without a conscious trigger or intention, then the PMA was facilitated by your subconscious mind. However, if your conscious mind realizes the PMA happened as a result of your conscious intention, then your PMA was initiated by your conscious mind. If your subconscious mind frequently or repeatedly performs consciously unwanted activities that cause problems, overload your mind and make you tired, sick, or perform inefficiently, take unnecessary actions frequently, make mistakes during intentional work, feel anxious or mind disturbed, then you need to train your mind and spirit to improve the cooperation of subconscious mind with your conscious mind.

§6.4 Cooperation of Conscious Mind and Subconscious Minds

Through a good energy practice of mind-body-spirit, your conscious mind should be able to sense the subconscious activities, get involved in the process of the subconscious activities and accrue support from the power and talents of the subconscious mind. At the same time, your subconscious mind will have good energy to play its roles; smoothly cooperate with your conscious mind and efficiently support it. As a result, you can achieve a clearheaded energy effective performance through the smooth cooperation between conscious mind and subconscious minds.

When your conscious mind has good energy and spiritual characteristics and is in a clearheaded mode and relaxed state, it can naturally, spontaneously and positively influence, work with, cooperate with, pay attention to, look after, or even partially guide or involve in your subconscious mind characteristics, behaviors and activities even on-the-fly. This way, you will be able to sense the current moment mind activity or physical actions even though these are being partly driven by the subconscious mind. In other words, even though your conscious mind cannot purposely and completely control the subconscious activity, your conscious mind can stand next to the subconscious mind, and watch, suggest or partially get involved in the subconscious mind while the subconscious mind performs its actions. In such a case, every CMA is actually the result of co-performance from both subconscious minds and conscious mind – and good mindfulness.

On other hand, at an even higher level of mindfulness, when you practice mind-body-spirit by following the universal spiritual law and energy principle and upgrade the level of both your conscious mind and subconscious mind, your subconscious mind in the higher dimensions will have good energy, spiritual characters, powerful talents, wisdom and creativity. Therefore it can more smoothly cooperate with your conscious mind and empower your whole being to perform the tasks effectively, energetically, and spiritually, mentally, physically at multiple dimensions. Your conscious mind influences and joins the subconscious mind activities, and at the same time frees your subconscious mind to optimize its power. What you do not want to do is to narrow the conscious mind such that it locks your powerful subconscious mind. Vice versa, it is not good to allow your subconscious mind to perform random, unnecessary, unwanted, and incorrect behaviors, activities and habits. An ideal balance can be achieved by a good mind-body-spirit cultivation practice. Consider the following example.

When you are writing an article, for instance, typing on your computer, your body and mind are relaxed. Your conscious mind takes the lead of your writing, and your subconscious mind is free, and activating and maximizing its talents, knowledge, imagination, intuition, spirituality, and creativity while focusing on the progress of your work, in cooperation with your conscious mind.

Your conscious mind requests the memory of knowledge and words stored in the subconscious mind. Your subconscious, on the other hand, unconsciously and naturally outputs the memory, further explores the higher dimensions, provides intelligence, wisdom and creative ideas, and then commands your hands to type the words. As such, you can progress your writing, through a smooth cooperation of conscious and subconscious mind.

Here both conscious mind and subconscious mind are working together interactively to accomplish the action. As long as both your conscious mind and subconscious mind are relaxed, and in a good energy state and at a higher spiritual level reached by your daily cultivation while synchronizing with all positive characteristics such as peace, love, beauty, truth, compassion, passion, etc., your working process will be an energy-effective, time-efficient, result-oriented and achievement-creative performance. Such subconscious mind activities during the process of your work are necessary actions, performed under the primary guide and involvement of the conscious mind, but optimally and naturally empowered and facilitated by the free, intelligent, and unlimited super powerful subconscious mind in cooperation.

Another similar example for such cooperation between conscious mind and subconscious minds is playing piano. Together with the musical knowledge, training, skills and intentional guide of the conscious mind and the powerful subconscious mind's intuitions, imaginations, visualizations, autosuggestions, auto-inquisitions, musical skills, and creativities, and all inborn, genetic and after-born musical talents, geniuses and intelligences or wisdoms, a piece of music is produced. Containing the energy and messages of your conscious mind and subconscious mind, your musical performance can weave and manifest all your living energy, at its various levels of mind, body and spirit, depending on your life experience and cultivation. This is why two musicians of equal talent and disposition can play from the same score and yet the performances contain certain nuances which may render one good and the other great. Consciously, both musicians hit the same notes. What they hear, feel, intuit and so on unconsciously, however, is making the difference in the quality of their performances.

In all of above examples, however, if the conscious mind did not involve itself in the process, the subconscious mind may still commandeer the entire event, but the result would be totally different. If your performance, per se, is interrupted by random thoughts bubbling up in your mind or if your conscious mind becomes tired, confused, low in energy, and your subconscious bubbles up randomly, without clarity, mutual (or any) purpose, and runs away with what you are doing, the activity albeit writing or playing the piano, another instrument or whatever will at best turn out happenstance and at worst lose all sense of unity, purpose and communication. Physiologically you will feel fatigued afterward because of the overabundance of randomness in the subconscious mind – which burns a lot of your energy. In contrast, if the conscious mind too tightly controls the process, and subconscious mind is locked and cannot naturally and optimally explore its power in other dimensions, then the work will be very tiring as well and the result won't be good at all.

An integrative person has both a clear conscious mind to lead the whole being and a powerful subconscious mind to explore the powers in other higher dimensions, cooperate with the conscious mind, and at the same time expand or extend the space and strength of the conscious mind. This balance is the hallmark of a flowing and centered mindset and also a long-standing aim of mind-body medicine and holistic arts and sciences.

§6.5 Relationship of Conscious Mind and Subconscious Mind

You may wonder how your conscious mind is associated with subconscious mind and what the relationship is between them. As indicated by the original Chinese terminology, the conscious mind is called *main conscious mind*, and the subconscious is called *assistant conscious mind*. Obviously the conscious mind is the major feeling of conscious that is responsible for the whole being, and the subconscious mind is the assistant of the main consciousness.

Some parts of the memories, talents, genius, wisdoms, creativities and spiritual powers in the subconscious mind are obtained through conscious process of study, education, training, experience and cultivation and assimilation with higher spirits in this life, and some parts of these came from the original life spirit and experience and Virtues of previous lives and genetic influencers.

Therefore the subconscious mind assists the conscious mind in daily performance by outputting the memories and wisdoms stored in the subconscious system that can help you (or not) in achieving your goals.

As assistant of conscious mind, the subconscious mind naturally and automatically integrates the activities, actions or behaviors to accomplish the goals of the conscious mind. The main conscious mind, at this physical dimension, can lead and train the subconscious mind to cooperate with the whole being. Balance is key.

When we learn to drive, for instance, the conscious mind intentionally learns and remembers how to operate the car in detail, step by step. At the same time, the subconscious mind cooperates with the conscious mind to get used to the driving techniques and processes. The conscious mind passes details to the subconscious mind to remember, mastering the wide range of necessary driving techniques and guiding the body (hands, eyes, ears and legs, etc.) while the conscious mind then goes on to operate other aspects of the driving with focused intention – consciously. Therefore, the subconscious mind gradually remembers the process and works with the conscious mind, unconsciously, in order to drive smoothly.

Eventually as you get used to driving, the subconscious mind will become more cooperative with the conscious mind naturally and smoothly. This is an example of how conscious mind leads the subconscious mind, learning skill and gaining experience in this physical life, and then how the subconscious mind outputs the memories and skills with its freedom and powerful energy from other dimensions to help conscious mind achieve the complete performance in this physical dimension. Without subconscious mind's great powers from higher dimensions, the driver will forever drive like a beginner with a lot of hassles, while without the conscious mind to intentionally learn driving, he will never know how to drive.

In fact, other learning and education processes such as schoolwork, science and technology, athletics – really all types of training programs in this life – operate the same way.

For higher wisdom and spiritual character, however, the main conscious mind also can lead the subconscious mind to learn, cultivate and assimilate with higher spirits and wisdoms. For example, intentional consciousness can initiate good spiritual cultivation practice, moral quality improvement, spirituality practice, Virtue and personality improvement, self-improvement, intelligent education, meditation, energy practice, health and beauty and longevity practices, artistic and cultural training, and so forth. These practices involve the initial intention of the conscious mind access to the higher spirit and the spiritual energy source through the subconscious processes. The mind-body-spirit practice needs an intentional goal and persistent efforts from the clear and consistent conscious mind while involving unlimited powers of the subconscious mind and spirit.

If one has a good quality from inborn or genetic influencer or after-born environment or spiritual education (not necessarily the education in the schools), he/she may wake up spiritually and initialize a spiritual cultivation.

Someone may have a good quality of subconscious mind in other dimensions from inborn experience, and after coming to this life he/she believes many spiritual things and wants to cultivate spiritually, but the conscious mind in the maze of this physical dimension may refuse to do so. For such reason that individual's subconsciousness will keep searching higher teaching and practice. One day a faith may come, for example, reading a book of higher teaching, meeting a friend who helps make the connection, a or via a dramatic occurrence (e.g., a trauma or health issue) that wakes the individual up and he/she starts thinking of the true meaning and improvement of spiritual life. Within this context, the role of the subconsciousness is powerful not only because it helps perform tasks in this physical life but also because it can help cultivate to higher level of life, of course, if the main consciousness agrees to do so and persistently practices mind-body-spirit cultivation.

A practical problem is that some people meditate with a busy mind having a lot of thinking unconsciously. Such meditation is not beneficial because the subconscious is too busy, and a lot of unconscious thinking inputs much "noise" into your mind, making your mind attach on the lower dimension and human attachments, and burns a lot of energy. As a result, the mind gets confused, anxious, and tired. This is a common meditation problem that needs to be addressed.

The key to improvement is to stop the random subconscious mind activities. You can do this by quieting the mind and reeling it back into the peaceful focus of the meditation. It may not be easy for some people who have already formed the pattern of subconscious activity into a habit of allowing the mind to drift into random mind chatter and racing thoughts. This problem is usually due to the mind's becoming used to attaching on certain issues or repeatedly thinking of the daily issues, sending your mind the repeated message that you want to go there so that it starts going there automatically (and usually unconsciously) "for you."

Sometimes issues such as worry, concern, fear, or compulsivity, too much care about certain things or combinations of these situations set you off in the circle of thought that leaves your mind stuck in rumination. Initially this pattern of mind activity may be facilitated by the conscious mind with intention, and subconscious mind gets involved, and eventually the subconscious mind (getting a message that you want it to go there) takes over, generating an endless circle of interruptive thoughts that can dull your presence or sweep it away entirely.

The solution to stopping this subconscious circle of thoughts from invading your attention is to have a strong, clear and righteous conscious mind that will in turn train your subconscious mind, cultivate the body-mind-spirit, enhance the positive energy, simplify both subconscious and conscious minds, and establish a healthy and meaningful lifestyle, daily activities, and clear-headed thinking pattern, quiet and cooperative subconsciousness. We will discuss this solution more in the following sections.

Your conscious mind is a part of your true Self that is associated with this physical dimension in this life, and your subconscious minds follow and cooperate with the main conscious mind in other dimensions. Therefore, the true Self in this life takes the responsibility for the whole being to live in the way of harmony with the original life nature. Otherwise, if the true Self as well as the whole being of body-mind-spirit have conflicts with the peaceful nature of its original Self, the mind and body will get sick and at the very least experience discomfort. Sickness is the conflict and constriction of the mind and body with both (1) the original spiritual characters of the being, such as peace, harmony, truthfulness, compassion, love, kindness, tolerance, forgiveness, and detachment as well as (2) the energy nature of the balanced Yin-Yang and The Five Elements.

We often see that the conscious minds of people who are sick physically and/or mentally are unclear, confused, in conflict, wondering, noisy, fighting, frustrated and experiencing difficulty concentrating.

In such cases, most of them will tell the doctor that their minds are always busy and get tired. However if you ask them what is on their minds, they sometimes cannot clearly answer or they often will tell you that all things in their minds are random, clouded, confused or conflicted.

To heal the mind and body and stay healthy, balanced, energetic, clear headed, and take good care of all issues for your whole being, your conscious mind should take the lead and stay clear, righteous, peaceful, positive, focused, relaxed, connected with the peaceful and energetic spiritual energy source, balanced in the energy of Yin And Yang and The Five Elements or stay Beyond The Five Elements (after cultivated to extreme high level), and take care of the health of the mind and body through a consistent practice of body-mind-spirit on a daily basis. This is the center focus of mind-body health practice for any one at any age, in any field or profession, and from any level of our society. When the conscious mind is strong, clear, and stays peaceful and at ease, then subconscious mind will become quiet, peaceful, and cooperative with and under the guidance of your main consciousness.

Good practice of mind-body medicine works with both the conscious mind and subconscious minds. The practice has many modalities such as meditation, hypnosis, psychological consultation, spiritual teaching and communication, energy healing, oriental medicine, music sound therapy, biofeedback, Qigong, Taiji, and more. These practices not only work at the subconscious level, but also importantly on the main conscious mind. The processes of total healing involve finding the problem, incorrect thoughts, negative mentality, unhealthy lifestyle and habits, rigid notion, wrong beliefs and value systems, and relearning and regaining the healthy ways of living, thinking and acting, of course with your willing and in a friendly way suitable to you.

§6.8 Healing the Subconscious Minds and Conscious Mind

Clinically many health issues are caused and accompanied by conscious mind and subconscious mind delusion, confusion, cloudiness, noise, incorrect cognition, human notions and attachments, in addition to unhealthy lifestyle and habits. These health issues are not just mental problems such as ADD, ADHD, anxiety, depression, bipolar, insomnia, but also many physical health issues or their combinations such as chronic pain syndromes, fatigue, TMS, FCS, MCS, high blood pressure, diabetes, over-weight, obesity, male and female sexuality problems, cancers, and the list goes on.

The mind is the bridge, linking the energy source and body. It is the original source of health, but also the core cause of the sickness.

Physical and mental health problems are the final and superficial expression of internal noises, conflicts, contradictions, ignorance, rejections, and imbalances of energy, in the deep dimensions of mind, spirit and body. Causes for these internal noises, contradictions and imbalances can be originated from many courses, regarding, for example, genetic factors, childhood developmental factors, family issues, school education, social environment, relationships, job, working environment, self-education, stress, emotional factors, habits, addictions, lifestyle, living schedule, foods and eating habits, nutrition, culture, belief system, value systems, living and working condition and environment, social environment and social conscious influence, sometimes even involving Karma or negative/sick messages carried on from past lives, etc. In most cases, it is the combination of multiple issues of these as described above.

Remember, the conscious mind leads the entire being and is in charge of all these experiences in this life, therefore, establishing all these factors in the life experience and creating the memories in the subconscious mind and/or triggering, restoring or activating the wisdoms, talents, creativities, and spiritual characters and powers in the subconscious minds at other dimensions.

The subconscious minds store, manage and output these memories and energy powers in all these aspects during the life experience in cooperation with the conscious mind.

Therefore, the clear, correct, and harmonized contributions of the conscious and subconscious minds and its resulting activities are vital to the whole person.

To heal, one needs to go through the main conscious mind to see how all these factors are related to health issues. And at the same time, the wrong and unhealthy memories, habits, messages, thoughts or notions created in the subconscious mind need to be removed, cleaned up and then reinstalled with new and healthy messages into the individual's memory and energy system.

Thus healing process is actually the process of healing the conscious mind and subconscious minds in order to restore your original state, your true Self, within a peaceful, loving, compassionate, forgiving, and balanced, Yin-Yang and Five Elements energetic state. In other words, healing is the process of re-recognition and rejuvenation of your original Self at all levels of mind, spirit and then body.

§6.9 Fundamental Mission And Ultimate Guide for Life Journey

In this life journey, we need a clear ultimate guide about lifetime mission and purpose to live on the earth. Without this clear guide, you will be lost in your life journey and get into a maze of darkness and meaningless cycles, and finally burn out your energy, feel anxious, frustrated, depressed, worried, fearful, tired, and even get sick mentally, physically and spiritually. Without a clear mission and purpose in this life journey, it is just like you have no idea about where to go when driving, or have no a map or GPS to direct your driving. Then, as a result, you completely lose your direction or perhaps never have a direction, but just keep driving around anyway without destination. Eventually you run out of gasoline and end the journey without any satisfaction of purposeful achievement. In fact, today in our modern life, people get sick just because of this reason – loss of true Self – easy to do when the mind is confused and everyday life becomes too busy. We all need the highest guidance for our lifetime mission, purpose and final destination. With such guidance, you can focus and simplify your mind and lifestyle on the major goal, and then as a result, you will stay on course and live meaningfully, work efficiently, with joy, peace and a much higher quality of life.

To have a clear ultimate guide, you need to know your fundamental life mission. But what exactly is a lifetime mission? Before we answer this question, let's look at how people live in this life at modern time. Today, people are used to being busy for their entire life in many things – starting with preschool, elementary school, then many more years of education from high school to college, some through graduate school and postdoctoral trainings, working hard for degrees, career, job, income, boyfriend/girlfriend, marriage, husband/wife, kids, house, money, and then they get old, sick, and finally on one day leave this world, finishing this life journey.

Can just these things be the mission and purpose of this life? Is the end of this lifetime just simply the end or finishing of your life? Many of you probably answer no. And of course, they are not our life mission and purpose. In fact, they are just basic needs, processes and activities for surviving this life in this physical world, in this lifetime.

So what are the mission and purpose of this life?

The mission and purpose of this life are to improve, strengthen, purify, cultivate and elevate the quality of the spirit, mind and body, in order to achieve a better quality and higher level of the life itself, but not anything else besides, and then to live healthy physically, mentally and spiritually in this life and finally to be able to go back to the highest final destination, the original Self in the future life at other higher dimensions.

This statement is not what someone else or I myself have made up based on personal preference or imagination, but it is told by many thousands of years of human civilizations, experience, enlightenment from the divine spirits, sages or spiritual masters as we mentioned in early chapters in this book. It is also implied by a range of modern sciences and researches such as those regarding near-death experiences, past life regression, religion science, brain studies, consciousness researches, and neuron sciences.

This mission and purpose is the highest guide for the entire life process. Based on this, you can clearly and intelligently design your life. As an ultimate goal, it can help you determine and associate all activities in the process of your life. Additionally, it must be very clear in your conscious mind and established as a top priority in your life, so you can have clear intentional planning that guides your entire life journey and daily living on a daily basis. With such clear lifetime mission and purpose, you will not focus on gains in this physical world and attach on solely material life issues. You will not see and try to understand yourself and others and all things in this world with narrowed viewpoints and mindsets and will not "only" care about short term interests of your own Self without considering long term goals in the bigger scope of your entire life, personality, Virtue, moral quality, or finding the truth of life and universe, health of body-mind-spirit, your own internal and external quality and beauty (and that of others, people, and the world, including the Universe itself), longevity and destination of life – that of your own and that of future generations of human beings.

With such a lens and goal and mission in life, you will live in much broader, yet deeper, more satisfying spaces with greater energies, not only in this physical dimension, but also all over the lovely, peaceful and happy worlds of the mental, spiritual, artistic, and mystical dimensions. Your life will not drown in busy-ness and you will not become blind to your greater goals and purpose, and will not be stressful and struggling with material gains, relationships, families or others, but you will live in much higher quality of life with wonderful compassionate, blessing and loving energy surrounding you, and feel, relate and interrelate to all things and all people much more simply, lovingly, fluidly, positively and genuinely.

This mission and purpose will benefit you in both this life and your future life. I am sure that you want to have a healthy body, mind and spirit in this life. It is the most important thing in your life. Otherwise, if you get sick or mentally blocked in anything or any issue in your life, then, no matter how many other things you may have in this life, your life will be very miserable and difficult. And, in terms of your future life, no matter whether you believe in a future life after this life or not, you will still be wondering whether death is your ultimate end or whether there may be something else beyond this space.

Many religions and belief systems talk about this topic. No matter. You may already have your own belief or you may not have one. Here we are not talking about just a belief system or religion; we are talking about how to achieve a healthy life, clear-headed mind, and peaceful energy state in this life. We are talking about achieving such purpose through a cultivation practice or self-improvement effort on our mind, body and spirit for this life and future life in terms of the actual energy from within the body, mind and spirit. While we cultivate the whole being, the energy will be purified, strengthened, and elevated to a higher level, therefore in this life you will stay healthy, energetic, peaceful, and with wisdom, and in the future life your spirit will be able to enter the higher and fascinating spiritual dimensions of the eternal life.

Many people go to church or temple to pray for fortune and luck, asking God or Buddha to give them all kinds of desired things, such as money, a job, house, relationship, health, children, and so on. They read the Bible or Buddhist scripts, but do not take it into personal cultivation practice, so it does nothing to them. What you do or believe in, if you do not actually practice cultivation and improvement of the mind, body and spirit and work on greater Self awareness inward and external mindfulness, will help nothing and may, in fact, increase one's desires and attachments, and as a result, negatively affect health of mind and body.

Today, modern people sustain a busy lifestyle because of all their physical attachments and desires, but barely think of the most important mission and purpose in this life regarding their whole being of mind-body-spirit and how to design a daily living schedule to achieve this mission and purpose. Many have scheduled 365 fully busy days a year; working very hard for all things toward a better material life, pleasures as well as all related issues such as money, jobs, degrees, careers, entertainments, relationships, family, and so on, but never or barely ever have their own quiet and peaceful time to focus on the practice of mind, body and spirit for health, self-improvement, spirituality, and good high quality energy.

In such an outward lifestyle and mentality, their soul or spirit is scattered all over other places, but is not adequately communicative with their core Self, their own spirit, body and mind, and their mind is exhausted with its busy-ness in this physical dimension. After years of such activity, people finally age and become sick mentally and physically. The integration of your mind, body and spirit through a practice such as meditation, energy music healing, mind-body-spirit cultivation, Qigong and Taiji movements, or other health practice and spiritual cultivation, is extremely important thing to do for your whole being in this life and future life. This is supposed to be the number one, most important thing to do and care for in your everyday life. You should choose one cultivating system to practice for your whole being health and give it top priority throughout your entire life journey.

Some people may ask a question like this: "I do have my belief system or religion and understand what you talk about in terms of the mission and purpose of this life as described above, but why I am still sick?" My answer to your question is: No matter what belief or religion you have, do you really cultivate your mind-body-spirit by following the original teachings, do you truly practice it in your daily life and improve your mind nature, spiritual character, moral quality, compassionate heart and kind and peaceful personality, as well as overall energy and health at all levels of mind, body and spirit, and do you really let go of human attachments and complicated human mindset that burns your energy in the material world? Your answer to this question is vital to your overall health and development.

You may ask me another question: "Are you really telling me that as long as I have a spiritual belief or religion, then I should automatically have a good health?" My answer to your question is similar as above, again, the answer is: No, it was not what I meant, and no matter what religion or belief you have, if you do not actually put effort into the practice of cultivating your mind, spirit and body by following the true teaching, then you can still get sick and age.

Here we are not talking about religion or just believing in God. We are talking about the actual daily cultivation practice for your mind, spirit and body, and not about any religion, and we will never affect whatever religion you may already have. We will gradually and further explore the body-mind-spirit cultivation science in the following chapters. In the following section, however, we will first discuss how to choose a daily practice for you.

§6.10 Youth Mental Development to Avoid Violence And Crime

While at this juncture and we are talking about the ultimate purpose and true meaning of this life, I have to insert this section to address the mental development of children and youth, so that we may help prevent them from participation in violence and crimes. This is an issue that is worthy of all our attention. Every time a criminal incident involving our youth – e.g. gun shooting or mass killing – occurs, our entire society is shocked. These acts always trigger big waves of discussion, concern and thinking about why such incidents happen and how to prevent the likes of them in the future. Nonetheless, we never seem to find a practical and effective solution to avoid this kind of behavior.

After a while and as things calm again, we start forgetting the problem exists. But then, it happens again, a similar (or even worse) act of youthful violence manifests again. This scenario keeps repeating over and over.

Although each individual incident has different elements and reasons that lead to the tragedy, many of them continue to involve shooters of relatively young ages. For example:

April 16, 2007, the Virginia Tech mass shooter was a 23-year-old Virginia Tech senior, killing 32 people and injuring 17.

December 5, 2007, Omaha shopping mall gunfire was perpetrated by a 19-year-old man, killed 8 people and wounded four others.

February 14, 2008, a 27-year old man shot into a classroom, at Northern Illinois University, killing 5 and injuring 21.

July 20, 2012, a 24-year-old man shot inside the movie theater in Aurora, Colorado, killing 12 and injuring 58.

June 7, 2013, an unemployed 23-year-old, killed 5 people in an attack that started at his father's home and ended at Santa Monica College.

There have been so many. The most recent gun shooting (as I write this book) occurred on May 23, 2014, Friday, the last weekend of spring semester at UC, Santa Barbara. At about 9:30 pm, Elliot Rodger, a 22-year old college student, went on a shooting spree, killing six people and injuring thirteen in the neighborhood of Isla Vista near the campus. At the end, he was found dead with a gunshot wound to the head, which appeared to be suicidal.

Of course not all gun shootings involve younger shooters, but the criminal psychological mindset often involves the shooter's mental development, particularly in early childhood, teen, and young ages.

After looking into the details of these shootings and others, it is clear the shooters had fundamental problems within many areas of their life. As well, there was a lack of good guidance and education across the board that could have helped them onto a different path, one of peaceful, mentally balanced living and with a deeper understanding and appreciation of life, and a cultivation of healthier practices and good, positive attitudes imbued with more consideration for others, kind manner, tolerance, compassion, and caring as well as a deeper understanding and appreciation for spirituality, culture, the arts or traditional values, and their own personal life - free of the energetically negative effects of computer games, heavy metal music, guns, drugs, smoke, alcohol, sex, gambling, and money.

Let's face it, computer gaming attaches a person to the likes of a machine – for certain individuals occupying them almost every day for hours of time, and even late into the night, minimizing the person's contact with either humanity and/or the natural environment, leaving the person drained, negatively detached, and dys-associated from positively invigorating life resources, as well as from their true Self and spirit, and the Universe itself.

Many such individuals attach to and flood themselves with dysfunctional messages from a variety sources including, music and other forms of what they perceive as "entertainment." As a result, their conscious mind gets blurry, and their subconscious mind has too much random noise. They play with various guns (digital, real, etc.), take drugs, drink alcohol, and have sex at an early age and with random people without caring about love or not. They are basically into only self-centered entertainments, enjoyments, satisfactions of their own desires, but lack the combination of knowledge and experience of other more positively nurturing activities, or have come to know of these only from a selfish, narrow-scoped and negative angle.

Such individuals are, at times, not necessarily handicapped mentally, sick psychologically or psychiatrically, or of low IQ. In fact, sometimes they even have a good IQ in certain narrowed areas, mostly involving left brain activity – which may also shed light on why they are attracted to some of these aforementioned harmful behaviors. In fact, they attach so much to a few areas that they easily develop addiction, isolation, autism, loneliness, depression, anxiety, selfishness, self-centeredness, carelessness, and even violence, hate, jealousy, vengefulness, etc. Their soul or spirit is lost, and their personal life and their mindset are confused, messed up, or against normal humanity. The original pure natures – which young children are supposed to have – have been destroyed.

You may wonder why they become like this. Of course, at the point when they have already developed such bad character and criminal mindset, we can say that such criminals do have an evil spirit or soul that carries dark Karmas. They do not have a kind heart and basic human nature nor do they take responsibility regarding their life and others' lives, nor understand that killing lives will create Karma and they will have to pay for it with a lot of pain and suffering either in this life or future lives.

On the other hand, we need to consider the causes of their behaviors in a broader and deeper way.

Think of this: How do people, parents, families, schools, teachers, doctors, mental health practitioners, social workers, governments, and our societies teach and influence our children or young people in their mental development processes? Do these methods have something to do with those violent and criminal mindsets developed in our society? Is there something we can do to prevent such outcomes?

Nowadays, most parents, families, schools, teachers, doctors, including health providers, individuals as well as our entire education system and society provide the children's needs at a superficial level, such as their material life, physical health, entertainment, satisfactions, the development of a so-called happy childhood, as well as providing background in: science and technologies for future careers, degrees, other credentials, employment, finance and having the "good life" (all of which are fine), but not enough.

We need care for the young person's mental development as well, greater support for their daily emotions, relationships, personal ideas and thoughts, their troubles in understanding others, society, parents and themselves, and more deep guidance about the meaning of this life and their own spiritual connection with true Self and higher Spirit and plenty of conversation capable of feeding their soul's needs with higher spiritual energy.

In fact, many adults are also very much attached to a superficial path as well. It is a road of one-way driving on an imbalanced course - physical living without developing spirituality or understanding and cultivating life purpose and not knowing where to go to find these, or why and how to cultivate the mind, body and spirit for a balanced quality life as well as their future eternal life path.

Whole person cultivation is not set as a priority in our society in general, so how can our younger generations in general understand its concepts? Facing such conditions, some young people can completely lose their soul, go to an extreme, and skid onto a path that rages against humanity and god's nature.

Some of them, at such point, may still run under the radar of parents, family, school or communities, so their dangerous behaviors grow and intensify until the worst happens.

Some of them may be noticed and sent for mental healthcare, which is supposed to be able to help make positive change in the subject. But in most cases, mental healthcare cannot help improve their condition. This is because mental healthcare nowadays is basically an emotional treatment at the human level, but not spiritual teaching and enlightenment. It is not able to touch the soul of the individual, waking up the spirit, and moving the heart. Instead it is just superficially diagnosing what kind of symptoms the subject has and then giving it the name of a disease or condition, and then prescribing its various forms of treatment, including pharmaceutical.

By following such rigid procedures and not the highest spiritual teaching and guide for enlightenment and without profound and strong energy produced by the practitioner, of course, there is no way to truly reach deep enough into the person's heart, soul and spirit in a godly way. Therefore, it will never change the person at all. Using the human way (the superficial) cannot heal the human problem. Using emotional psychology cannot heal emotions. The reason for this is that these treatments are at the same levels, often causing confusions and conflicts logically and emotionally. If the higher Self is not waking up to lead the whole being, then the lower human being will lose its direction, drop down to the lower level or even become evil. Often we see such a pattern: in the session when the subject is with his mental health practitioner, social worker or police, the subject behaves normally, he can hide his bad spirit character very well, but afterward the subject's evil side still drives him to take bad action. This is because his higher Self, true Self was never awakened to lead his whole being. It means the treatment has no actual positive effects to make change in the person.

As a result, children are not taught about what is good, what is not good, what you are supposed to do as a good person and what you are not supposed to do as a good person, what is Karma, and what is Virtue, why we are here, where to go in this life, why we human beings have some difficulties in this life and how we should view these and deal with them in a positive way through the cultivation of our mind-body-spirit, how others are energetically related to us and how we should treat them, and what is the most valuable meaning, purpose, goal, and beauty of this life, and so on. This is a large part of the problem. As such, children are not provided with such deep guidance and soul-touching instruction that helps them understand that their life itself is important and should be treasured, and others' lives also should be treasured. So these children can have a good material life, but they are so hungry for mental and spiritual foods.

Therefore, many young beings wind up estranged of their True Self, the higher Self and don't know how to get back and consciously connected to it. Some may never have awakened their True Self at all. This is why they behave as they do – as a low or even evil spirit; self-centered, desired-driven, mentally confused, money or material oriented, and quite isolated from family, school, society, humanity, nature and the universe.

Somewhere along the line, they reach the extreme point, get frustrated, angry, disappointed, depressed, ungrounded, hopeless, seeing no light in the future, having no clear direction and meaningful goal in their mind, or finally intend violence against society. They feel completely in the dark and have no hope left in their life, so they are finally committed to suicide or want to destroy others' lives before ending their own.

Giving hope, light, love and shining spirit can save these lives, as it is more needed than giving foods.

Of course, there are many other factors also involved in the mass killing incidents we are discussing. Some of these are lawful issues, mental healthcare procedure and policy issues, and other medical and social factors, including genetics, parents, family, marriage, relationships, neighborhoods, friends, social environments, and so on. But here we are talking about the fundamental understanding of human life, its meaning, as well as the importance of cultivating the mind, body and spirit as the most basic and important task in this life, and with that kept in mind, our education system, schools, teachers, parents, families and society can provide a positive, balanced, child / teenager/ young adult and growing adult a suitable format for the development of mind-body-spirit which will include: inspiring, uplifting, cultivating, and nurturing advice, support, and environments.

All are related as a whole. If all or most of the people within our society become materialistic, are not positively and actively putting effort into or even aware of cultivating the whole being of mind, body and spirit, how can our children know it is important to improve their mind, soul and character?

If our schools from kindergartens and elementary schools to colleges and graduate schools, as well as our society are just focusing on science, technologies, skills, and business but are not also teaching individuals the practices for cultivation and enlightenment of mind, soul, moral value, character, mental health, spirituality, internal strength and energy, we will continue to seed the future with potential violence and superficiality. Yet, by forming such environments to nurture the "higher practices" of holistic learning and cultivation, our children and students in these schools will grow on a balanced path mentally, physically, spiritually, academically and professionally.

It is so painful every time when I hear of a mass shooting. I especially feel deeply sad for those who lost their loved ones. As mental health practitioners, however, we are not just experiencing sadness as most people do, but we also have to think – deeply and broadly – about the causes of such violence as they are rooted within our families, schools, communities and societies.   We need to find the solution to help prevent such violence from reoccurring in the future.

We need to ask: What made such a killer hate people like that? Through what process did he develop such terrible mental character that is totally opposite against the god's will and original human nature? When this happens to a particular young college student, are there still other young people of his age having a similar mentality and hiding out somewhere in our society like undetected bombs? Yes, there are some of them hidden there like undetected bombs. And do we have a reason to say no to this violent mentality? Probably you will agree that the answer to this question is that we do have reason to say no to this violence. It is dangerous to us all. We have had enough of it, we don't want anymore, and we want to stop it now from ever happening again.

Someone may say; the shooter in the recent UC Santa Barbara incident seemed to be diagnosed with Asperger syndrome (AS)[11] or Narcissistic personality disorder (NPD)[12] or

---

[11] Asperger syndrome (AS), also known as Asperger disorder (AD) or simply Asperger's, is an autism spectrum disorder (ASD) that is characterized by significant difficulties in social interaction and nonverbal communication, alongside restricted and repetitive patterns of behavior and interests.

some other mental / psychiatric diseases. So people say, there is nothing we can do because his mental illness drives him to act that way. If only looking at his symptoms, then yes, it could be true that he has the AS and/or NPD or whatever mental problems, but the original cause(s) before he became like this and correcting such cause(s) are the central issue with which we should concern ourselves.

As you can see, this individual may have a good enough cognitive ability and is smart enough in most things. His brain functions normally. What he is lacking is a clear, higher quality and broader view of soul - higher spirit, which seems something he never got from anyone or anywhere.

Let's ask the following question while keeping this case in mind. However, by "he" as mentioned below, you can consider anyone in general:

If a young man practices his own energy through a daily meditation and energy movement such as Qigong, Taiji or Yoga, cultivates his mind, body and spirit, energizes himself mentally and physically, feeling confident about himself, feeling at ease to communicate with people and that he can understand others and all issues of life in a positive and balanced way, feel himself becoming attractive not only physically and financially and most importantly spiritually and energetically, and

If he knows who he is, why he is here on the earth, what is the meaning and purpose of his life, why and how he should cultivate his mind-body-spirit, what are his valuable life purpose and the beautiful destination and

If he knows that money, fame and desire (including desiring heterosexual relationship or attraction between a man and woman) are just a (small) part of his life at the physical and emotional level, but are not everything, thus he should not attach on it "only," and on the other hand, he knows his broad compassionate heart, peaceful shining soul, and manly caring character are the most honorable values that a man (human beings in general) are supposed to have, is, in fact, the most attractive nature a man has, and will result in all good things in this life and future lives, but may or may not become a visible form in this physical world, and

If he understands that everyone can have some hard times, difficulties or even suffering or tribulations (including loneliness mentally and physically) in this life, but the key is to learn overcoming them and looking at them in a positive way, which cultivates our mind and spirit better, makes life meaningful and happier, and

---

[12] Narcissistic personality disorder (NPD) is a personality disorder in which a person is excessively preoccupied with personal adequacy, power, prestige and vanity, mentally unable to see the destructive damage they are causing to themselves and to others in the process.

If he knows that he can and should look into himself, improve his own personality, character, Virtue, eliminate his own Karma, helping others, giving to people, serving the society that can result in his long-lasting happiness,

Then he will not hate, be jealous or vengeful towards others, and he will not take such action as to gun down other people, nor kill himself either.

It is the positive characteristics and mind nature that should be established from his early childhood through the guides and influences within his growing environments.

If we know all these mind-body-spirit cultivation concepts, as a parent, brother, sister, teacher, doctor, psychologist, social worker, government leader, or just a friend, neighborhood, or any individual, we can help him stop killing and turn him into a good man, happy man and true man, which is forever good for himself, his family, friends, school and our society.

Most people, of course, grow up naturally with the original good natures of humanity, but if the families, schools, education system – as a whole – and social environments are not intentionally adding spiritual guidance and humanity cultivation efforts to form a strong spiritual energy atmosphere, there will always be some children, teenagers and youths who fall down and cause problems.

We can comfortably say that most of such cases regarding teenager/youth mental problems are preventable – if our family influences and guidance, education system and social environments improve – with exception to the small numbers of true illness due to problems related with brain biochemistries and genetics.

§6.11 Choose A Mind-Body-Spirit Cultivation System

There are many cultivation practices available today. Some of them have a long history and some of them are created in more recent times. Some are good and some are not that good. Choosing a good practice system and truly learning the good cultivation is extremely important.

We have to point out that some of today's practices are not that good because the teacher or so called master may not have that much good Virtue, GONG (a Chinese word, meaning Energy Power of Spiritual Character from High Spirit) or higher teaching principle to give to you, but instead be filled with too much human desire and attachment toward achievement at the physical (human) realm. They created a practice to attract your involvement and desire to learn from their class(es), pay for their program and products, but do not really care about how you will achieve your health and how you will grow mentally and spiritually. Some practices only teach physical forms to practice, but have no principle to improve mind nature. Even though some of these practices may have such a principle, it is often at a very low level. As such, these practitioners take advantage of your human desires to get you involved or donate money to them, but will not really purify your mind and improve your character and energy, and benefit your health and spirituality.

A good practice for your mind, spirit and body is a high level of teaching system that guides you based on the universal nature and Yin-Yang and Five Elements energy system for your whole being. In original Chinese it called Xing-Ming double cultivation (性命雙修), meaning mind nature and longevity health double cultivation.

As an exceptional example of high level practice, in recent years, the most popular and well-known practice called Falun Gong or Falun Dafa as mentioned early in this book has received attention of, and benefited a large number of practitioners over the world. This practice is the most complete and profound teaching based on the original ancient practice and guide of both the spiritual growth and physical strength for your whole being.

Spiritually, it teaches you to cultivate the mind and spirit to meet the universe's characteristics; truth, compassion and tolerance, and then physically the practice teaches five forms of meditation and movement exercises, covering all meridian systems in your body to open up all energy channels in order to achieve physical health and mental strength.

Medically, psychologically and spiritually speaking, this practice makes a lot of sense because its teaching focuses on your mind nature practice, helps you detach the strong human attachments, opens and frees your mind, enlightens your spirit and relaxes your emotion, gives you a new and broad view of life, so you are no longer locked on so many difficult issues in this physical life. This is called letting go of attachments. This makes your mind healthy and connected with the high spiritual energy source, activates the energy generating system, and limits or reduces the human attachments-based energy consuming system. Therefore this practice reaches out to the most important fundamental issue and resolves the core cause of sickness or disease. This is a spiritual teaching that helps you understand a lot of issues about life, the meaning of life, and the mind and body, health and sickness, and so on. In addition to this spiritual teaching, it teaches an energetic mechanism – five sets of physical practices including 4 sets of standing exercises and one set of sitting meditation. These physical forms are truly powerful. All together Falun Gong provides a complete practice system of spiritual nature and energy mechanism.

The four forms of standing movements open up all energy channels, relieve sick Qi (Chi), and promote circulation of blood and energy within your body and mind. The movements are effective in improving your energy, strength, immune system, functions of all your organs such as kidney, liver, stomach, spleen (digestive system), lung, gallbladder, heart, and intestines, etc. These movements will balance your hormones, automatic nervous systems, and emotions. They especially help people who have back pain, spinal problems, leg weakness, chronic pain syndromes, constipation, short breath, insomnia, stress, low energy, fatigue, anxiety, depression, and many other mental and physical issues. You will gain good mental and physical health, and feel much relaxed, clearheaded, energetic, and your appearance and skin quality will be dramatically improved.

The sitting meditation will let you experience an extreme quiet conscious state where you are surrounded by all peaceful and powerful energy, and you feel the eternal peace and lighting world. This practice integrates, purifies and energizes your mind, body and spirit and elevate your whole being to a high level mentally, spiritual and physically.

This is just giving you an example of a good mind-body double cultivation practice and a brief review on how the practice will help you in mental and physical health. For the detailed original teaching and practice guide, however, you need to read the original teaching book and listen to the original teaching lecture for Falun Gong. This book is not the teaching itself, but just a recommendation from point of view of mind-body science and health practice.

§6.12 Break: Healing Music • Memorization • Meditation

Sit cross-legged and visualize yourself as two parts: consciousness and subconsciousness. Differentiate them. Keep your conscious mind clear, relaxed and upright, and integrate all thoughts and subconsciousness together by following the peace of your main conscious mind. Review the contents of this chapter, test yourself to see if your mind is clear, and be aware of who you are, what is the purpose and meaning of this life, what is the guide for your life journey, and if your subconsciousness is quiet? Ask: What is the true health of your whole being and realize the importance of mind-body-spirit cultivation in your answer.

And then listen to the following energy music and meditate with empty mind, no activities in your conscious mind or subconscious mind, and go deeper and deeper as long as you can.

EHM06: Calm And Comfort You *(Yin, Metal, Earth)*

This music is composed with focus on the relatively yin energy of metal and earth elements to strengthen your lung and stomach energy. However if you feel you are weak, cold, have low energy, or unhappy, unconfident, or at a low mood emotionally (yin type of condition), then you can choose the following CD (yang type of the healing music) to practice: *EHM05:* Heavenly Song Purifies You *(Yang, Metal, Earth)*

[*Play Energy Healing Music #6*] You are a remarkable cultivator with great compassion, love, passion, spirit, and having the highest goal of beautiful eternal life destination. Now for achieving such wonderful lifetime mission, slow down your living rhythm, ground your mind, rebuild everything on the ground firmly with the highest law of the universe, its character and energy foundation, and then you keep this in mind everyday and every moment, and you are happy, positive, grounded, confident, fearless, patient, loving, giving, open minded, and energetic, no attachment, simple living but clearheaded and efficient in everyday performance. And then you grow day by day more and more mature, more and more close to the perfect, towards your eternal success of life transformation.

§6.13 Exercise Questions

1. What is conscious mind and what is subconscious mind? What are the differences between them?

2. Can you differentiate *your* conscious mind from *your* subconscious mind and how?

3. Do you have random mind chatter and racing thoughts in your conscious mind and/or subconscious mind during the day and your meditation time? If yes, how do you deal with it and do you have a strong intention and the confidence to stop the busy mind? Practice training your mind with the tools offered in this book. Improve your meditation quality by letting go of attachments, negative addictions, human thoughts, notions, as well as thought patterns and habits to which you have become accustomed.

4. What is the relationship between conscious mind and subconscious mind, and how are they cooperative in daily performance?

5. What is the ultimate goal and guide of your life journey and how does it help you keep a clear mind and a simple, focused and simplified life?

6. Why do we need to practice mind-body-spirit cultivation, and how do you do your cultivation?

7. If you are a healthcare practitioner as well as a self-improvement cultivator, how do you help your patients or clients have a clear mind, clear lifetime guide, and understand the importance of mind-body-spirit cultivation?

8. What we (you) can do in everyday life to help prevent youths' mental problems that may lead to the violence and crimes in our society? As we study the mind-body medicine and healthology, how do you understand this problem in terms of mind-

body-spirit cultivation, true Self wakening, positive energy vibration creation, healthy personality and character development starting from each individual, parent, family, child, school, and society?

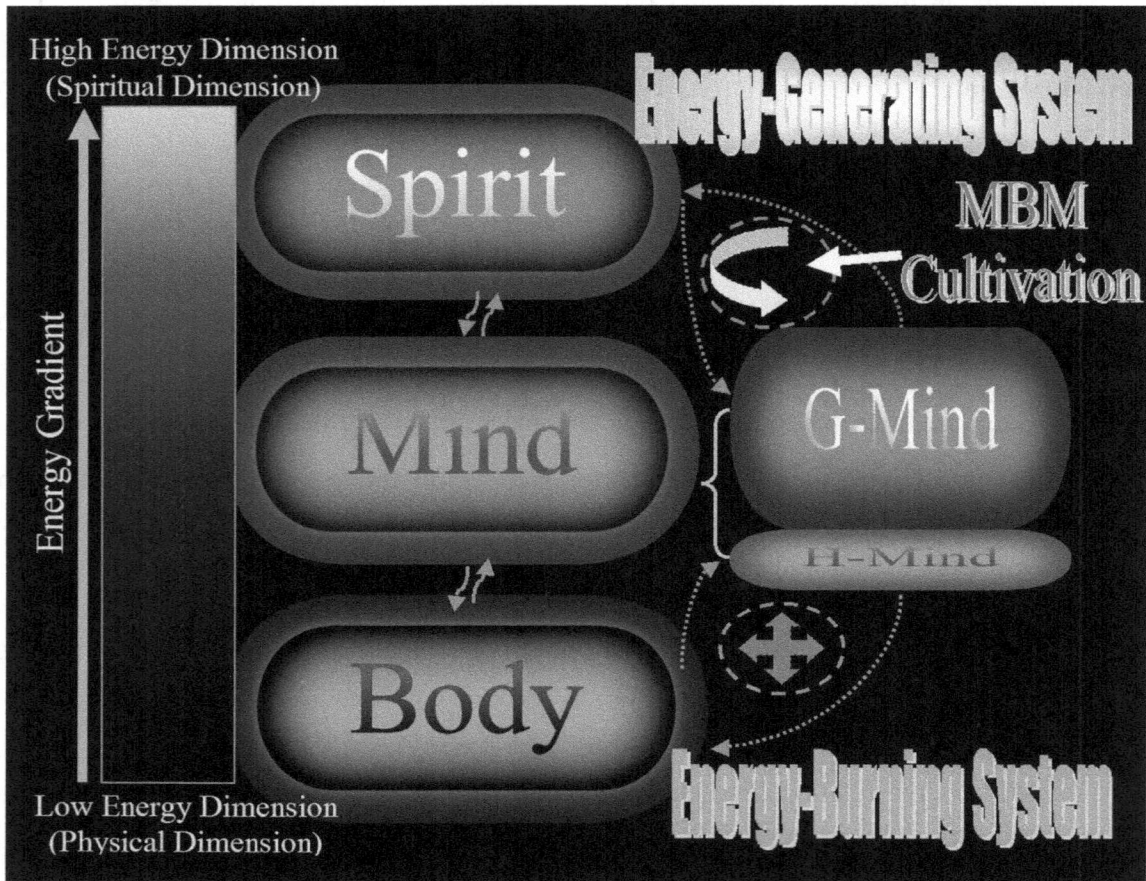

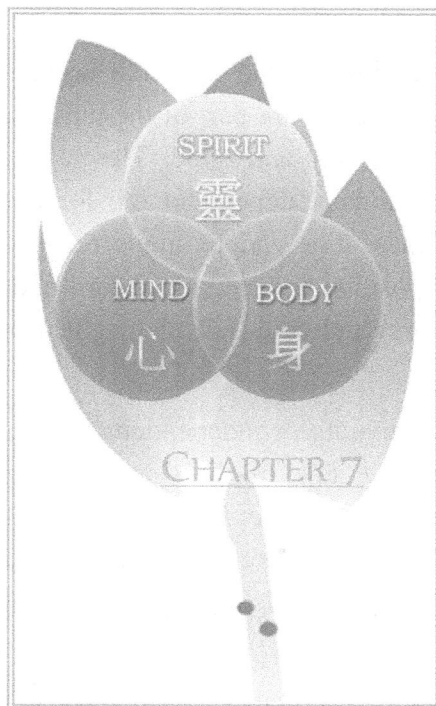

Energy Mechanism: Yin-Yang and Five Elements

As a part of the universe in the three realms, the physical world – and as part of it, your whole being as well – is made of a balanced energy system of Yin-Yang and Five Elements (earth, metal, wood, fire and water). Staying in a balanced state within this system is extremely important for the health of your entire being – mind, body and spirit.

You may, as well, be able to go Beyond The Five Elements, if you reach a highly advanced spiritual level and energy level, but before reaching such level, your practice within The Five Elements is necessary. In this chapter we will deepen our discussion and understanding of Yin-Yang, and Five Elements and how to apply this core principle of energy mechanism to our daily health practice.

§7.1 The Yin and Yang of Your Mind-Body

Every day, the sun rises in the morning and sets at the end of the day, and then the moon rises and sets when sun rises again next morning. Similarly as such natural phenomenon occurs each day; human beings also have a biological, emotional and spiritual clock. It operates by switching between Yin-Yang rhythmically as the universe's energy vibrates.

Based on the original teaching of Lao Tzu, the universe is made of two primal energy forces, Yin and Yang. Because we are part of the universe, human beings also have these two energy forces within our body and mind. The yang and yin represent the two primary, relatively opposite but mutually dependent life forces. The natures of these life forces are called yang and yin: masculine and feminine respectively, active and inactive, light and dark, plus and minus, positive and negative, hard and soft, up lifting and down going, creative and receptive, warm and cold, left and right, fast and slow, in motion and still, and so on.

These two forces are not separate or independent from each other (that is why we hyphenate them, yin-yang, when we talk of them together), nor are they opposites in conflict with each other. Indeed they are interdependent to each other, forming a mutual supportive, promoting, restricting and balancing pair in one unified system.

Maintaining balance between these two energy forces is critical for a human being to stay healthy at all levels. For example, during the night yin energy period, sleeping is the process for you to restore the yin energy that helps your body, mind and spirit stay calm, peaceful, quiet, grounded, clearheaded and stable. Night meditation and sleep restore the yin energy of all organs and retain healthy status of their functionality. Daytime is the active and energetic yang energy time. So during the day, your body, mind and spirit have the great opportunity to be properly and relatively active, doing exercise, practice, study, work, and activities that enhance their yang energy and allow you to stay positive, active, happy, and bright, alert and energetic in order to balance with the peaceful yin energy.

Following the universe's energy daily clock each day and night to arrange your living schedule, your body, mind and spirit will gain their optimal healthy energy and stay in balance between yin and yang at all levels and all time. This will result in the best health and optimal functions of your organs, tissues, hormones, brain chemicals, emotions, thinking and learning ability, intelligent creativity, daily life and overall performance.

§7.2 The Five Elements of Your Mind and Body

Under the ultimate principle of Yin-Yang energy system, interaction between yin and yang further generates five elements of energies. Based on their energy nature (property), they are named as earth, metal, wood, fire and water. These elements do not only refer to the five kinds of matters, but also refer to the five types of energy systems.

All material matters (ordinary matters) fall into these five categories of energy systems. As a part of the universe, human beings are also made of these elements of energies in the body (e.g., organs, meridians) and mind (emotions) accordingly. In traditional Oriental medicine, because of the concepts of energy meridians, the fire element is subdivided into two, which are called fire and ministerial fire. Therefore there are six pairs of organs / meridians, and each pair of organs/meridians is composed of one yin organ/meridian and one yang organ/meridian, belonging to yin and yang of the corresponding element and related emotion, respectively. They are Wood (gallbladder-liver/anger), Metal (lung-large intestine/grief), Earth (stomach-spleen/worry), Fire (heart-small intestine/joy), Water (bladder-kidneys/fear), and Ministerial Fire (pericardium-triple burner/love, happiness and overall essence, Qi and spirit), as the yang organ, yin organ, and related emotions, respectively.

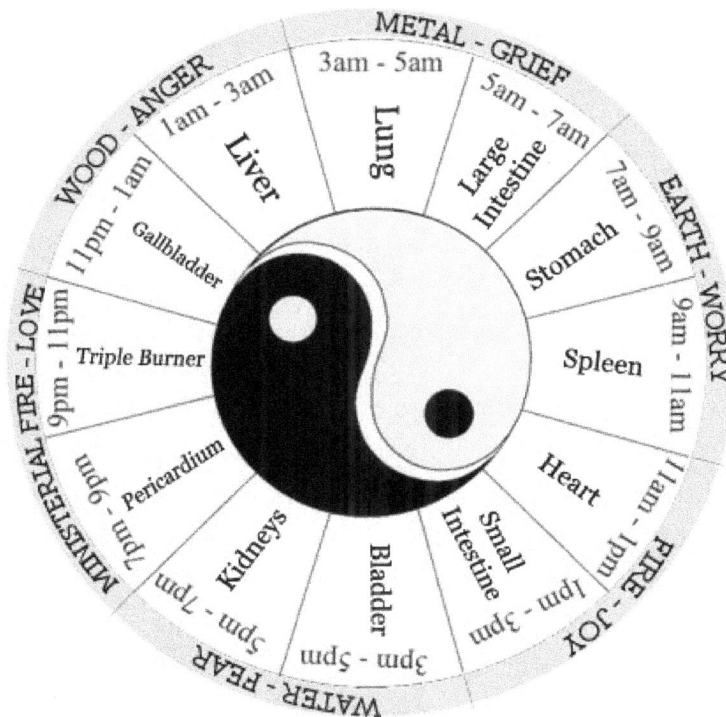

Fig. 7.2. Five Elements and Energy Clock. Each day, 24 hours can be divided into 12 time periods. Each time period covers 2 hours, and every four hours are grouped as one element, associating with two organs – one belongs to yin and the other belongs to yang. For example, 11 p.m. to 3 a.m. is the wood element, within which 11 p.m. – 1 a.m. is the wood yang time, covering the wood yang organ, gallbladder, while 1 a.m. – 3 a.m. is the wood yin time, covering the wood yin organ, liver, and so on.

The pericardium organ and triple burner (also translated *triple warmer*) are not organs recognized by modern anatomy, but they are conceptually important organs as energy meridian systems in energy medicine. The last element "Ministerial Fire" belongs to the Fire element, called life gate fire (*ming men fire*), which is yang vital energy (kidney yang) as opposed to the "Sovereign Fire" of the heart and small intestine.

The yin organ of Ministerial Fire is pericardium, of the heart, that is the tissues surrounding the heart organ, playing the roles of (1) protecting the heart from external sick Qi invasion and (2) regulating Qi or dissipating the excess Qi from the heart and directing it to the Laogong cavity/acupoint, which is located in the center of the palm. While the yang organ energy system triple burner includes three parts, upper burner (chest, neck, head, heart, lungs, and functions of heart and lungs), middle burner (the area between the chest and navel including functions of stomach, liver and spleen), and lower burner (below the navel including kidneys and bladder). The triple burner energy integrates all major organs and energy meridians together and helps them stay balanced and in communication, playing a backbone role for the life and health.

As shown in Fig. 7.2, the 24 hours of a day are divided into 6 time periods (4 hours for each), representing the corresponding elements, and the elements of organs/meridians and emotions as described above. Each period is subdivided into two time frames (2 hours for each), corresponding to the yin and yang organs/meridians/emotions, respectively.

For instance, for the time period of 11 p.m. – 3 a.m., it is the wood element, within which 11 p.m. – 1 a.m. is the wood yang, corresponding to the wood yang organ, the gallbladder, while 1 a.m. – 3 a.m. is the wood yin time, corresponding to the wood yin organ, the liver. From 3 a.m. to 5 a.m., it is the metal yang organ, the lung, and while from 5 a.m. to 7 a.m., it is the metal yin organ, the large intestine. From 7 a.m. to 9 a.m., it is the earth yang organ, the stomach, while from 9 a.m. to 11 a.m., the earth yin organ spleen. During 11 a.m. through 1 p.m., it is time for the fire yang organ, the heart, while 1 p.m. to 3 p.m., is the time for fire yin organ, the small intestine. In the late afternoon, 3 p.m. to 5 p.m. is the time for water yang organ, the bladder, while 5 p.m. to 7 p.m. is the water yin organ, the kidney. Lastly, from 7 p.m. to 9 p.m., it is the time for ministerial fire yang organ, the pericardium, while from 9 p.m. to 11 p.m. is the time for triple burner, which is the yang organ of ministerial fire.

This entire breakdown is listed in the table below. As we understand from this natural clock in which we live, our organs are functioning along with the energy process of the universe, especially our home solar system and earth world. Ancient cultivators used to practice meditation at a certain time period to accumulate energy from the universe (e.g., 11 p.m. to 1 a.m.), because of this natural law. For sleep and rest time, as a longevity health practitioner or cultivator, you also should practice this energy clock in daily life. We often see many people live in a disordered living schedule that goes against this natural law of energy process, resulting in physiological and mental dysfunctions.

Element	Yang		Yin	
Wood	11pm – 1am	Gallbladder	1am – 3am	Liver
Meter	3am – 5am	Lung	5am – 7am	Large Intestine
Earth	7am – 9am	Stomach	9am – 11am	Spleen
Fire	11am – 1pm	Heart	1pm – 3pm	Small Intestine
Water	3pm – 5pm	Bladder	5pm – 7pm	Kidney
Ministerial Fire	7pm – 9pm	Pericardium	9pm – 11pm	Triple Burner

§7.3 Teaching from The Ancient Medicine – Original MBM

Earlier we discussed the ancient medicine book titled, *Yellow Emperor's Classic of Internal Medicine* [1]. We reviewed a conversation between the Yellow Emperor and the heavenly teacher, physician Qi Bo (or Chi Bo) in which Qi Bo explained that people of ancient times had lived much longer lives, as long as one hundred and twenty years with no signs of weakening movements. He, on the other hand, also said that people "nowadays" (and remember this was many, many years ago) become weakened in their movements at an age of less than sixty years old. Of issue in The Emperor's and Qi Bo's exchange was an attempt to figure out whether this change in average life-span was "due to a change in the natural environment or due to man's faults?"

Qi Bo replied: "The ancient people who knew the proper way to live had followed the pattern of Yin-Yang which is the regular pattern of heaven and earth. They remained in harmony with heaven-earth's natural follows which are the great principles of human life, ate and drank with moderation, and lived their daily lives in a regular pattern with neither excess nor abuse. For this reason, their spirits and bodies had remained in perfect harmony with each other, and consequently, they could live out their natural life span and die at the age of over one hundred and twenty years."

Recall how Qi Bo went on to explain that people "nowadays" (back then – but also applies to us now) are quite different, because they intoxicate themselves exorbitantly, replace a normal life with a life of abuse, have sexual intercourse while intoxicated, exhaust their pure energy through gratification of their desires, waste their true energy through careless and prolonged consumption, fail to retain their energy in abundance and to guard their spirits constantly, rush to the gratification of their hearts to the contrary of the true happiness of life, and live their daily lives in an irregular pattern. He held this as the main reason why they can only live half of their life span.

The teaching of the ancient sage was such that one should avoid the deficiency vicious energies and the stealing wind (that of energy consumption) constantly, that one should live a quiet life with few desires so that he could retain his true energy and his internal spirits that are the effective weapons to head off the attack of disease.

Consequently, Qi Bo offered that an individual should be able to maintain an easy-going attitude with fewer desires, to sustain a peaceful mind without fear, to work without fatigue, to retain a smooth energy circulation, to satisfy his desires naturally, and to obtain the satisfaction of every need. Therefore, he felt, we should be content with whatever delicious foods as available to us, with whatever customs of our society, with whatever class we belong to. This is what we call the truly satisfied individual.

This was the teaching of ancient medicine, the original mind-body medicine as it addressed daily lifestyle and encouraged people to live in the natural way, by letting go of attachments and desires and following the principle of Yin-Yang and Five Elements. It is a very different lifestyle and ideology from the way people live and think today.

In the ancient times, people preferred the simpler lifestyle with a more focused mind, internal peace and happiness, and strong connection to true Self internally and the beauty of nature, universe and spiritual realms. People nowadays, in contrast, are more focused on and influenced by things outside of true Self. These things often include various aspects of material life, excitements, desires, busy-ness and rapidly changing lifestyles with addictions to computers, drugs, overwhelming information and distractions, and so on. Modern people are surrounded by outward-pursuing (material world-focused) activities that distort, mislead, pollute, overwhelm, overload and confuse people. As such, people's minds are full of these distracting messages, and their lifestyle is disturbed by too many factors.

People have become used to working so hard and devoting more efforts and time toward material life, at the neglect of daily health of body and mind. Therefore, their living schedule is messed up, often keeping them up late into night. Some young people (as well as adults) drink alcohol at late night hours and sometimes don't return home from such binges until the a.m. Many individuals stay up late (or get up in the middle of the night) and work or surf around on their computers for hours on end. Some teenagers attach to computer games to the point of addiction and do not get enough sleep and overall mental downtime, leaving little to no time for introspection. All these elements affect people's health of body and mind, as well as their understanding of Self and others and the natural world they are part of and in which they live.

§7.4 Living Schedule for Balance of Yin-Yang & Five Elements

Based on the teaching mentioned above, we should have a good daily living schedule in order to synchronize the energy vibration frequency of mind-body-spirit with the cycling vibration of the universe's energy (earth-solar system). Such a healthy routine lifestyle will balance the mind-body energy of Yin-Yang and Five Elements through a harmonious interaction, synchronization and resonance with the cosmic natural rhythms.

As an example, I would like to recommend the following daily schedule. This daily routine timetable is just for your reference based on a general 8 hours of daytime working schedule.

1. 10:00 p.m. – 11:00 p.m. meditation for 1 hour

2. 11:00 p.m. – 6:00 a.m. night sleep

3. 6:00 a.m. wake up

4. 6:00 – 7:00 a.m. morning practice (Qigong, Taiji / exercise)

5. 7:00 a.m. – 8:00 a.m. breakfast, prepare to leave for work

6. 8:00 a.m. – 5:00 p.m. daytime work or activities

7. 5:00 p.m. – 7:00 p.m. free time, dinner, walk after dinner

8. 7:00 p.m. – 10:00 p.m. free time, arts, entertainments, family time, relaxation, reading, etc.

The above is just an example for anyone who just wants to be healthy and keep a good habit of daily health practice and living schedule. If you are a healthcare practitioner of any type of practice, especially holistic medicine or mind-body medicine, I would like to suggest that you put more time and effort into the practice of daily meditation and movement exercises like Qigong or Taiji.

As another example, the following is a typical schedule I personally live with in my life.

1. 10:00 p.m. – 12:00 p.m. meditation and advanced Qigong cultivation 2 hours

2. 12:00 p.m. – 5:00 a.m. go to bed and sleep

3. 5:00 a.m. wake up

4. 5:00 a.m. – 7:00 a.m. morning practice 2 hours (advanced Qigong cultivation)

5. 7:00 a.m. – 8:00 a.m. breakfast, prepare to leave for work

6. 8:00 a.m. – 6:00 p.m. daytime work and activities

7. 6:00 p.m. – 8:00 p.m. free time, dinner, walk after dinner

8. 8:00 p.m. – 10:00 p.m. free time, art, news, relaxation, reading, etc.

Your actual living schedule may be different because each individual has a different job, personal life, living environment and living conditions. The idea here is to suggest that you sleep on time at 11 p.m. or not later than 12 p.m., and have at least one hour in the morning and one hour at the night of meditation, energy practice and exercises each day. If you are able to do something like this, you will have much better energy, effective daily performance, higher quality of life, overall health and longevity, and less or no sickness.

Do not skip your daily meditation, energy practice and spiritual reading no matter how busy you are. In fact, the time you spend for meditation, energy practice and mind-body cultivation is never a waste and will not shorten your daytime working. On the contrary, you will realize that your daily performance becomes much more efficient, things become much simpler and easier, life is more joyful, and relationships are improved, due to your energetic mind and body, clear-headedness, better focus, and stable and positive emotions achieved by the daily practice. Once you form this habit of daily health practice, you will have much more unexpected good quality of life and health mentally, physically and spiritually.

§7.5 Disordered Yin-Yang Five Elements of Modern Lifestyle

Changing one's habits and lifestyle is not easy. People today seem to have so much work to do, and so many activities and entertainments to enjoy every day. They stay up very late. Some people even stay up to 1 a.m., 2 a.m. or 3 a.m., missing the time needed to restore energy for major organs such as liver, gallbladder, and lung, and they often cannot wake up until 10 a.m. or even later the next day, missing the active functioning time of the organs such as large intestine, stomach, and spleen in the morning. Sometimes people do not get enough sleep and force themselves to wake up to go to work in the morning. Due to this lack of rest and energy in all these major organs, the individual cannot perform energetically in the daytime and cannot feel peaceful emotionally.

The liver and gallbladder are wood element organs, storing energy for emotions, courage, blood and Qi creation and circulation, as well as digestion. Due to a lack of energy in these organs caused by missing sleep at the best time, under the night yin energy condition, daytime activities won't have the support you need from an active, positive and peaceful emotional network and the strong yang energy you need to perform activities.

Such an unhealthy living schedule engenders sickness – mentally and physically. A myriad of illnesses commonly manifest. These can include: depression, anxiety, bipolar disorder, anger, loss of appetite, bad digestion, lack of concentration and slow response, mistakes in daytime performance, even physical diseases such as liver, heart and kidney problems, high blood pressure, and diabetes, and accelerated aging.

The daytime belongs to yang and helps you to be active and perform your activities such as exercise, study, work and other activities, favoring yang life force and energy, and exercising the sympathetic nervous system in balance with parasympathetic nervous system.

The nighttime is yin and helps you calm, rest and restore peaceful yin life force and energy, and favoring the parasympathetic nervous system in balance with the sympathetic nervous system. Lacking sleep at night, however, makes you have low energy at the daytime, which you need to normally stay clearheaded, active, passionate, efficient and positively functioning. As such, you do not have good energy in the daytime or you may even feel tired and sleepy. It becomes easy to get anxious, angry, worrisome, fearful, depressed, unhappy, and joyless with regard to daytime activities. Because your daytime is not performing actively, and your yang energy does not serve to support it, as a result, at nighttime (the yin time) your body and mind do not comply with the clock to stay quiet and sleep. Instead, you stay up until late night after night. This forms a very unhealthy cycle of biological and psychological rhythms that result in negative outcomes to both body and mind.

Eventually the yin and yang of your mind and body are totally flipped or reversed, and all five elements are messed up. Many diseases including depression, anxiety, chronic pain, heart failure, kidney failure, liver diseases and other mental and physiological function disorders are caused by such a disordered lifestyle. No matter how good and expensive the supplements you take or how wealthy your living condition may be, these problems cannot be easily healed until the wrong daily schedule is corrected.

Throughout history, there have been many long living cultivators. Even though because of historical reasons the records are sometimes difficult to find or have never been recorded, we still can list some of their names and ages. These include individuals such as Pengzu, 800; Lao Tzu, 160; Sun Simiao, 孫思邈, 541-682, 141; Li Qingyun, 李清雲 or Li Ching Yuen 李慶遠 1677-1933, 256; and Wu Yunqing, 吳雲青, 160. Here we learn two good examples of longevity practitioners, Li Ching Yuen and Wu Yunqing, and will introduce other longevity cultivators in other following chapters.

On May 15, 1933, TIME magazine published a report titled "CHINA: Tortoise-Pigeon-Dog" [99] to introduce the story of the 256 (based on investigators) or 197 (1677-1933, based on his own story) years of long living Chinese medicine physician (herbalist), martial art master, Qigong cultivator, longevity practitioner and educator Li Ching Yuen. He wrote a book called *Knack of Longevity* (長生不老訣). The book was written in well-organized poetical style of Chinese, sharing 10 secrets for longevity living: (1) meditation, (2) quiet mind, (3) cultivating mind nature, (4) letting go of attachments on desires, lust and human sentiments or emotions, (5) firm belief and sincere faith, (6) unmovable mind staying still and peaceful, (7) inward cultivation, (8) simplifying lifestyle and daily things, (9) clearheaded to see through the truth, (10) deep stillness developing wisdom.

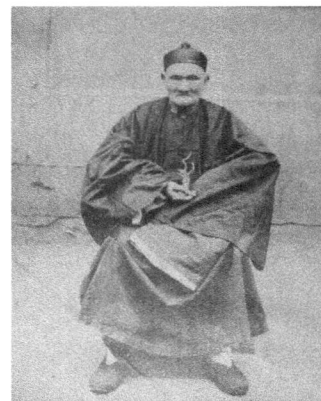

Li Ching Yuen further summarized his longevity principle into four words:

慈 (ci) - Kind heart, never harm others and surroundings, cultivate peaceful energy, live to the maximum length of natural age.

儉 (jian) – Simple foods that does not harm the stomach, less desires to remain internal vitality, cultivating mouth (talk with clear mind never say things meaningless by subconsciousness) to remain energy, meaningful yet less social activities that keep mind and body clean and avoid being contaminated by bad energies, and having simple thoughts and no worry and anxiousness.

和 (he) – Peaceful to others in family, friendship and society.

靜 (jing) – Quiet, calm, peaceful and cheerful mind, unmovable heart (not frivolous), never over work to harm your body.

When people asked him what are the secrets of his long living life, he told "Keep a quiet heart, sit like a tortoise, walking sprightly like a pigeon, and sleep like a dog," meaning mind, body and spirit stay still, focused, relax and quiet. It said that his longevity lifestyle includes three factors: vegetarian foods, peaceful and cheerful mind and drinking teas of lotus leaf, cassia, mangosteen, and wolfberry, keeping good circulation of blood and Qi (energy), and preventing difficult urination and constipation.

In his 100th birthday he received award from the government due to his excellent achivement in Chinese herbal medicine, and when he was 200 years old, he could still often give lectures to the universities. During that period of time he was actively interviewed by western media.

Another long living example is Wu Yunqing. His living schedule is a good example of following nature's energy clock.

The Tao and Buddhist cultivator Wu Yunqing was born in Dec. 13, 1838. He started his practice of Taoism and Buddhism when he was 18 years old. At the age of 100, he still looks young, energetic, and healthy. His heart rate 72, blood pressure 140/80, height 1.59 meters, weight 53 kg, good eyesight and hearing ability, muscles and skin are still strong, climbs a mountain like a young man. He does not get sick even in the hot summer and cold winter. He often walks in the mountains without shoes. He does not eat meat but many varieties of vegetables. October 12, 1996 he taught cultivation to over 1000 students from all over the world, he made a joke, "Chicken, duck, fish, meat, and eggs, are big villains" (egg is pronounced as Dan in Chinese, and the word for villain is Huai Dan, meaning bad Dan). All the people were laughing. In fact, he really meant that eating no meat is his way to stay healthy and live long. After he shared his secret of long living life, he recited the following poem:

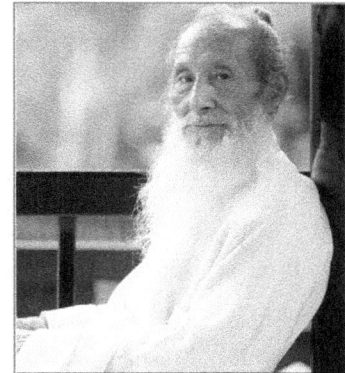

酒色財氣四堵牆 *Alcohol, lust, money and emotion are the four walls,*
世人都在牆裡藏 *People are caged inside the courtyard.*
有人能跳牆外去 *If someone can jump over the wall and go outside,*
不是神仙也壽長 *He will be either an Immortal or have a long life.*

He shared his cultivation practice in another poem:

練精化氣氣化神 *Practice essence to develop energy which uplifts spirit,*
練神還虛保自身 *Cultivate spirit to return to the emptiness and true self,*
自身自有靈丹藥 *One's own Self has the immortal medicine,*
何需深山把藥尋 *Why need to search long life medicine in the deep mountain?*

His day starts at 5 clock in the early morning, and his first thing activity of the day is two hours of *Lian Gong* (cultivation meditation and energy movement), followed by breakfast, field work, noon cultivation practice, afternoon field work, cultivation practice, dinner, walk, then sleep, then middle of the night cultivation practice, and then night sleep.

Wu Yunqing eats very simple and ordinary, never fussy food. His main foods are millet porridge, rice, noodles, and Chinese bread (*Man Tou*), buns, dumplings and the likes. He eats more common vegetables such as Chinese cabbage, cabbage, pumpkin, winter melon, cucumber, potato, tomato, babe cabbage, etc. Wu Yunqing has three meals a day, no meat and no onion, green onion or garlic because he think they produce turbid (aggregate) Qi as he told his disciples. He works with his disciples in the field like a villager, 3 hours in the morning and 3 hours in the afternoon, and meditates in between four times each day (*see* his daily life schedule at the end of this section).

Wu Yunqing lives happy and enjoys his cultivation life. Even though he is over 100 years old, he is so energetic and passionate about what he does, cultivating every day, teaching students to cultivate, and encouraging people to practice cultivation. When he gave the big lecture to nearly 1000 students from all over the world, he repeatedly told the audiences: now is the last chance to cultivate during this law's wheel spinning period, otherwise you have to wait 120 thousand of years.

Time	Activity
5 am ~ 7 am	Morning practice
7 am ~ 8 am	Breakfast
8 am ~ 11 am	Field work
11 am ~ 1 pm	Noon practice
1 pm ~ 2 pm	Lunch
2 pm ~ 5 pm	Field work
5 pm ~ 7 pm	Afternoon practice
7 pm ~ 8 pm	Dinner and then walk
8 pm ~ 9 pm	Taiji and activities

9 pm ~ 11 pm	Sleep
11 pm ~ 1 am	Middle night practice
1 am ~ 5 am	Sleep

Table 7.6. Wu Yunqing's daily life schedule.

§7.7 A Clinical Case of Depression and Fatigue

One day, Cherry's husband David called in and made an appointment for his wife. He said that Cherry was diagnosed with severe depression with the possibility of Schizophrenia. This, he said, was diagnosed in accordance with her symptoms of random non-communicative speech, cursing people, losing interest in activities, etc. Her condition seemed to be getting worse and worse of late. She had no improvement with conventional medicine, psychotherapy, Chinese herbal medicine, and acupuncture.

This brought her to our clinic. She wanted to try something alternative and integrative. She and her husband were in their early 40s and very nice. Her husband was caring and she is a nice looking wife. After I heard about her condition and history in the first half of the initial session, it was obvious that Cherry had very severe depression and fatigue.

She told us that she had stayed in the bed all the time – every day. For the past year, she explained, she never woke up before 3 p.m. At night, she said, it always took hours to finally fall asleep and sometimes she'd find herself up until 3 or 4 a.m.

Scientifically there is no clear clue about what causes depression and schizophrenia. Some researchers suggest these may be caused by an imbalance of brain chemicals that result in dysfunctional messages in the brain. Even assuming this is true, however, nobody knows what causes the brain chemical imbalance. Commonly, scientists in these fields believe that schizophrenia as well as depression, like many other illnesses, seems to be the result of a combination of genetic, environmental, psychological factors related with each individual's life. Conventional medicine often uses psychiatric drugs to try to balance the brain chemicals, but in holistic natural medicine, we question those drugs because we know that there is no such precise way to really identify which and how to what extent various brain chemicals are imbalanced and how to balance them. Our body is a complicated and dedicated self-balanced system. Brain chemicals are dynamically generating, cascading and consuming constantly and automatically.

As we trace over Cherry's entire life journey, it seems Cherry did not have a well-parented childhood. What was missing was the parental care and advice that provides appropriate guiding posts and helps establish good personality, peaceful attitude, healthy thinking pattern, value system, good and necessary living habits and lifestyle.

Cherry grew up in her own way, without a cultivated regular daily schedule and organized lifestyle. Additionally, her communication skills were under-developed, which snowballed into an overall lack of finesse in fitting in and getting along with others, as well as getting her own needs met. As a result, relationships, for Cherry, were often difficult.

Others perceived her as self-centered and difficult to live and work with. On other hand, she very much wanted to be loved and cared for. Her need for love may have partly been driven by the lack of love and care from her parents. It was what she'd missed from the beginning of life and, in fact, what had left her wanting – and needy.

Cherry had no clear self-awareness. Her character seemed immature and her thoughts and actions often appeared random as well as driven by random ideas and random people. Nonetheless, she does not really follow others and is not a team player.

She jumped from one job to another a lot, many times re-locating from one living place to another. At the beginning of whatever she does, she shows excitement, but after a while, she gets bored and quits on it, then starts searching for something else – it's a constant search, for Cherry, for that something else.

She kept repeating the same dysfunctional patterns over and over. She would feel very confused, anxious. And this would eventually spiral her into depression, coupled with an increase in her use of violent language and behaviors. She often cursed people, threw away things of significance, broke furniture, fought with and even beat her husband.

She was finally diagnosed with chronic depression by her clinical psychologist, but her psychiatrist had already begun medicating her for schizophrenia. As she took those drugs, however, she only got worse. Now, she developed symptoms that involved the drugs themselves – e.g. she felt tired, numb, she started getting headaches, chest tightening, and felt sleepy all the time, yet, was unable rest well even though she would get over 16 hours sleep. She had been like this for about a year when we met.

How do we understand this case, and where and how do we start to help Cherry?

Although her family doctor and psychologist diagnosed Cherry respectively with typical chronic depression and schizophrenia, in mind-body holistic medicine, we try to understand her case with a different lens, looking for *root cause,* from the concept of energy – in fact, all energy – associated factors such as: overall health, history of personal development, lifestyle, psychological factors, family and social factors, living environment, and daily schedule. Of major focus will be the energy imbalance, which will allow us to understand and improve her condition.

By reading her pulses, both kidney yin and yang deficiency, liver Qi overheated and blocked, heart yin deficiency and internal heat in spleen and stomach, are observed. It is not surprising because she does not sleep at night and is always lying in bed for long periods of time during the day, so yin and yang are completely reversed and messed up, causing an overall yin Qi deficiency for the major organs. Her yang Qi cannot grow because the yin is low. As a result, the internal heat built up over a long time period, and her calming, soothing and, at the same time, the cooling yin energy (she needs to balance this heat buildup) is very low.

As known in traditional Chinese medicine, the Three Treasures (Essence, Qi and Spirit or in Chinese called Jing, Qi and Shen, 精氣神), are the most important energy forms at different levels (physical, mental and spiritual, respectively). Qi is the energy within the body and mind that drives blood and physical or biological substances moving and circulating throughout the body. Essence is the fine biochemical substance obtained from food and nutrients, and Spirit is the highest spiritual form of the life origin.

These Three Treasures are related, influencing and dependent upon each other. They have to comply with the original law and energy principle of yin and yang and five elements. When yin and yang are reversed, as in Cherry's case, and energy is deficient, Qi gets messed up and runs low, and functions of the body and mind are disturbed and disordered. It's why Cherry cannot eat well, digest well, and cannot intake good nutrients, which in turn, is causing her essence to be totally deficient.

Without rich Essence and Qi, of course, her spirit becomes blurry, scattered, weak, and caught in a downward cycle. It is why her pulse tells that her kidney yin and yang is deficient (Kidney Stores Essence), her liver Qi (Liver Stores Soul) is overheated and blocked, heart yin (Heart Stores Spirit) is deficient, and the internal empty heat in the spleen and stomach is high, digestion and appetite are bad. She, therefore, cannot obtain Essence from foods, and all this is forming into the negative feedback circle. The heart stores the spirit (spiritual and mental energy - vitality), so when its energy is low, the spirit cannot be held within her mind, and her spirit becomes scattered and blurry, making her crazy, and uncontrollable, generating huge blocks and heat that affected her liver, and causes a lot of anger. It is why she behaves so angry, anxious and even crazy.

To heal Cherry's problem, the key is to rebalance her yin and yang energy, cool down internal heat/fire, as well as harmonize her energies at all levels, restoring her Essence, Qi and Spirit.

Cherry did see a regular Chinese medicine doctor, but this doctor's only using Chinese herbal medicine as a stand-alone treatment did not work on her mind, spirit and energy, simultaneously (which is what she needed) from all levels. It is important to note: The reason why regular Chinese medicine does not heal all of Cherry's problems of body, mind and spirit is its lack of attention to the multiplicity of the problem and its causes which are rooted at **all** levels: physically, mentally and spiritually.

Cherry's health issues demand a truly integrated holistic treatment that deals with body, mind and spirit – simultaneously – to restore Jing Qi Shen (Essence, Energy and Spirit).

In our clinic, we successfully helped Cherry's condition by using Brainwave Meridian Therapy (BMT) with a combination of therapeutic Yin-Yang-Five-Elements energy music healing, meditation, hypnotherapy, and spiritual and psychological teaching and conversation. We will introduce the details about BMT and its associated healing system in later chapters, where we will fully explore the mechanics of this entire aforementioned regiment in detail, by using Cherry's case as example.

The key to helping Cherry heal was to focus on her main conscious mind, help her find her true Self, correct Yin-Yang reversed lifestyle, correct the negative thinking mode, help her use higher Self and principle to guide her thinking, emotions, behavior, activities, healthy diet, and daily living schedule.

BMT successfully helped her restore and rebalance her energy, so she could relieve the internal fire in the liver, restore kidney Qi and heart yin. Therefore, she could now sleep better at nighttime and have some (positive energy producing) activities and exercises during the daytime. Meditation, hypnosis and spiritual conversation and teaching together helped her step back and become more aware of and find her true Self, so she gradually became clearheaded, and her stable conscious mind could now take start "leading" into the better, healthier, positive direction at all levels. Her negative thinking, hate, anger, violence, hopelessness and feelings of non-confidence were eliminated.

Therefore, she felt much more positive, hopeful and joyful. She could wake up early and go to park to do exercises and meditation. She is now also able to involve herself in some community and family activities she had not participated in for a long time. She no longer needs all her former medications and has started her normal healthy (and healthy feeling) cultivating life.

§7.8 Proposed Model of Mind-Body-Spirit

After the theoretical and practical discussions about the mind, body and spirit, and before we get into actual applications of these principles and practice, we propose the following model of mind-body-spirit as a summary to this point. This proposed model describes the mechanism by which the mind-body-spirit operates as a whole living being.

The spirit is an energy form that pervades the whole being, and its surrounding spaces with bigger or smaller area range depending on cultivation energy level. This energy field can be as big as the entire universe if a high level of cultivation is achieved. An ordinary person, however, may just have an energy field within and surrounding the physical body. The energy field has a central point and its energy particles are spread surrounding the central point. We name this central point of the energy field as the Spirit Energy Center (SEC).

During this physical lifetime, the SEC is supposed to stay with the body and mind, positioned at the Dantian point (around belly area). The energy within and surrounding the body and mind is circulating surrounding the Energy Center and along the pathway networks (meridians), and connects to and communicates with the universe's supreme spirit, in order to sustain its energetic state, its integrity, unification and cooperative functionalism of the whole being.

The centralized degree of the Spirit Energy Center within the living being and the size, quality, purity and power of this energy field depends upon the person's cultivation level of the spirit. The higher his/her cultivation level is, the more centralized the spirit is, the bigger the size of its energy field is, the higher quality and purity it has, and more powerful it is, the better the energy circulation within the body and mind is, the stronger the connection and communication of the person's spirit with the higher supreme spirit is.

Otherwise, if the Spirit Energy Center shifts away from the original central point within the whole being (Dantian area), goes around outside the living being, scattered over different places outside the body and mind, and is driven far away from the spiritual connection by material attractions and desires, or if the energy pathway (meridian) is blocked, energy is not smoothly circulated or has low, negative or impure energy or a small energy field, if one lost spiritual and mental clarity and righteousness, stays in a clouded or confused state, or if the life energy is contaminated by lower dimensional energy or evil spirit energy, then the Oneness of the human being will be deteriorate, and the body and mind at this physical dimension will lose support from the higher energy, higher spiritual guide and the higher power to integrate the whole being. This results in sickness, disease, discomfort, premature aging, and/or loss of life.

Therefore, in this life, cultivation through higher spiritual guidance and energetic meditation practice will help centralize the Spirit Energy Center within the body and mind; energize the spirit, body and mind; keep the energy pathways open and allow the energy to circulate smoothly within the body, mind and spirit. The practice helps connect the Spirit (SEC as well) and whole being with the universe's original Supreme Spirit and energy source, and ground the whole being and stabilize the mind-body-spirit as one unified, living being. This is why cultivation requires the cultivator to focus inside his or her own mind, improving the inner self, yet not for the purpose of attaching to the materialism of the physical world

After this physical life, however, the Spirit Energy Center goes to other dimensions at it certain level, depending on the life's spiritual quality. It can go to a higher dimension such as the Buddha / God's kingdoms, stay at human level for next reincarnation, or fall down to a lower place such as hell. If one is cultivated well and achieved high Virtue during past lives and this life, and reached consummation of cultivation, then he/she can reach higher places such as Buddha / God's dimension. If one is not cultivated or not cultivated well, or has created a lot of Karma, then he/she will have to go down to a lower level.

To cultivate to a higher level, one should have a high standard of spiritual guidance to assimilate with the universe's characteristics: having a great compassion and forgiveness, being truthful, and being energized with the universe's energy vibration frequencies: Yin and Yang and Five Elements or Beyond.

The mind-body medicine and healthology is the science, teaching, guidance and practice to help its scientists, practitioners, patients or any individuals understand, study, research, learn and practice this mind-body-spirit model as described above.

§7.9 Meditation: Balanced Yin-Yang and Five Elements

EHM07: Let Go and Stay High *(Yang, Earth, Fire)*

This music is composed with focus on the relatively yang energy of earth and fire elements to strengthen your stomach and heart energy. However if you feel you are over heated, anxious, overwhelmed, have too much heat internally or feel too excited and ungrounded emotionally (yang type of condition), then you can choose the following CD (yin type of the healing music) to practice.

EHM08: Assimilate with Earth & Heaven *(Yin, Earth, Fire)*

This chapter discussed the universe as a balanced energy system of Yin-Yang and Five Elements. At the same time, the universe has a great spirit with the characteristics of peace, compassion, love, truthfulness, forgiveness and tolerance. Now [*Play Energy Healing Music #7*], I invite you to meditate with me on this profound energetic system – the whole universe. With your clear conscious mind and quiet subconscious mind, imagine you are sitting on the great land, meditating under the sky, let go of human mindset and thoughts, being one with the universe, and assimilating to its characteristics and its great energy. Keep your mind still, righteous, and clear as you luxuriate in this crystal clear, transparent and enlightening world. Your true conscious mind peacefully and clearly guides your entire life journey into cultivation, balance, purification, focus and groundedness with the energy, spirit and character of the universe.

Feel your mind, body and spirit are integrated, balanced and elevated to a much higher level. All are in the Whole One, unified and purified.

Carry this great and restorative energy into your daily life. Let it re-vitalize you. Let it re-organized you and perfectly balance you with the energy system of Yin-Yang and Five Elements. Tap into this energy and mindset often. Use it to stay calm, confident, positive, active, clearheaded, humble, grounded, intelligent, productive and creative in the daytime and sleep peacefully in the evenings. All unhealthy habits, living schedules, imbalanced nutrition, random unconscious thoughts, addictions and attachments can be eliminated, and you can nourish and re-charge yourself in the profound, deep, creative, intelligent, meaningful and spiritual wisdoms from the heavens and reach a high level living within this life and your eternal future life.

§7.10 Exercise Questions

1. What is the Energy Mechanism of the Universe at this material dimension?

2. How is the energy mechanism of the universe applied in the mind and body, and what are the characteristics of Yin-Yang in within the mind and body?

3. What are the Five Elements of the mind and body, and how is the clock of the earth-solar system associated with the natures of The Five Elements and their corresponding human organs? How are 24 hours of a day correlated to The Five Elements and, as well, the organs of the human being?

4. How do you understand the information cited in this chapter regarding the Ancient Mind-Body-Spirit medicine and *The Yellow Emperor's Medicine*, regarding healthy lifestyle? What are the inspiring teaching points you can acquire from these that are applicable to people's contemporary lifestyles and living schedules? How can lifestyle and living schedule affect people's health issues? Base your answers on the principles of Yin-Yang and Five Elements and the natural clock of the earth-solar system.

5. What is your daily schedule so far? Is your schedule the best for your health or may you want to make modifications after reading this chapter?

6. How does this chapter help you check your patient/client health issues with better understanding of his/her lifestyle or living schedule?

7. Can you give an example from your own experience, or a family member, friend or patient's, and describe how the balanced energy of Yin-Yang and Five Elements play a major role in generating a healthy lifestyle/living schedule for the health of mind and body. Conversely, can you supply and a real life example of how the imbalance of these and bad lifestyle/living schedule affects the mind-body health?

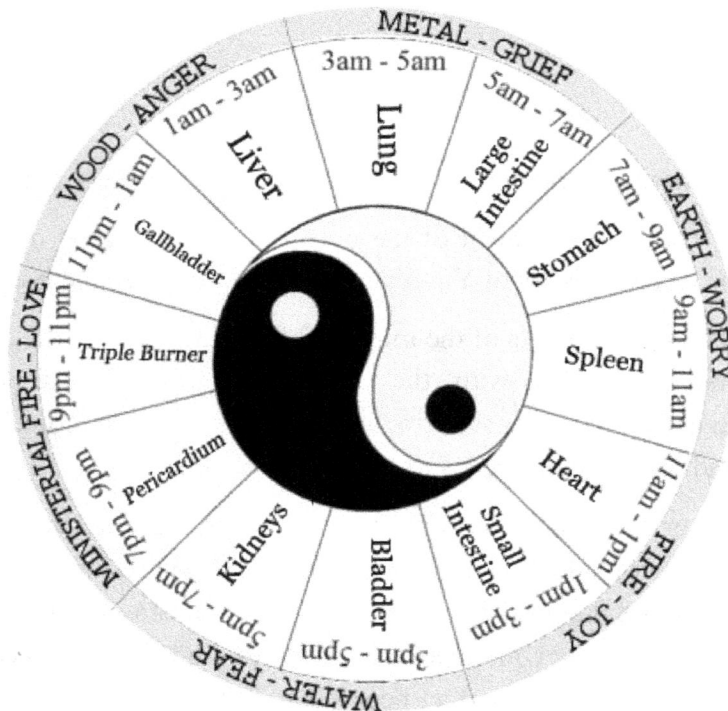

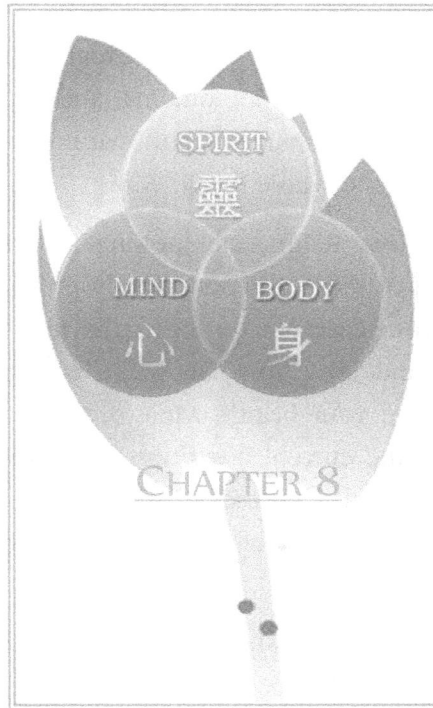

Modern Life Needs Integrated Mind-Body Medicine

Nowadays there are many mind-body healthcare modalities. Each of them has a different set-up, ranging from methodologies to the facility, procedures, advantages and disadvantages. For example, Chinese medicine, naturopathic medicine, psychotherapy, and psychiatric medicine, these are all working on the mind and body. We are not going to address all details about all these modalities because it is impossible to cover all these therapies in one book, and it is also not the purpose and focus of this book. However, we can principally and conceptually discuss some basic differences in characteristics between these practices, so that you can better understand the reason why a deeply integrated medicine is indeed needed for healing modern diseases and improving the health condition of modern people.

As known commonly, Chinese medicine today mainly uses approaches such as needle acupuncture and natural herbs, and other naturopathic medicine practices such as clinical nutrition, physical therapies, and homeopathy, in addition to Chinese herbs and acupuncture. Each of these modalities has their own facility, method, procedures and great benefits as well as limitations.

When visiting most of these doctors, you will realize that they are experts in their techniques of: needles, herbs, nutrition, supplements, and hands on therapy, but most of them rarely talk about mental issues, consider emotional and mental factors and the mind-body connection as part of healing the whole being.

After the typical TCM four diagnoses; looking at, smelling and questioning the patient, and reading pulse, most of these doctors directly proceed to their treatment, but do not explain how they look at your case nor do they offer any further communication with you about why you get sick and how you can make changes in your mind, thinking, cognition and lifestyle to improve your health. Most of them do not teach you systematic mind-body practice to improve the current condition and prevent future health problems. Modern naturopathic medicine and Chinese medicine do not make these mental or psychological issues part of their practice and think it is the business of psychologists or psychiatrists.

From the point of view of mind-body health practice, the problem is how an acupuncture treatment or herb formula (as an example) can simply help heal your mind, emotion, lifestyle, relationship, and energy that are the original causes of your health problems, including physical health problems.

As with the case of Cherry, which we addressed in the last chapter, her sickness resulted of multiple causes: spiritual, emotional, mental, physical and energetic. With only herbs, acupuncture, nutrition, and so on, which would have been the course in Chinese medicine or naturopathic medicine, the treatment would not have been effective enough to heal from the root.

What Cherry needed was a fundamental transformation of her energy, mind, thinking, and lifestyle. The reason why Chinese medicine could not help her fundamentally is because the cause (rooted in her mind, mental energy, and spiritual clarity) was left untreated. In other words, the mind, body and spirit were not integrated, and Essence, Qi (energy) and Spirit were not taken care of, at all levels. Spirit and emotion were ignored.

Some Chinese doctors may think that as Qi blocks were eliminated and essence improved, then spirit would be automatically restored. Actually this is not correct because the Qi blocks were at all levels including mental and spiritual levels. Needles and herbs could not reach deep enough into mental, emotional and spiritual levels, could not touch their daily unhealthy thinking pattern, notion, desires, attachments, habits, relationships, could not really wake the patient's soul, true Self to help her/him understand what is good and what is bad, and so on. Therefore the core causes and energy blocks in other dimensions of mind and spirit remained unchanged. This is why regular acupuncture and herbs could not heal the case like Cherry's.

So why were her psychologist and psychiatrist unable to help in Cherry's case? In fact, psychotherapy and psychiatry therapy follow their way of verbal conversations – and in psychiatry drugs as well. These approaches and ideology are totally different from those of energy medicine and mind-body-spirit medicine, which we are addressing in this book. Psychotherapist talks to the patient but does not focus on energy and does not use concepts such as Yin-Yang, Five Elements, Essence, Qi /energy, and spirit, cultivation of the spirit and mind by following clear principles such as the spiritual law and energy principle of the universe. Psychology is the science at human level, which addresses the life issues based on human logics, ideas, emotions, and biological science, so it only addresses some issues from surface but not really the real cause in the deep level of the mind and spirit with energy transformation.

Psychiatrists mainly rely on drug treatment, manipulating brain chemistries and forcing the patient to a mood of lowered energy. This form of treatment is very different from energy focused healing that crosses multiple dimensions of the body, mind and spirit integratively at the same time to restore and rejuvenate the original life force mechanism.

Both psychologist and psychiatrist are relying more on modern medicine such as brain science, neurology, and psychiatric drugs. These approaches are more involved with taking care of the issues that appear on the surface, but are not reaching into core causes.

Cherry had already lost her energy and interest for daily life performance, so her day and night completely reversed, she did not feel good, and lost hope about her own health and life. Under such a condition, psychiatric drugs only desensitized, numbed and inhibited her nervous system and make her sleepy all the time, so she stood to lose even more energy, and her Yin-Yang energies stood to become even more locked into their reversed cyclical positions. As well, the drug she was prescribed had a lot of negative side effects, further complicating her condition. Regular psychologists could not help her because her main conscious mind was so weak – had no energy to support clear thinking – so no matter how much her psychologist talked to her and tried waking her up or making her more aware, her spirit and conscious mind had no energy with which to listen or understand the conversation, They still remained clouded, had no uplifting strength to wake up, therefore as a result, she could not respond with the necessary clarity.

Without energy, sometimes the logic inspired through psychological conversation can even further confuse and irritate the patient. What she really needed was a peaceful, compassionate, comforting and enlightening energy in her mind, body and spirit that could resonate with her original internal vibration, energize her life force and uplift her spirit and conscious mind. But conventional psychotherapy and psychiatry do not have such energetic power.

Through the case addressed above, it is clear that mind-body health problems like Cherry's need some work dealing in the areas of body, mind, spirit, energy, lifestyle, eating habit, living schedule, thinking, personality, and general habits in order to improve all these aspects of her profile and help her turn the corner toward better health and happiness. The key is to integrate the body, mind and spirit *at the same time* through a practice that involves powerful energetic vibrations to resonate, synchronize, harmonize, balance and transform the whole being to a new energetic level. Such practice is where the integrative medicine is supposed to come from.

Integrative medicine is not simply putting different therapies together to treat a patient.

Integration is not equal to sum or adding together. The integration of mind-body health practices or so called integrative medicine means to integrate the mind, body and spirit into one unified life system through an internally integrated practice that may or may not involve multiple therapeutic modalities, but that covers multiple levels of healing work mentally, physically, spiritually and energetically, ***at the same time***.

With the burgeoning popularity of integrated medicine, you may have noticed an increase of integrative medicine centers or holistic medicine centers. Many (if not most) of these are simply putting different treatments or different fields of doctors together to treat patients. In such cases, a patient simply goes through different types of doctors to receive different types of treatments. As such, a patient may see one healthcare practitioner for acupuncture, another for herbs, another for nutrition, another for message therapy, chiropractics, hypnosis, psychotherapy, naturopathic medicine, and the list goes on. This system commonly referred to as integrative leaves the patient busy seeing all kinds of doctors and therapists, one after another. This is fine in terms of holistic medicine that treats patients in different approaches such as natural medicine, psychological therapy, etc. But it does not mean doing these different therapies are integrative medicine. In fact, putting all therapies together is doing nothing in terms of integration of the body, mind and spirit. The key is to integrate multiple levels of healing in order to achieve the true integration of the mind, body and spirit simultaneously. It can (but does not have to) involve multiple approaches. Nonetheless, they must be internally integrated into one smooth healing protocol to meet the needs of a patient. In fact it can be just one single approach, or a few of them, the simpler the better as long as it can integrate the mind, body and spirit into one to heal from the root.

Like Cherry's case, if only working on her body, such as using drug, herb, acupuncture, physical therapy and exercise, such an approach won't completely heal the individual because, as with Cherry, the mind and spirit are still confused, blurry, depressed, negative, anxious and angry, and keep leaking energy and sustaining her condition – which without a truly integrative approach will remain unchanged or even worsen. No matter how many efforts are made on her physical being, as long as the core cause in her mind and spirit remains unchanged, the energy within her whole being won't be improved, and the treatment – whether drug, herb, acupuncture and/or physical therapy won't take effect.

Conventional psychotherapy, for Cherry, is ineffective because under such an exhausted condition, she sustains no interest or energy or the physical and mental strength to understand and absorb the session's talk and consultation. As a result, she will not resonate with the doctor's talk and will not cultivate more positive thoughts and spirits. Even though she may agree with the doctor in the session theoretically, intellectually or logically, afterward she will go back to her condition again because she has no such energy to actually improve her whole being, and the Yin-Yang cycle is still reversed, imbalanced, and her Five Elements energy is still messed up. Therefore, she remains unchanged in her behavior, energy, lifestyle and condition even after psychotherapy sessions.

In addition, talk and teaching that focuses only on philosophical principles or psychological concepts but disregards working on her physical and emotional energy and taking care of her mental feelings won't work either, as she won't have the intention and interest to listen to the session and resonate with the spiritual teaching.

Her energy is low, her emotions low, her mind depressed and negative, and her true spirit is deeply suppressed and tightly masked by the darkness of negative energy. Therefore to really open the door of her mind and introduce a good healing energy into her whole being of mind, body and spirit, the key is to provide a high, pure, deep, strong, powerful, righteous, compassionate, caring, inspiring, effective, and soul-touching therapeutic energy vibration in an integrative mind-body-spirit, multi-level therapy that immediately and effectively makes her feel good mentally and physically, and deeply resonates emotionally and spiritually, and then heals the whole being of body, mind and soul at the same time. We will further discuss such a model, the true Integrative Medicine.

§8.3 True Integration of Mind-Body-Spirit

To truly integrate the whole being of body, mind and spirit and achieve a complete healing, total health and high quality of life performance by an integrative practice, we need to have a complete model of mind-body-spirit holistic therapy. What we don't need is just grabbing some different existing healing modalities and putting them together as a kind of snack pack.

In mind-body integrative medicine system, we look at a patient in a holistic way from all levels of body, mind, spirit and energy. We need to understand the case from an integrating, interacting and multi-dimensional scope of insight into the entire being of mind, body and spirit. As well, we need insight into the person's growth, personal development, parents, family, education, work, relationship, social experience, personality, character, habits, lifestyle, and psychological, mental, physical, nutritional, genetic and existing environmental factors, and sometimes even extending to the deep understanding of energy vibrations, spiritual life and past lives in other dimensions. Of course, this does not mean that such an integrative medicine doctor has to take so much time and efforts to very carefully research or analyze into all these aspects, one by one, as within other modern sciences. A good practitioner of true integrative medicine should be a good mind-body-spirit cultivator who can immediately sense all these aspects about the patient and design a suitable healing protocol right after a short contact and brief conversation with the patient.

Based on the information regarding all of the above aspects, we simplify the case and find the most important cause from the root to get started with the treatment at all levels of body, mind, emotion, spirit, energy, personality, lifestyle, and so on, simultaneously in one integrated therapy.

Again, we use Cherry's case as example. After acquiring a profile at our initial session and reviewing her own (and family's) as well professional reports on her condition and case history and evaluating her energy status based on the conventions of traditional Chinese medicine, we understood the following factors:

1.   Physically she is not diagnosed with any physical disease. She cannot, however, function well because of low energy, bad sleep and living schedule, unhealthy eating habit and imbalanced nutrition, depression, fatigue, pain all over her body, no interests in anything, not getting along with people including family members, fearful of meeting with people, and trying to hide herself from the public all the time – typical symptoms of severe depression, and some negative symptoms of schizophrenia.

2.   From Chinese medicine diagnosis (energy status checkup), obviously she is dramatically deficient in kidney Qi (both yin and yang), heart yin, high spleen

and stomach heat and fire, and blockages in liver Qi. Her soul or spirit is scattered all over other places, but is not harmonized with her Self.

3.   She did not have a good childhood experience with enough care from parents to develop a good mature personality, lifestyle, communication skills, social contact skills, and living habits.

4.   She is a young and smart lady with a master's degree education. She is a spiritual person believing in god and has the intention to be a good person in general and a good cultivator spiritually. She also has some Eastern and Western beliefs such as Karma, Virtue, past lives, fate, Buddhism, and cultivation.

5.   She never really fell in love with her husband to whom she was introduced by a friend, but for some reason she got married. This is what she typically does for many things in this life; without clear self-awareness.   Instead she rather unconsciously and randomly falls into the things that happen to and for her. When she finally realized her marriage was a regrettable mistake, she felt it was too late to make any correction.

6.   She thinks negatively about most things including life, her relationship with family, friends and others. She easily gets mad, generally expressing herself and behaving with anger, hate and disappointment.

After looking at all these factors in Cherry's case, where will we get started? As we addressed in the previous section, her Chinese doctor treated her with herbs and acupuncture to improve Qi status over her kidney, liver, spleen and heart meridians, while her psychologist tried to work on her depression and help her improve the negative emotions and behaviors. However, these treatments did not work for her.

As an example of applied mind-body medicine, the following describes the approach we took with Cherry in our clinic. The immediate difference in approach was our focus on her mind, body and spirit as a whole unit. Our mechanism was energy therapy at multiple levels.

First of all, we suggested that she not think that she has a depression or schizrenia that can never heal or that will be difficult to heal. She had gotten so many negative or hopeless impressions of her mind with regard to severe depression and schizophrenia from the diagnosis and treatment process of conventional medicine in the hospital. Her family, nervous themselves about her situation, increased the pressure she felt about getting healthy again.

> ***Her mind and living environment were inundated and suppressed in negativity and this became the first negative energy vibration we had to get rid of, if we wanted to heal her.***

"Cherry, do not worry, you can be healed," we told her at the very first session. We explained to her with very positive encouragement: "The reason why you get sick like this is simply because you do not have enough of good (high quality/higher level) energy to ward off the difficulties. Your living schedule is messed up; your day and night are essentially reversed, meaning that the yin and yang of your body and mind are reversed and energetically imbalanced. Your mind is noisy and confused."

> ***Very importantly I told her: "All these factors are just at the energy level, and I can help you improve them, so don't worry, you can get healed soon."***

We could see that Cherry is an understanding person and still had strong intentions of getting herself better. Further, we strongly believe that as long as a doctor is positive and encouraging, it will create strong positive energy to empower a patient to heal. This positive thought and angle to our approach were applied throughout the entire process of Cherry's healing journey. In fact, we did more than just encourage – we made sure to energetically display confidence in her healing. After our explanation regarding her condition, she felt more hopeful about her health, and emotionally she felt a lot of better and positive. Actually, this had been what she really wanted.

She never had someone in her life helping her create a healthy lifestyle, positive thinking and optimistic personality. She highly looked forward to a new and healthy Self at the end of her healing journey.

Our conversation made her understand that human beings get sick for a reason, and the healing process of a disease is a good opportunity to learn a lesson that we missed somewhere along the line. If one can consider healing as an opportunity, then sickness and its healing can be a good thing for the future.

At the clinic, we encouraged Cherry with the idea that we would all work together and make this a positive change. She fully agreed.

We used Brainwave-Meridian Therapy (BMT) combined with hypnosis, Yin-Yang and Five Elements energy sounds, meditation, exercises, spiritual teaching, and Qigong to improve her energy, empty her mind, stop her negative thinking and negative subconscious activities, balance hormones, improve sleep quality (in fact she could sleep much more deeply and restfully during the session right away). The key was to work on her energy at the physical, mental, emotional, and spiritual levels – again, at the same time (all these were integrated into her treatment session) and follow with a combination of teaching her self-improvement practice, self-recognition about her own problems, unhealthy habits, negative thinking over the long years, and giving her activities to practice at home.

All these steps were taken at the same time. Of course, we were careful not to overload her. We further helped her improve her energy and strengthen her emotions by deeply hypnotizing her with positive inductions, suggestions and powerful energy vibration of the energy healing music. Her conscious and subconscious mind could get quiet during the session. Therefore she felt good and was able to get the deep sleep she so needed.

After that, she restored a lot of energy, looked much better, with peaceful eye contact and nice smiles. During our session meditation, we combined guided imaginary therapy with energetic induction of relaxation and positive spiritual teaching while both she and the doctor's eyes closed with the energy music in the background.

The teaching talk naturally went deeper and deeper while her feelings got deeper and deeper. As the patient progressed and her emotional mood improved, the talk in the sessions reached a point where she could respond with perfect clarity and comprehension. The teaching brought her into the great energy field of universe produced during the doctor-patient joint meditation. Note: The talking was a teaching about the universe, about the Yin-Yang and The Five Elements, about the human body, mind, and spirit resonating with the universe's natural law to live healthy and comfortable. Then naturally the session proceeded to points on how she could restore a balanced, peaceful, healthy energy state by changing her thinking mode positively, her lifestyle and schedule into a healthy time-frame, sleeping and waking up on time, and participating in activities and exercise in the daytime, as well as reading spiritual books and meditating with empty and peaceful mind. Our sessions became longer than other treatments. They always ran for a minimum of two hours and sometimes went two and half hours, like the initial session.

§8.4 Key Elements in Integrative Health of Mind-Body-Spirit

You may say, well, it seems nothing too special based on what we just described above about the session as compared to other psychotherapy treatment or holistic medicine sessions. From the superficial level, staying only on the surface of words of this text, it may not be dramatically different. Yet, in fact, it is different.

The major difference is that the doctor, the talk (the content of talk and the way to talk), the energy music and entire treatment process carry a deep healing energy vibration and spiritual principle, and that goes into the deep part of the patient's soul, spirit, heart, emotion, and body at the same time. Additionally, the session combined several key components into one treatment to work on body, mind, spirit, emotions, cognition, behaviors, lifestyles, and habits, all together.

Here are some of the key elements in the integrative treatment not readily visible in its overall, general description:

1. The doctor's energy and approach to the patient as well-personal cultivation is a very important influencer to healing the patient. It can immediately and effectively calm down the patient, gain the patient's trust and cooperation, and make the patient feel hopeful, think positive and open to positive changes. This is always the most important factor for the successful integrative medicine treatment that transforms the patient's mind, body and spirit.

2. The balanced vibration energy of the Yin-Yang and Five Elements music compositions directly and quickly improves the energy state, substitutes for needle acupuncture, but goes deeper than regular acupuncture in working on the body, emotions, mind and spirit simultaneously. This energy music was created and customized for the patient, in a meditated state, and previously to or on-the-side during the session.

    The healing vibration, melody and energy with combination of spiritual conversation together help the patient clean up a confusing mind, empty the busy subconscious mind, stop the negative thinking, feel fresh and positive, and open energy meridians, again simultaneously. Therefore the patient feels energized, stronger and transformed to a higher level – physically, mentally and spiritually. This further helps the doctor better communicate with the patient in the mental and spiritual dimensions. At the same time, it helps the doctor perform the session induction and teaching more easily and smoothly.

3. Brainwave sounds combined with the Yin-Yang and Five Elements music helped the patient empty the mind and get into a deep trance state faster, and absorb the energy more quickly. The hypnotizing effect of brainwave vibrations added to the energy music is very helpful in the session in order to quickly stop the patient's busy conscious mind and subconscious mind – especially in the very beginning of the healing process before the patient gains energy, feeling better and becoming clear-headed enough to proceed to deeper healing conversations. At this juncture, the combination of brainwave sounds, Yin-Yang Five Elements energy music and hypnosis is very effective in order to stop a busy confused mind and quickly allow the patient to receive a positive healing result. The energy music balances the energy and autonomic nervous systems. The combination of brainwave frequency and the powerful energy music work

together to enhance the healing benefits, making a faster transformational and integrative improvement for the patient's body, mind and soul.

4.   As the patient has improved mental, physical and spiritual energy and overall strength to some extent, we started to teach self-improvement practice and spiritual growth, helping further awaken the spirit, strengthen conscious mind, improve the condition, and stabilize the healing result. This is one of the important parts of the healing. Without improving conscious mind clarity, and deeper understanding, self-awareness and introspection into her inner self, mind, attitude, thinking mode, personality, character, relationship, lifestyle, and clear awareness concerning what is good and bad, healthy and unhealthy, the patient will still have the negative messages and sick energy vibrations deeply buried inside the mind and spirit. Therefore, the bad attitudes and dysfunctional thinking mode and unhealthy lifestyle cannot be changed, the Karma cannot be eliminated, and the sickness cannot be removed from the root.

In subsequent sessions as the patient acquired better and clearer mind, the doctor introduced the principle of the universe's characteristics such as compassion, peace, love, forgiveness, tolerance, open-mindedness, etc., and meditated with the patient while taking an inner look into herself and making corrections on her own. The patient resonates with these higher energy vibrations, and, for others, as for Cherry, true Self begins to waken and grow.

5.   Calming, cleansing, and purifying the subconscious mind is another very important component in the treatment sessions. As the positive energy balanced and enhanced, righteous Qi rose up, the patient's mind and spirit got clearer, quiet, and awakened, and the subconscious mind also quieted. Through energy music, conversations, meditation, hypnosis, and energetic exercises, we helped her train the subconscious mind with clear and strong conscious mind, and stop the random, clouded and bad subconscious thinking and habits.

These treatments follow the principle of "Uphold good and suppress evil (idiom)" in traditional Chinese medicine. We believe that the noises and confusions within the mind and body are the sick messages, which can be eliminated by upholding good energy – compassionate, love, peaceful, and balanced yin-yang-five-elements energy. This energy is provided by the energy healing compositions and doctor's energy produced in the session as well the conversation and teaching. Therefore the doctor's good cultivation in energy and spirituality is absolutely required in order to have the powerful healing result.

6.   Another important component is the patient's involvement in the entire process of healing treatments, conversation, teaching, consultation, meditation, hypnosis, energy music, daily health practice and healing homework.

As the patient's mind and subconscious mind became clearer and more energetic, and her physical body became stronger, we started to teach her energy practices such as meditation and energetic movements, and also give her homework, which included daily meditation, exercises and self-improvement in living schedule, lifestyle, food habit, relationship, communications, and involvement in family and society. We encouraged her and motivate her to get involved with these healthy practices with her own interest and joyfulness. This is one of the very helpful and important steps in the healing process. Changing a person must have that person directly involved. As the healing progressed, and with her agreement, we suggested the patient practice meditation and exercise in the morning after wakeup and during the evening before sleep, for at least 30 minutes.

As the patient gets used to it, the meditations can be increased to 1 hour each in the morning and evening, or even add one more hour during the day. For most patients who have depression, morning wakeup is always tired and unhappy, so doing the meditation and/or energetic movement is very helpful toward a positive mood change. These patients do not easily fall asleep and/or have bad quality sleep, so doing meditation before sleep will help them clean up the mind and subconscious mind, balance the autonomic nervous systems, and sleep will become easier and deeper.

For those patients like Cherry, we also suggest trying to improve daily performance in matters such as relationships, family and society activities and communications, and ask for feedback in the following session, which helps further conversation and improvements while implementing musical healing, meditation and other mind-body healing approaches. All these are done with the patient's own interest, joyfulness and motivation while the doctor gives encouragement, teaching and suggestions.

Coming to this point, we can actually see the true transformation of the entire person is made through a true integrative healing practice.

In the subsequent sessions, based on the changes and improvements after each session and the patient's own practice, we continued the treatment by following the principles and procedures as described above.

Even though the procedure for each session may be different or may be similar from session to session, the healing result and transformation progress further and further, going deeper and deeper, and therefore sessions are never quite exactly the same because the patient grows more and more after each as the doctor guides the patient into a deeper healing state.

§8.5 Healing Energy at Multi-Levels & Integrative Teaching

Through the previous sections above, we discussed the integration of the healing at multiple levels of body, mind and spirit especially for our current times as people's sicknesses are caused by multiple complicated causes. The doctor cannot easily heal the patient by only working on the mind or only on the body, separately. However, simply putting different healing modalities together is not the optimal effective approach either.

As with Cherry's case, although the Chinese doctor, psychologist and psychiatrist worked on her at the same time with separated healing protocols or procedures, improvement still could not be achieved. The reason is that integration is not equal to a simple sum of different disciplines put together superficially. The healing practice must be an internal integration. This means that in one treatment system, the healing practice contains multiple techniques at all levels of mind, body and spirit and with simplified procedures to work on the vibration energies resonating deeply into and widely within body, mind, spirit, emotion, conscious mind, subconscious mind, relationship, lifestyle, living schedule, eating habit, thinking mode, attitude, character, spirituality, family and social environments, all together, at the same time.

In BMT treatment as described above and in the later chapters, we are able to work on the physical, mental or emotional energy and spiritual energy with Yin-Yang and Five Elements composition and brainwave sounds combined with meditation, exercise, hypnosis, psychological and spiritual teaching conversation, and daily self-improvement practices.

The most important key in this integration of healing practice, using BMT as example, is the healing energy produced by the music sound frequency and the doctor, as well the doctor's cultivated energy, his/her essence, heart, composition, healing expressions (in all possible forms such as talk, manner, voice, tone, body language, or even a smile, eye contact, with or without sincerity, compassion, and all vibrations in the session and its environment settings, etc.), conversation, teaching, and all treatment performances based on the higher spiritual teaching of universe characters and the energy nature of Yin-Yang and Five Elements, and daily practices of healthy lifestyle, mentality, letting go of attachments and open mind.

The procedure progresses with a simplified model combining energy vibrations produced by energy music sounds and brainwave vibrations, meditation, hypnosis, emotional and spiritual conversation and teaching, exercise, and daily self-healing and improvement practices. The energy may be in visible forms, but also in invisible forms based on the doctor's cultivation and experience, and dynamically designed upon the patient's situation and extent of his/her acceptance ability while the healing progresses.

This healing energy is much more powerful than regular acupuncture, herbs, massage therapy, psychotherapy, hypnosis, imagery therapy, and general relaxation, meditation, Qigong / Taiji , yoga, and physical therapy, in their separated forms. The healing energy in this practice carries the profound energy of the universe's compassionate and peaceful powers, and reaches the original true Self, the life origin of the patient, resounding all over his/her body, mind and spirit to waken, restore and rejuvenate the patient's soul, vitality and life force. As a result, the patient becomes clearheaded, spiritually enlightened, emotionally calm and energetic, physically active, sleeps well in the evenings, and performs well in the daytime.

An important note: all these teachings and conversations are not given at once to overwhelm the patient. On the contrary, they are indeed always naturally approached, as the patient gets more and more awakened. From high level (such as universe's characteristics) to low level (such as daily living schedule) of issues, they always come out automatically and naturally in each session to perfectly meet the patient's need and level of acceptance. It seems the healing system itself has an automatic driving force to lead the healing process deeper and deeper. I believe the law and principle as well as the healing music energy vibrations together have a systematic mechanism that drives the healing treatment dynamically toward the positive transformation and enlightenment of the patient who has such fate and is ready for such a blessing – healing.

§8.6 Highest Healing Principle Instead of Human Way

There are many truths at different levels with different levels of energy in the universe. The truth and energy of life, health, healing, beauty and longevity are the same way; there are truths at many levels with different qualities of energy.

Healing results are dependent upon what level of the truth and energy the doctor has reached and cultivated, what level of the truth and energy the doctor used in the treatment, and what level of the truth and energy the patient resonated, and practiced. The reason why a treatment is effective, and another is not is absolutely because of this. No matter mind-body medicine, psychological consultation or energy healing for mental health issues, physical or a combination of both, the level of the healing principle, theory, logic, method, presentation, expression, procedure, and the doctor or therapist him/herself, and his/her energy determines the healing result. Even though the same doctor or therapist may use the same treatment on more than one individual, the healing result can be different, depending upon the level of the truth reached and the energy produced by the doctor during the particular healing session in his/her existing cultivation state in the spiritual energy realms.

In order to heal the whole being, the treatment must deeply touch, awaken, activate and resonate with the true nature of the patient's soul with a high level of truth and energy produced by a well-cultivated mind-body-spirit health practitioner. This true nature is expressed in multiple forms of energy vibrations within the body, mind and spirit.

The vibration energies crossing all dimensions are associated, influenced, transformed, and transferred to each other. It's why when one of the life components (body, mind and spirit) is sick, then other components can also get sick.

The spirit and mind are at the higher levels and have the greater energy. If the spirit and mind are healed, then the body will also be healed accordingly. The healing energy depends upon the spiritual healing principle. The high healing energy comes from the spiritual natures – e.g. peace, compassion, kindness, harmony, truthfulness, righteousness, and forgiveness and energy natures of the vital life force – the energy of Yin-Yang and The Five Elements or even Beyond The Five Elements (the extremely high powerful healing energy).

Using the human level of healing ideas, theories, logics, understandings, sciences, techniques, methods, principles and/or concepts won't truly heal the person because these have much lower energy vibrations. In fact, these human level or even lower levels of vibrations have impure or even bad or negative energy frequencies such as noises; confusions; selfishness; ego, imbalanced energy messages; human desires; attachments; random, misleading, conflict or contradictory thoughts, ideas and information or messages; random unconscious messages; narrowed mind; unspiritual mind; fear; depression; worry; non-confidence; anger; hate; revenge; violence; jealousy; dishonesty; suspicions; paranoia or even bad, evil or demon characteristics and so forth. These messages within the human mind and body are at conflict with thus disturb the original natures of true Self. These bad or low energy vibrations are indeed the original cause of sicknesses and discomforts physically and mentally. The healing process is to eliminate these negative factors.

If a doctor or therapist of integrated mind-body-spirit medicine does not have a higher and clear spiritual guide and compassionate righteous thought in understanding of (1) what the original spiritual natures of a human being are, (2) what good energy vibrations and their reflections, expressions or existing forms and manifestations at the physical/human realm and other dimensions beyond this physical world are, or (3) the confusion or misunderstandings about these fundamental issues regarding human beings, or (4) the problems with use of human level or even lower level concepts, notions or logics to try healing the patient, then the healing work will not touch the soul of the patient deeply, will not resonate with the true Self of the patient, and will not be able to have a deep communication with the patient at the higher level of mind, spirit or soul. Therefore as a result, the patient cannot be healed or may even get confused or wondering, and the condition may remain un-improvement. This can even disappoint the patient so that he/she will lose hope of healing.

The doctor or therapist must keep in mind that all patients have the same true natures of original spirit as the universe has, which can be summarized with some words such as love, compassion, peace, kindness, harmony, truthfulness, forgiveness, giving, sharing, unselfishness, tolerance, patience, opened mindedness, and spirituality. At the same time, we understand that these good natures can be suppressed, blocked, masked, contaminated, mutated, or hidden temporarily by the darkness, noisy or disturbing energy vibrations in the human world – the family, school, community, society, etc. where the person has been contaminated during this human lifetime and past lives (the spirit carries the vibration messages even from past lives), to different extents, depending upon the individual. Therefore, spiritual and mental healing is to wake up and resonate with the true nature of the person, and activate, balance and strengthen the original vibration energies within the body, mind and spirit through the doctor who produces such healing energy vibrations based on the highest spiritual natures and energy principles, but not on the lower levels of human thoughts, logics, notions, emotions, sentiments, and methods.

In our previous example of treating Cherry's case, throughout the entire process from the very beginning to the end, we held onto this highest principle and worked with her accordingly throughout her healing progress. The energy vibrations we utilized resonated with and awakened her true Self, and so we encouraged her and guided her to cultivate herself spiritually, emotionally and physically, step by step during her healing journey.

She was very happy and encouraged to know that, the same as others, her original life was rich in high values of spirit, soul and character, but that these good values are contaminated, influenced and mutated in this life; however, they can be restored through the healing process. Cherry's forte was that she wanted to be such good person. She wanted a clear mind, a beautiful spirit, and an organized lifestyle. She very much wanted to end her existing health condition, messed up lifestyle and confused mind, so she could have a healthy, happy and normal or even meaningful life. Her hopes were attractive to her. Therefore, she was quite cooperative as she worked toward acquiring her goal during the entire healing process, including not only the sessions, but also with regard to the self-healing work she did outside the clinic, such as time she devoted to meditation and gentle movement exercises as well as all other aspects of mind-body-spirit cultivation.

236

As mind-body medicine healthcare practitioners, we stand at the highest level of healthcare by putting forth the highest spiritual principle to work at all levels and dimensions. Nonetheless, people get ill. When the body and mind get sick, however, we maintain they have been energetically contaminated by too much noise, confusion and weakness – mentally and physically. The patient's conscious mind and subconscious mind are always blurry, clouded, weak, blocked, and confused. The sick energy or bad message in the body and mind is like an evil being which attaches to the person and does not want to go away. It's why sometimes the person doesn't want to change him/her self, and refuses to listen to suggestions from the doctor, or doesn't even want to continue the treatment.

Sometimes the conscious mind may want to change, but the subconscious mind unconsciously fights against the conscious intention, stays stuck in the old way of thinking, feeling and doing things, and doesn't want to change. It is not easy to wake up the original Self and at the same time to shut down the bad messages or sick vibrations in the conscious mind and subconscious mind.

Modern people, especially, are influenced by science that adheres only to the physical dimension, so some of them do not really believe in the spiritual power and secret of other dimensions. In such a case, the patient sometimes only pursues the immediate relief of their physical suffering and emotional discomforts, but they do not have the patience to listen to the doctor's explanation about their mind, emotions, or spirit, nor do they want to hear their doctor talking about introspection and changing their lifestyle and bad habits, much less about having to practice meditation and exercise.

For such reasons, the process of spiritual awakening and positive emotional transformation has to involve multiple modalities – we favor sound (good, simple, practical and effective) forms and higher levels of energies that work dramatically and quickly and are simultaneously effective not only spiritually, but also physically, mentally and emotionally. This approach helps the patient absorb the energies at all levels and feel better right away, even if it is just "a-quarter-of-a-turn" better. Sometimes that's all you need, just a-quarter-of-a-turn to get someone going and keep them progressing in a positive direction. This is important affectively. This way, the patient can have more trust in the doctor and the treatment, and more confidence and interest in the healing approach. Therefore, the most effective, fastest and beneficial way to heal multiple causes at all levels is through an energy balancing program (such as BMT we have mentioned above and will introduce in detail in the later chapters) that addresses all levels and dimensions of health – physical, mental and spiritual – and unifies these into one smooth healing system, making the patient feel physically good, mentally relaxed and energized, and spiritually awakened and enlightened.

§8.8 Suggestion For Young Health Professionals

The healing work we are talking about here with regard to mind-body-spirit medicine is not quite same as some of psychotherapies or oriental medicine practices nowadays. Except for some comprehensive holistic psychotherapies and energy psychology approaches, psychotherapies today are working on emotion, cognition, behaviors, relationships, and performance, but not on the fundamental causes and the solution, energy practice and cultivation. As a trend, experimental psychology and brain science or neuroscience lack in their focus on connections such as those of mind, emotion and energy; body, spirit, and whole being – in a holistic sense – and higher spiritual energy. Of course, again, we are not talking about those well-cultivated energetic holistic mental health practices or psychotherapies. If the communication, dialogue, cognition and behavior treatment, teaching, induction, instruction, and so forth in the mental healing or psychotherapy are based solely on concepts at human level or at the level of limited science, which is (1) not able to eliminate human thoughts, noise, messages and disturbers within the patient's body, mind and spirit, (2) not able to enlighten the patient to a higher spiritual level, and (3) not able to extend the healing energy to the mind, emotion, body, daily lifestyle, thinking mode, personality, self-awareness and self-improvement practice, then as a result, the treatment will not go deep enough to eliminate the root cause, fundamentally improve the condition, and achieve a long-term healing benefit.

In summary, many traditional oriental medicine and naturopathic medicine practitioners have achieved, however, with long years of spiritual cultivation, a high level of practice in mind-body-spirit connection. Yet, younger professionals always need more efforts in their personal cultivation and more years of practice experience. In fact, oriental medicine and naturopathic medicine practices today are not quite the same as the holistic mind-body medicine practice as we have discussed in this book. These practices focus more on needles, herbs, nutrition, massage or other hands-on treatments, but do not put enough effort in the connections of the mind-body-spirit.

In addition, if the practitioner in this field does not practice self-cultivation such as high level of Buddha Law or advanced Qigong cultivation as we mentioned in this book to improve his/her own energy and spirituality, then the practice cannot produce high level of energy to heal patients. No matter what health problems you focus on, including many physical diseases, they always involve mental and spiritual causes. Therefore, at times, the modern oriental medicine and natural medicine still cannot eliminate the original cause and heal from the root.

As a practitioner of psychotherapy, oriental medicine, naturopathic medicine, or conventional medicine, especially if you are a student or young professional in these fields, besides your existing training and practice, we highly suggest that you diligently cultivate your spirituality, mind nature and energy at all levels of mind, body and spirit, deeply understand and practice the higher spiritual natures and energy principle of the universe as we addressed in this book, so you will build a strong foundation for your practice and elevate the level of your healing work.

§8.9 Intermediate Break: Story • Healing Music • Meditation

The healing story for this chapter is from a successfully healed patient who had severe depression and physical pain.

"My 9-Year Pain Gone!"

- An Elephantiasis and Depression Case

Alice suffered from chronic pain in her lower back, legs and feet for the past 9 years. She could only sleep for 2 hours each night. Her conditions have complicated factors, including elephant legs (elephantiasis), depression, anxiety, anger, insomnia, and severe pain. Her daughter, who is a nurse, took her to all kinds of the doctors she knew, including pain management specialists, psychologists, neurologists, acupuncturists, but she was told they couldn't do anything to help her.

When Alice came into the clinic, she was in a wheelchair. Her posture was bent over, and she was very tense. Her legs and feet were swollen so badly that she could not take off socks. After 30 minutes of BMT treatment, she found that the pain in her feet was gone. Her screams of joy and the scene of the mother and daughter embracing each other were so touching. Alice could stand straight and walked to the bathroom by herself. Vera told us that she found us through one of her co-workers, whose mother had been healed by BMT.

A few more sessions continued and she felt a lot better, but she had to go back to her home in Texas.

Six months later, Alice called and said thanks while telling that she had continued to heal after the sessions. The healing had automatically progressed by itself and as a result of her ongoing efforts. Her pain was completely gone, depression healed, and her sleep was very good, weight balanced, and she was totally transformed to another person. "My 9-year Pain gone!" Alice told everyone. Her families and friends saw how dramatically she had changed her condition and could not believe she could be so happy.

Healing Meditation For Chapter 8

EHM08: Assimilate with Earth & Heaven *(Yin, Earth, Fire)*

This music is composed with focus on the relatively yin energy of earth and fire elements to strengthen your stomach and heart energy. However if you feel you are weak, cold, have low energy, or unhappy, unconfident, or at a low mood emotionally (yin type of condition), then you can choose the following CD (yang type of the healing music) to practice.

EHM07: Let Go and Stay High *(Yang, Earth, Fire)*

[*Start to play Energy Healing Music #8*] Meditate and cultivate the concept of Being One with the Universe. Let go of all thoughts and peacefully resonate with the vibration. Feel yourself merged with the universe and its wonderful spiritual characters: love, compassion, truthfulness, and forgiveness. Whether you are a mind-body health practitioner or self-improvement cultivator, you now understand the most important law of the universe and the most fundamental principle of the life energy. You have truly realized how important it is to cultivate your mind-body-spirit. You have made up your mind to cultivate your whole being, helping yourself and helping others.

§8.10 Exercise Questions

1. Briefly describe the natures of Eastern and Western medicine, psychology and psychiatry in terms of their practice and their differences. What are their limitations in healing multiple causes of modern diseases?

2. Is integrative medicine simply the sum of different kinds of therapies and why?

3. What is the true integrative medicine for mind-body-spirit holistic health?

4. What are the key elements in the integrative health of mind-body-spirit?

5. What is the highest healing principle and why does mind-body medicine use it instead of the human way?

6. What is the most effective, quickest, and beneficial way to heal at all levels of mind, body and spirit? How do you make the patient feel good quickly and gain his trust and confidence about you and your treatment?

7. Why do you need to seriously practice mind-body-spirit cultivation and energy improvement as a healthcare professional?

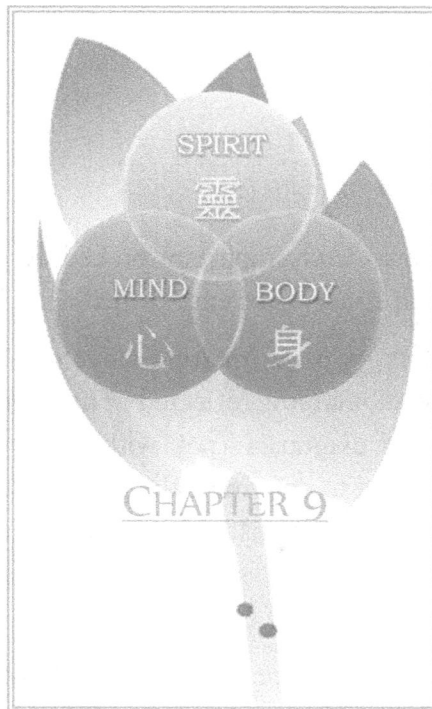

SPIRIT
靈

MIND   BODY
心   身

CHAPTER 9

Energy Checkup Based On Chinese Medicine

We have discussed previously that mind-body medicine practice works with energy in multiple dimensions of body, mind and spirit. Therefore, knowing the energy condition of the person is critical in the healing treatment. In fact, the energy state of a human being can be diagnosed by using the methods of traditional Chinese medicine (TCM) or traditional oriental medicine (TOM). This chapter will introduce you to how to apply the energy diagnostic methods based on traditional Chinese medicine to the practice of mind-body medicine.

In mind-body medicine practice, however, we do not exactly follow all procedures as TCM does, but instead, we employ a simplified protocol based on its basic principles and methods. These simplified diagnostic methods are naturally incorporated into the mind-body medicine practice. The information on an individual's energy status as obtained from our diagnostic helps us understand and treat the entire being of mind, body and spirit from the energy aspect, which reaches into the root causes of a health problem.

An important note: In mind-body medicine we do not diagnose disease (either mental or physical) or give a name of any disease as the conventional medicine or Chinese medicine does, but we diagnose (check to know) energy state of mind-body-spirit as cause of the health problem(s) and in attempting to improve the patient's energy condition, to foster - positive healing.

So, checking energy status is an important procedure in mind-body medicine. We do this by using the principle and concepts of energy medicine. Let's look.

We know that life energy is at multiple levels, including the physical level, emotional level and spiritual level, and it is reflected in many aspects. In traditional Chinese medicine, the four methods of diagnosis (not within conventional Western medicine diagnosis) are typical and well used to determine the patient's energy. These four diagnostic methods refer to (1) looking diagnosis (observation), (2) listening and smelling (auscultation and olfaction) diagnosis, (3) asking diagnosis (inquiry), and (4) pulse reading diagnosis.

In our mind-body medicine practice, however, we do not follow this practice exactly as the Chinese doctors do because of practice nature differences: (1) We mainly focus on the mind-body-spirit connection, emotions, lifestyle, relationships, social connections, thoughts, notions, habits, behaviors, true Self/main consciousness, subconsciousness, mind-body-spirit cultivation, and we attempt to heal the whole being through working with the individual's mental and spiritual energy, (2) We do not use or mainly use herbs, needles, cupping, and other oriental medicine tools, but we use energy music, hypnosis, biofeedback, psychological conversation, brainwave vibration, meditation, energy movements, etc., and these approaches target mental and spiritual levels, higher than the direct body treatment, so the energy vibrations have the dynamic flexibility and multiple levels of power to automatically balance the entire being in all aspects at the same time, instead of treating one part or one single issue at a time, (3) Due to the first two reasons as described above, we spend longer time (e.g., 1.5 hours or 2 hours in each session) directly working with the patient (instead of using needles) for 30-45 minutes and giving herbs to be taken to home, so that our diagnosis occurs simultaneously with the conversation, instead of at a separate time before, during, or after the session.

For these reasons, therefore, we do not need to diagnose the person in every detail like the oriental doctors do, but we do need to know the status of the person's energy state, for example, if it is Yin or Yang, hot or cold, deficient or excess, dry or damp – note: we will define these terms as this chapter continues.

Thus we simplify the TCM procedure based on these diagnoses, and incorporate it into the mind-body healing session, making the practice easy, practical and effective.

Usually we incorporate the first three diagnoses (observation, auscultation/olfaction and inquiry) together in the initial conversation. If you have learned Chinese medicine and are able to perform pulse reading, you can do so during the initial conversation. However if not, it will be good enough to only do these three diagnoses. During the first session with our patient, we pay attention to the patient's body tone, fitness, gait, motion, skin, facial expression, eye contact, emotional expression, and mannerisms, talking voice and its volume and clarity, manner of speaking and use of words, body language, conversations (questions and answers with the patient), etc. to know his/her energy status, spiritual state, mental and physical conditions. We will introduce these methods in each of the following sections in details, but when you actually practice them, you can simply combine them with the initial conversation, and then follow-up will include tongue diagnosis and pulse reading if you want.

Again, we are using the principles and concepts of TCM regarding energy medicine to observe the patient's energy state as vibration frequencies within the body, mind and spirit. Based on this diagnostic information, we can understand the patient's body, mind and spirit in multiple dimensions, helping to determine the energy pattern and nature – e.g. the elements of energy music – to use in the treatment.

§9.2 Diagnosis by Asking

In general oriental medicine practice, the doctor always asks the patient 10 standardized questions or has a questionnaire form for the patient fill out. These questions were developed by the Ming Dynasty doctor Zhang Jiebin 張介賓 (also known as Zhang Jingyue 張景岳, 1563-1640), and have been passed on until today. The ten questions are as follows:

1. Cold and Heat, Chills and Fever – Are you always feeling cold, have cold hands and feet, or unable to tolerate cold? Or are you generally feeling too warm? In an acute illness, what are your severity of chills and fever? And does your fever fluctuate with time of day?

2. Perspiration – Are you experiencing night sweats or spontaneous perspiration without physical activity, a high fever with no perspiration, or sweating of palms and soles of the feet?

3. Pains in Head and Body – Do you experience pain: lower back, knees, chest, front, sides or back of the head; is there any dizziness; is there an uncomfortable feeling of fullness in the chest or abdomen; what type of pain (sharp and piercing or dull and

aching); and does the pain recede or worsen with the application of cold, heat or pressure?

4. Urination and Bowel Movements – Are you experiencing a frequency of urination and bowel movements (times per day), constipation, diarrhea, frequent copious clear urination, scanty dark urination, incontinence, or the need to get up one or more times during the night to urinate.

5. Diet and Appetite – Are you experiencing a lack of appetite, constant insatiable hunger, bloating after eating, desire for hot or cold foods, craving certain tastes such as sweet, sour, salty or spicy, habitual intake of sugar, caffeine or alcohol? Or are you often experiencing a particular taste in the mouth such as metallic or bitter.

6. Thirst – Are you experiencing excessive thirst, lack of thirst, thirst with no desire to drink, or constant desire for cold drinks?

7. Mental or Emotional State – Are you experiencing any negative emotions?

   TCM recognizes that the emotional and physical are interrelated, and emotional states such as grief, anger, worry or fear can affect the patient's physical well-being. Conversely, physical disharmonies can bring about emotional responses. Is the patient experiencing any of the above negative emotions?

8. Hearing tinnitus, ringing or other sounds in the ears – Are you experiencing any ringing in his or her ears or any sudden or gradual hearing loss?

9. Sleep – Are you experiencing an excessive desire to sleep, difficulty falling asleep, or waking in the middle of the night and feeling unable to fall back asleep, nightmares or dream-disturbed sleep?

10. Gynecological Issues – If the patient is female ask: Are you experiencing menses early or late or irregularly – e.g. is the flow light or heavy, the color too light or dark, or accompanied by pain or cramps during menstruation?

§9.3 Diagnosis by Looking

During the initial session while you talk to your patient, you can perform the looking diagnosis (observation). This includes observing the patient's appearance, facial expression, skin tone and color, as well as tongue, hair, and movements.

§9.3.1 Eyes, Face, Appearance, Fitness and Complexion

Vital Energy Level can be diagnosed by looking at the patient's eyes, appearance, facial expression, fitness, complexion, and so on. By looking at these factors, you should be able to quickly know whether the patient has good vitality or has a lack.

I. Good Vital Energy

If the person appears in the following ways, it indicates a good spiritual, mental and emotional vital energy. These give a conceptual picture of how a healthy person is supposed to look – appearing otherwise may indicate that the individual has some health issues to deal with.

Eyes

Bright and shining, energetic, peaceful, calm, friendly, honest, warm, responsive, lively and expressional, naturally and confidently inviting eye contact with people.

Face

Bright, lighter, pink, shining, smooth, delicate, and transparent skin, peaceful, relaxing, smiling, confident, expressional, with happy facial expression, and slightly plump, rich and balanced healthy look in facial shape.

Appearance and Body (Fitness)

Fit body tone, balanced weight, energetic, smooth, natural, peaceful, active, balanced and flexible movement.

Complexion

Skin tone, texture, quality, and color are reflections of the person's vital energy. These factors of the skin as well as the impression or feeling from the energy beyond the surface are collectively called Qi color (Qi se) in the terminology of Chinese medicine. When one is healthy, and has good cultivation energy in the mind, body and spirit, the complexion tone color and quality should be bright, lighter, clear, smooth, shiny, pink or light red in color, relaxed, peaceful, positive, elastic, energetic, beautiful and attractive.

If the above has been observed, the patient is healthy, or health problems are minimal because his/her vital energy is still at a good level and has not been diminished. In such a case, a health problem (if any) can be easily and quickly recovered from. Otherwise (see the following section II), the problem needs deeper healing work to take care of.

II. Low Vital Energy

Eyes:

If the eyes are listless, lethargic, dull, not shiny, have no energy, have no or little expression, direct no or little eye contact, the indication is low energy, fear, depression, low or lack of vital energy and its related conditions such as anxiety, worry, fear, nervousness, low/no self-confidence, tiredness, and lack sleep. Note: Eyes that avoid contact with you may indicate fear, autism, depression, low energy, and/or anxiety.

Face:

If the facial expression is rigid, no expression, unhappy, worrying, wandering, confused, has dark color or unusual colors (see below), then the person is sick mentally and also may be physically. Especially if face or lips are dark color, this usually indicates a low circulation and/or blockage of energy flow.

Appearance and Body (Fitness):

Not fit, imbalanced weight (skinny or over-weight), low energy, rigid, slow and/or imbalanced movement, this indicates such diseases as neurological disorder, stroke, metabolism problem, hormone problem – e.g. hyperthyroid, hypothyroid, etc.

Complexion:

Human's life force energy is always clearly reflected on the Qi color (*Qi se*), the skin tone and color and the expressional image from the energy beyond the surface. When one is lacking in good energy or sick, his complexion will appear darker in color or an unusual color. The complexion colors are classified into five types:

- Blue

  Caused by wind and cold, sign of pain, tightness of muscle and nerves, low energy, blockage of blood and energy circulation. Complexion in excessive blue color may be a sign of liver problem.

- Yellow

  Caused by dampness or heat wetness, sign of deficiency of vital energy (Qi) and blood, low body resistance (ability to prevent sickness) or immunity. Complexion in excessive yellow color may be a sign of spleen problem such as deficiency of spleen Qi.

- Red

  Caused by heat or fire, sign of cardiac vascular problems, yang over yin; deficiency of yin, and excess of yang. Complexion in excessive red color can be a sign of a heart problem.

- White

  Caused by deficiency of vital energy (Qi) and poor blood circulation. Also as a sign of cold Qi. Note: white here means pale, but not the bright and shiny whiteness of face that indicates a healthy and energetic state. Complexion in excessive white color may be a sign of lung problems.

- Black/Dark:

  Caused by cold, deficiency or blockage of Qi and blood, sign of pain, fluid retention and blood clots. Complexion in excessive black color can be a sign of kidney problems.

It's necessary to point out that a woman with makeup may not show her true complexion (Qi color). Especially if the makeup is heavy and covers up the original complexion, you may not fully rely on the out-look color. As an experienced mind-body practitioner, you may be able to look at her Qi color or energy aura behind and combine other information together to determine the diagnosis result on the energy state.

As we mention makeup in general, on other hand, we do see some women do not choose healthy color tone in their makeup, so the makeup itself makes them look unhealthy. This may also affect their emotional mood and health negatively – e.g. purple lips, dark cheeks or entire face that show no brightness and smoothness, making them look unhealthy and aged. Color is energy, and it influences the mind and body. From energy medicine's perspective then we suggest that a woman should choose proper makeup color based on their original complexion, but more brighter, lighter, and fresh colors towards light pink with delicate, smooth, and shining texture, so that it will not only make you look energetic, happy, positive, young and attractive, but also make you actually feel that way in your mind and help generate a positive happy mood throughout your day, bringing you more healthy energy mentally, physically and spiritually. As you train and improve your daily mind-body cultivation practices such as meditation and energy movement, your complexion or skin quality will also become healthier in color and texture: rosy pink, white, clean, and smooth, bright, and shining.

If you practice self-cultivation, you can know how you have progressed in your practice by performing a self-check based on the ideas as described above. In oriental medicine, the three treasures "essence, Qi and spirit" (*jing, Qi, shen*) are the life forces at different levels. The essence is the fine substance within the physical body that includes nutrient, hormones, blood, DNA, neuron transmitters, and brain chemicals, etc. And the Qi is the invisible energy life force within and surrounding your body which has the power to carry on the essence to circulate inside your body, and the spirit is the highest form of energy in the spiritual dimension that governs the entire being as a living spiritual life, which is the root source of your life force.

All these life forces at different levels of body, mind and spirit are reflected on the surface: eyes, face, appearance, and complexion. By observing these factors at surface level, you will see through all these critical life forces/essence, Qi and spirit, at a glance.

As you practice day after day and year after year, you will discover yourself looking young, feeling young, thinking young, and behaving young, but with great wisdom and creativity. Self-checking in this way while progressing in your practice will motivate you to improve and cultivate your mind nature and longevity successfully.

§9.3.2 Tongue Diagnosis

I. Vital Energy Level and Tongue Diagnosis

The tongue provides a lot of information about vital energy, internal organs, Qi and blood circulation, and metabolism. The tongue is the only internal organ you can see directly from outside the body, and it reflects all other internal organs' conditions. Its color, shape, and mobility indicate the person's vital energy, blood production and circulation. Through the information obtained from tongue diagnosis, you will know about not only the patient's overall vital energy level, but also each individual organ's status such as ability to digest food, breathe, eliminate toxins and fight diseases, and so on.

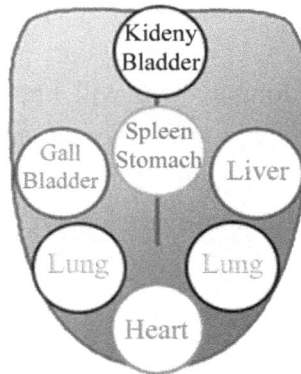

Fig. 9.3.2.1. Tongue diagnosis diagram shows the allocations of the tongue that are associated with internal organs correspondingly.

Life phenomena often have the holographic property – e.g. some parts of the body contain the information about the entire body. The tongue is such organ. It can be divided into several parts, which represent the vital energy states of the five internal organs (Fig. 9.3.2.1). We usually look at the tongue's color, shape, coating and distribution of cracks or spots to know any changes that may be related with some health conditions.

To diagnose your patient's tongue correctly, both of you should sit in a place where you have natural daylight (the light of a lamp including fluorescent lamp can alter how the tongue looks). Then, ask the patient to open their mouth and stick their tongue out fully.

The tongue should be relaxed naturally so that it shows its shape in a natural state. If your patient just had some foods, drinks, tea, medication, vitamins, herbs, or fruits, etc., please note that this may stain the tongue and change its coating color. In such a case, you need to wait an hour or longer until the color returns back to its usual state before you perform the tongue diagnosis. If the patient is a smoker, this may also change the tongue color.

II. What A Normal Tongue Looks Like

To diagnose an abnormal tongue of a sick person, we need to know how the normal tongue looks. A normal tongue should look fresh, pink uniformly with an even and symmetrical shape, and have no cracks or spots anywhere, but a layer of thin moisture coating the surface. You may look at a healthy child's tongue as reference for a normal tongue.

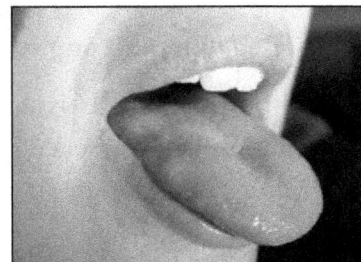

Based on the color of the tongue, you will know the energy status of corresponding internal organs. Tongue color refers to the color of either or both the tongue body and/or the coating of the tongue. Tongue body reflects blood status, and the tongue coating reflects Qi (energy) status, and, as well, the depth of sick Qi. The following are the major types of tongue coloration:

1. Pale Tongue

Pale tongue means the color of the tongue has a pale color, ranging from a slightly paler color than normal, to complete white color, depending on the condition. A pale tongue indicates a deficiency of Qi, blood and yang. It is a typical type of tongue for deficiency of Qi energy *(Qi Xu)* and blood *(Xue Xu)*. If you see your patient with a pale tongue body, then he/she has deficiency of blood, needing to supply (tonify) blood and/or improve blood circulation, while if you see a pale tongue coating, then he/she has deficiency of Qi, needing to supply (notify) Qi and/or improve Qi energy circulation. Both need to supply (tonify) treatment and promote circulation but never perform cleansing treatment. A patient who has had chronic disease for a long time or an elderly person may show a pale tongue.

2. Red Tongue

Red tongue means the color of the tongue is in red color. It indicates heat in the patient. The heat is located in the corresponding organ in the body based on the area where the redness appears on the tongue. The deeper the redness is, the worse the condition may be. If there is a tongue coating, then the heat is an Actual Heat condition (yang excess), while if there is no tongue coating, then the heat is an Empty Heat condition (not real heat, but appear as heat due to yin deficiency that causes a yang relatively excessive appearance). A patient who has fever, hot disease, hot flash, and cardiovascular diseases may show a red tongue.

3. Red-Purple Tongue

Red-purple tongue is an advanced stage of the red tongue and indicates that the condition has worsened. A purple tongue is a sign that the heat has damaged the blood and caused the stagnation (block) of blood.

4. Yellow Tongue

Yellow tongue is caused by dampness and heat stagnation, and/or phlegm retention with heat stagnation. It may combine with other colors when the condition becomes complicated.

5. Blue-purple tongue

Blue-purple tongue is a further advanced state of a pale tongue, as it is a sign of blood stagnation caused by cold, due to deficiency of Qi and blood. This is a symptom of severe deficiency and cold.

6. Blue tongue

Blue tongue usually appears in case of an acute life danger or emergency due to a lack of oxygen such as heart attack, epileptic seizures, etc. In some chronic diseases, the tongue may also become blue due to a long-term of cold that damaged the yang.

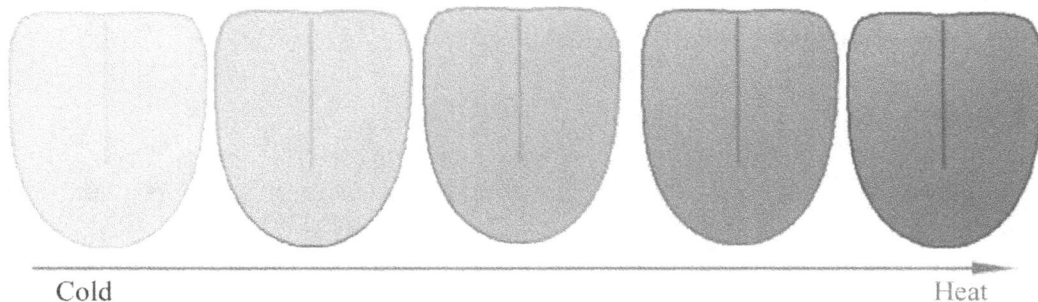

Cold ⟶ Heat

Fig. 9.3.2.2. The tongue colors ranging from normal (the third from left) to pale (the left most) and to red (the right most, note that it appears the more red the darker in black/white print), indicating cold, Qi blood deficiency, and heat (fire), yang excess, respectively.

In actual clinical practice, you may see many different combinations of tongue colors and coating types, showing complicated conditions. You can refer to more detailed traditional oriental medicine books for further progress in this practice. In mind-body medicine practice, however, the basic concepts and knowledge as described above will help you get started with some fundamental ideas about your patient's energy condition.

IV. Tongue Shapes

Swollen Tongue

Swollen tongue basically indicates a deficiency of Qi (low energy) or deficiency of yang, especially if the swollen tongue is pale. However if the swollen tongue is red, then it indicates the presence of heat or fire. Swollen tongue with rolled appearance in the sides may indicate 1) constipation, or 2) deficiency of spleen Qi or yang. Accompanying symptoms such as headaches, dizziness, anger or blurred vision indicate heat in the liver.

Sometimes you may see the tongue is swollen with tooth marks along the sides, this clearly indicates a deficiency of spleen Qi.

Thin Tongue

A thin tongue that appears thinner than normal or looks slightly shrunken indicates a lack of proper body fluids causing dehydration.

If the tongue is pale and thin, obviously blood deficiency is the problem. If it is a red and thin tongue, it tells the patient has yin deficiency. The tongue may also be dry, indicating some internal heat caused by yin deficiency.

Partial Swollen Tongue

Swelling in a particular part of the tongue indicates a health problem with the particular organ related to that region. Swollen edges, for example, can suggest a deficiency in the spleen, while a swollen tip of the tongue can indicate a heart problem or cardiovascular problem such as high blood pressure, heart attack, etc. Swelling between the tip and central area suggests a lung problem.

Indentation in One Area of the Tongue

A depression or indentation in a particular area of the tongue shows a deficiency in the related organ. A tooth-marked tongue, sometimes called a scalloped tongue, can be caused by spleen deficiency. If the tongue is abnormally stiff, it may suggest a heart problem.

Long Tongue

A long narrow tongue indicates heat and sometimes is seen as red in color. This tongue shape is often associated with heat in the heart, suggesting a tendency towards heart disease.

After the diagnosis by looking and asking as well as tongue diagnosis, you probably already have some basic ideas about the patient's energy status. Then you can analyze the symptoms and causes based on the Chinese medicine's Eight Principles: Yin and Yang, Cold and Hot, Interior and Exterior, Deficiency and Excess. These eight patterns of disease, symptoms and causes consist of four pairs, with each of the pairs containing two opposite aspects, categorizing the disease based on its nature, location, advancement and energy pattern or status. This is a very important diagnostic in that it allows you to develop a fundamental and ultimate strategy, based on the patient's energy type, toward a correct healing treatment.

Yin and Yang

Yin-Yang is the primary pair among all the four pairs / the eight patterns of diseases, symptoms, causes or energy types. In other patterns, Exterior, Heat and Excess belong to Yang, while the Interior, Cold and Deficiency belong to Yin. Yin is relative to Yang, while Yang is relative to Yin, and other pairs of the terms are the same, relative to each other.

Yin or Yang is not a specific or particular physical matter that can be found in this physical dimension, but are specific natures, properties, characteristics, qualities, or energy patterns seen within any substantial matters or living beings in the universe. A human being also has yin and yang, of course.

Yin

Yin refers to a nature that tends to be quieter, cooler, colder, lower, stiller, downward, more feminine, wet or damp, watery, softer, flaccid, reserved, relaxed, internal, inward, soothing, smooth, less colorful, less excited, etc. A yin type of person appears in the yin energy natures, such as: quiet, reserved, internal, supportive, careful, relaxed, and in preference of a quiet lifestyle. Yin is the natural quality or energy character of any matter or life in balance with the Yang (see next section).

However, if the yin goes to the extreme beyond the normal state and becomes an imbalanced or extreme condition of yin, then the person will manifest yin type of illness or disease. Yin type diseases are often chronic problems related with low energy; excess of yin or cold Qi; deficiency of yang Qi; pain; negative emotions and thought; less or no talk; depression; fewer or no activities; fatigue; pale face, dark, tired, no shining facial light; rougher skin; and pale or dark tongue and lips.

To heal a yin type of illnesses, we usually tonify yin, supplying yang energy, and provide the patient with positive, happy, encouraging and bright emotional and spiritual energy.

Yang

Yang refers to a nature that tends to be more active, warmer, higher, upward, more in motion, manly, drier, heated or fired, harder, faster, stronger, positive, outward, excited, external, colorful, etc. A yang type of person usually appears outgoing, extroverted, forceful, active, dynamic, working hard, in a career that displays their abilities, and having a lot of energy, not often feeling cold, with a rosy facial appearance, overall shining, smooth and energetic. Yang is the natural quality or energy character of any matter or life in balance with the yin (see previous section).

However when the yang goes to the extreme beyond the normal state and becomes an imbalanced or an extreme condition of yang, then the person will have yang type illness or disease. The yang illness often manifests with sudden or acute conditions – e.g., fever, feeling hot (hot hands and feet). Excesses of yang energy manifest in heated symptoms such as: anxiety, anger, over activity, hyper-reactivity, dramatic reactions, over excitement, difficulty calming the mind or difficulty falling asleep.

To heal yang illness, we supply peaceful and calming energy (yin), cleanse heat and the excess yang energy, detoxify and moisten the system, calm and harmonize the emotions and spirit.

Interior and Exterior

Interior and Exterior indicate place of the illness's location as being interior or exterior, and its extent as in worse or less worse, respectively. Exterior illness means that it is still located in the exterior of the body, in a light condition and easy to heal, while interior illness means the sickness has progressed to the interior part of the body and is not easy to heal.

In mind-body health practice, most cases are interior and chronic and have had their causes inside of the mind and body for a period of time, and as such, have further affected the mind and body. For this reason, the healing must be deeply reaching and resonating with the mind, emotion, spirit and body. Both the doctor and patient should understand this and put effort on the internal mind and body to cure the root cause inside the body and mind.

Hot and Cold

Hot and cold refer to the body type of a person. Hot is one of the yang symptoms, appears as yang over yin, with yin deficiency and yang excess, mainly manifesting as a body that is thermally hot. Cold is one of the yin symptoms and appears as yin over yang with yang deficiency and yin excess, mainly manifesting as a body that is thermally cold. The symptoms of cold are often felt in the limbs and appear as clear urine and pallor. The syndromes of hot often include hot flashes, warm or hot body, constipation, short temper and irritated mind. The following are some details about hot and cold symptoms.

Hot Illness

Hot illness often appears with characteristics as: redness, fever, thirst, dryness, strong symptoms, sudden and acute occurrence, and often (but not always) in the upper part of the body. Pain is burning or sharp.

The symptoms of hot illnesses can be one or some of the following: high body temperature, fever, constipation, short and red urine, sore throat, high blood pressure, heatstroke, inflammation, infection, hot flashes, pain with infection or inflammation, severe headache (but sometimes cold illness can also have headache), dry and/or bitter mouth, anger, and short temper.

The treatment for hot illness is to cleanse heat, tonify yin, and provide the patient with cooling energy, such as cooling diets, herbs and energy music. However if the heat is an empty heat (not a real heat) caused by yin deficiency as a chronic condition, the treatment should supply yin or treat with warm tonification, instead of simply cleansing heat with cooling energy.

Cold Illness

Cold illness is often caused by external cold Qi (sometimes along with wind) invading the body, causing an individual's blood to lose its yang warmth and circulation force, thus resulting in blocks, clogging or stagnating blood circulation, and therefore the patient often feels cold, gets cold easily, or becomes sick easily/often, as (with cold illness) the immune system is weak. Sometimes long-term sickness also causes deficiency of Qi and blood, and results in cold illness.

The symptoms of cold illnesses can be one or some of the following: cold limbs, fear of cold temperatures, sometimes feeling cold such that the muscles and tendons are contracted, feeling relaxed or tiredness, or many possible pain syndromes such as: joint pain, back pain, stomach pain, abdominal pain, headache, menstrual pain, frequent urination, diarrhea, cramping, twisting, stiffness or tightness of somewhere – e.g., abdominal area, legs or the body. Patients with cold illness often appear with darkened skin, lips or tongue, lack of thirst, skinny, weak, talk with low voice, are less active, do not want to move around, sometimes a couple of these appearances with depression, unhappiness, fear, worry, over-concern or over-carefulness, and low or no self-confidence. For females when the cold symptom worsens, sometimes there is vaginal bleeding.

The treatment for cold illness is to tonify warm yang, provide the patient with warm energy, such as warm or hot diets, herbs, and warm and yang energy music. However if the patient has internal heat coupling with the cold illness (it is typical case because the yin deficiency that caused cold illness as a chronic condition can result in excessive yang, appearing as empty heat or called internal heat), the treatment should be warm tonification to warm up the yin and uplift the yang, instead of simply supplying hot energy.

Deficiency and Excess

Deficiency (Empty)

Deficiency (also called *Empty* or *Xu* in Chinese) refers to deficiency in Qi, blood, Yin or Yang, which is classified as Yin illness. Deficiencies can additionally be seen in the different organs. As such, they can further be classified as: lung Qi deficiency, heart blood deficiency, liver yin deficiency, spleen Qi deficiency, kidney yang deficiency, kidney yin deficiency and so forth. Deficiency symptoms also appear as weakness of the body – e.g. loss of weight, lack of energy, or cold symptoms and other deficiency symptoms can manifest as pale complexion, listlessness, fatigue, heart palpitations, shortness of breath, cold limbs, heat flashes (internal empty heat caused by yin deficiency), spontaneous sweating, diarrhea, loose stools, frequent urination, incontinence, tongue having very little coating or no coating, and pulse force as empty, weak.

Both *Qi* (belonging to yang) *deficiency* and *Yang deficiency* (meaning lack in *Yang Qi*), show deficiency symptoms such as pale face or tongue, easy to fatigue, and spontaneous sweating especially during night sleep, but Qi deficiency does not show cold symptoms – e.g. fear of cold temperature, where as Yang deficiency does show cold symptoms – e.g. afraid of cold and slow pulse.

Both *blood* (belong to yin) *deficiency* and *Yin deficiency* manifest as a lack in body fluids, and show symptoms such as loss of weight, dizziness, heart palpitation, and insomnia.

However, the difference between Qi deficiency and blood deficiency is: blood deficiency does not cause excessive yang, so clinically it does not cause internal heat, while yin deficiency causes yang excess, generating internal heat which is empty heat, and not real heat.

Yin Deficiency $\Rightarrow$ Excessive Yang $\Rightarrow$ Internal Heat (Empty Heat)

Blood Deficiency $\neq>$ Excessive Yang $\neq>$ Internal Heat

For deficiency symptoms, treatment should use the method of tonifying. For example, for deficiency of Qi, blood, yin or yang, the way to treat the condition is to tonify Qi, blood, yin or yang, relatively.

Excess (Real or Full)

Excess (also called Full, Real or *Shi* in Chinese) refers to external sick Qi – e.g. cold invades the body or something inside the body accumulates to the extent of excess that causes sickness. For example, external cold Qi causes the body to have fever, which is real heat, called Excess Heat. The way to treat excess heat (real heat) is to cleanse the heat and eliminate the excessive Qi. However, sometimes a long-term deficiency of yin (lack in yin energy) cannot suppress yang, so that yang is relatively higher. This generates internal heat. Such heat is caused by yin deficiency, but not by real heat, therefore, it is called empty heat. Thus, the way to treat it is to tonify yin making the internal empty heat automatically disappear and balancing the relatively higher yang.

If the Excess illness is caused by external sick Qi invading the body, then the symptom occurs suddenly, and the condition develops fast and severe. If the dysfunction of internal organs caused the blockages of blood and Qi, it is often seen as blood stasis, phlegm, fluid condensation, parasitic diseases, food stagnation, and so on. Excess illness appears as a dramatic stage of struggling between the body's life force/positive energy and the sickness (sick Qi). It shows clinical manifestations such as: high fever, hot flashes, irritability, distention, pain, fullness of stomach, chest or abdomen, phlegm, dampness, constipation, or bleeding lumps, swelling, indigestion, parasites, thick tongue with greasy coating, and forceful pulse.

The way to treat excess illness is to cleanse the sick Qi. For example, if it is real heat, then cleanse the heat. If it is blocks of blood, then unlock the related meridians and then promote the circulation. Clinically you may need to do both: cleanse the excess *and* promote the circulation at the same time.

Up to this point, we have addressed the diagnosis procedures and methods based on traditional oriental medicine. As mind-body medicine practice, however, we need to further incorporate the mental or psychological factors in the patient's condition, so we will diagnose the patient as the whole being.

Different from general psychologists, we consider the mental, emotional and spiritual issues with more focus on (1) the energy mechanism (Yin-Yang and Five Elements) at multiple dimensions and (2) the spiritual natures of the universe, toward improvements in these two aspects in pursuit of a total healing from the root.

For example, if the patient has emotional anxiety and anger, then we will consider other conditions to figure out where the liver fire came from at multiple energy levels – e.g. liver organ and emotion. It can be due to kidney deficiency, liver yin deficiency, overwhelming liver yang, lack of sleeping or missing the liver sleeping time (11 p.m. – 1 a.m.), diet habit, stress, relationship, social environment, temperament, character, parental or family influences, genetic factors and so on or combinations of these factors.

Through the initial conversation combined with the energy diagnosis as described above, you will get a clear idea about the causes for such an emotional issue. At the same time, as a spiritual healer, we are clear that any emotional negativity – e.g., anger and anxiety as in this case – is karmic and is against the person's true nature, the universe's nature, and should be improved no matter what reason has caused it, otherwise it can cause further problems.

These causes at the energetic and spiritual levels should be taken into the complete diagnosis and dealt with in whatever treatment plan can be made (see the following section).

For other cases you will find out other energy causes and emotional/spiritual causes. In general, based on The Five Elements principle, the negative emotion fear (or positive emotions of courage, positive, motivated, confident) is related with the kidney (meridian includes kidney organ but this inclusion is not always necessary) energy status, grief (or calmness, peace) is related with lung system energy state, worry (or empathy, sympathy) is associated with spleen/stomach energy level, hate and over excitement (or joy, love and happiness) are related with heart meridian energy status, and anger (or patience and altruism) are coupled with liver Qi blocks and liver Yang (heat or fire) overwhelming, respectively. Because of the relationship of mutual generation and mutual restriction within The Five Elements, the energy causes can be combinations of these factors within multiple meridians and their associated emotional natures, but do not have to be associated with only one single meridian.

Element	Meridian	Negative Emotions	Positive Emotions
Water	Kidney	Fear, depression, negative	Courage, positive, motivated, confident
Wood	Liver	Anger, anxiety, short temper, impatience	Patience, altruism
Fire	Heart	Hate, negative, selfish, over-excitement	Love, joy, happiness
Earth	Spleen	Worry, anxiety, apprehension	Empathy, sympathy
Metal	Lung	Grief, sorrow, sadness	Calmness, peace

Table 9.5. Correlations of the five elements, meridian energy systems, positive emotions and negative emotions.

§9.6 Treatment Principles

Before we design a treatment plan, it is necessary to address the basic treatment principles. In addition to the principles of Yin-Yang and The Five Elements and highest spiritual law, in mind-body health practice the treatment principles also refer to and incorporate some traditional oriental medicine treatment principles, and the spiritual nature of the universe, and mind-body-spirit model. These principles are:

1. Uphold Goodness and Suppresses Evil (扶正祛邪). The life itself has its vital life force that is the most fundamental power to heal disease and restore health. This principle applies at both the physical energy level and mental/spiritual levels. The reason one gets sick physically and/or mentally is because the original life force and/or spiritual nature is weak, and taken over by the sick Qi and/or bad conscious noises. Sickness is evil that is against the goodness. To heal the sickness, the key is to (1) strengthen the original vital life force based on the Yin-Yang Five Elements principle and (2) return to the original nature/characteristics of the true Self, spiritual nature of the universe: peace, love, compassion, forgiveness, patience, etc.

2. Tonify Deficiency and Reduce Excess （補虛瀉實）. If the energy is deficient, then treat the patient with a reinforcing method (tonify) to restore the vital life force, while if it is in an excessive condition, then treat the problem with a reducing

method to dispel the pathogenic factors and eliminate stagnation, and help restore systemic immunity.

In mind-body medicine practice, we also apply this principle to mental and spiritual practice. If the patient has weakness, confusion, cloudiness or ambiguity in the mind/mental or spiritual energy state, then we treat the patient with a tonifying method by providing positive energies of higher spiritual clarification, reinforcement, enlightenment and cultivation. While if the patient has negative, bad and unhealthy emotions, blockages, noises, bad thoughts, notions, habits, addictions, or attachments, then we treat the patient with a releasing method to eliminate these negative energies while still strengthening the positive higher spiritual energy.

3. Mind-Body-Spirit Model. We have addressed the model of mind-body-spirit (dual energy switch) in earlier chapters. This is a very useful model in the treatment of many mental and physical health problems and energy issues. The patient gets transformed to a totally new person once they wake up to the truth that (1) the human thoughts, desires, notions, attachments, addictions, etc. are at the lower level, consuming energy (*Ec*) and causing problems including health problems, and (2) the original spirit came from the high level of spirit and can be cultivated to generate higher energy (*Eg*), assimilate with the higher spiritual source towards higher life level, true health and high quality of this life and future life destination.

4. Patients and Doctor Cultivating the Mind Nature and Vital Energy. The doctor's daily cultivation in mind nature, energy and spirituality strengthens his/her energy, belief and self-confidence, clarity of mind to help the patient truly wake up to the truth of life, learn meditation and mind-body cultivation, and quickly let go of negative emotions, attachments, addiction, unhealthy habits, and start a new healthy lifestyle, personal improvement and cultivation. As a result, the mind, emotions and energy truly become positive and healthy.

§9.7 Design the Healing Plan

Now upon an energy status and mental state diagnosis based on the eight principles, energy principle and spiritual law, as well as the treatment principles, we can come up with a clear picture about the patient's energy pattern, body condition, mental status, emotional mood, and spiritual nature, and we can treat the whole being with a clear goal, focus, and complete treatment strategy and plan.

The plan for the treatment comes naturally with the following components:

1. **Healing Energy Patterns Based on the Energy Diagnosis**

For example, if the patient has liver yin deficiency and liver yang excess, then choose the wood yin, water yin, of healing energy vibrations – e.g. Five Elements music – in order to treat the patient. After some sessions, if the condition improves and stabilizes, use the combination of Five Elements to strengthen the overall health, immune system function, Yin and Yang balance and emotional stability.

2. Mental and Spiritual Healing Practice

Based on the patient's mental, emotional and spiritual condition, plan a gradual improvement plan. After the energy healing improves the patient's feelings and overall health, such as sleep, appetite, emotional comfort, and peace of mind, start mental and spiritual healing based on the treatment principles (1 – 4) as described in previous section.

In the first session, however, you should not go too high in the spiritual aspects because you want to give your patient more time to get ready for self-improvement practice. The improvement can be started with the energy healing first, which you provided with the right energy vibrations for the blocked meridians – e.g., liver, kidney, and heart meridians in this case. This energy healing makes your patient feel good by soothing liver Qi, releasing liver fire, and enhancing the liver yin and kidney yin.

As the patient progresses smoothly in the positive direction, you can start the emotional and spiritual healing and teaching, in order to help the individual cultivate him/her self with peace, compassion, tolerance, patience, forgiveness, truthfulness, and positive mindset, healthy lifestyle, living schedule and natural diet, as well as with higher quality physical and mental energy while he/she learns about the true Self and the true nature of the universe (refer other chapters associated with meditation, energy music therapy, brainwave-meridian therapy).

§9.8 Intermediate Break: Story • Meditation

The healing story below is from a successfully healed 84-year old man.

Rejuvenated Vital Energy and Sex Drive

- David S.

Being an 84-year old man, I'm not afraid to tell you that I have a girlfriend in her 50's. I love her very much and would do anything to make her happy. But there was one thing I couldn't do because of my age. This really made me feel guilty sometimes.

By accident, I saw Dr. Jason Liu's advertisement on Vision Magazine. I felt a connection with this doctor. I called him to ask if he could help me at my age and was surprised by his positive answer and convincing explanation about his needle-free/drug free energy healing technique, so I immediately made an appointment with him.

After the pulse reading, Dr. Liu very confidently told me that his technique could rejuvenate my lost vital energy and kidney meridian function and may possibly improve sexuality. After he explained about vital life force, energy healing, Oriental medicine, the central neuron system, and the mind-body connection, which are all associated with the sex drive, he started treating me right at the first session. I really enjoyed each session with him. It was so relaxing and comfortable. Sometimes I would fall asleep. After the session, I felt relaxed, refreshed and energetic.

I need to share some surprising results: after the 6th session, my high blood pressure (usually around 180 / 110) returned to normal (118 / 75), and I could stop all five high blood pressure medications. After the 10th session, I was walking much easier and longer without any problem. I used to have weakness in my left leg and knee due to a stroke. After 12 sessions, I started feeling something that I haven't experienced for a long time - my sex drive returned!

I feel younger and happier emotionally, and physically, it's really an improvement to my overall health. I gained a lot of confidence about my relationship. I gained a lot of confidence about my relationship.

Meditation with Energy Healing Music

EHM09: The Sea of Happiness *(Yang, Fire, Wood)*

This music is composed with focus on the relatively yang energy of fire and wood elements to strengthen your heart and liver energy. However if you feel you are over heated, anxious, overwhelmed, have too much heat internally or feel too excited and ungrounded emotionally (yang type of condition), then you can choose the following CD (yin type of the healing music) to practice.

EHM10: Eternal life after many lives *(Yin, Fire, Wood)*

Meditate with the energy music as long as you can (for example, one hour), it will improve your vital energy, overall health and hormone balance, slow down your aging process and rejuvenate your body, mind and spirit.

[*Play Energy Healing Music #9*] Sit cross-legged or stand with relaxed posture, and meditate with your mind calm, positive, and happy. Deeply breathe and absorb the bright and positive energy vibration. Keep your shoulders down and entire body relaxed. Let go of all worries, no more depression, fear, wondering, confusion, anxiety, or any blocks in your mind, appreciate the peace of your every current moment, stay focused on your Dantian point (belly area) - your energy center. With this energy vibration, you are unified, harmonized and energized mentally, physically and spiritually. Eventually you are completely melted into the ocean of eternal peace and perfect happiness.

§9.9 Exercise Questions

1. Take a piece of paper or notebook, face a mirror and sit down to practice doing a self-diagnosis. Make sure the room has bright enough natural light. Start by asking yourself the ten questions as chapter 9.2 described.

    Mark each question with yes or no based on your own health condition. Give a simple explanation if needed. Then, start the diagnosis through looking: look at your eyes, face, appearance, fitness, complexion, and tongue (different parts of tongue). In each step, write down what you see and what health issues may be related with what you see.

2. Based on the Eight Principles of traditional Oriental medicine diagnosis, summarize the information you have just collected about your own health condition, and try to evaluate your own health status, energy pattern, or any possible issues you may think you would like to improve.

3. Do you identify any mental, emotional, or spiritual issues that concern you? Include these issues in your energy diagnosis above and associate them – e.g. the organ fear is associated with is the kidney, the energy imbalance is a kidney deficiency, and the cause is relationship difficulty.

4. Make a plan of treatment for yourself for any issue you have found in your diagnosis.

5. Follow the same diagnostic and treatment model (1-4 above), practice summarizing information and creating a treatment plan (if necessary) for anyone in your family or for, friends, classmates, or coworkers.

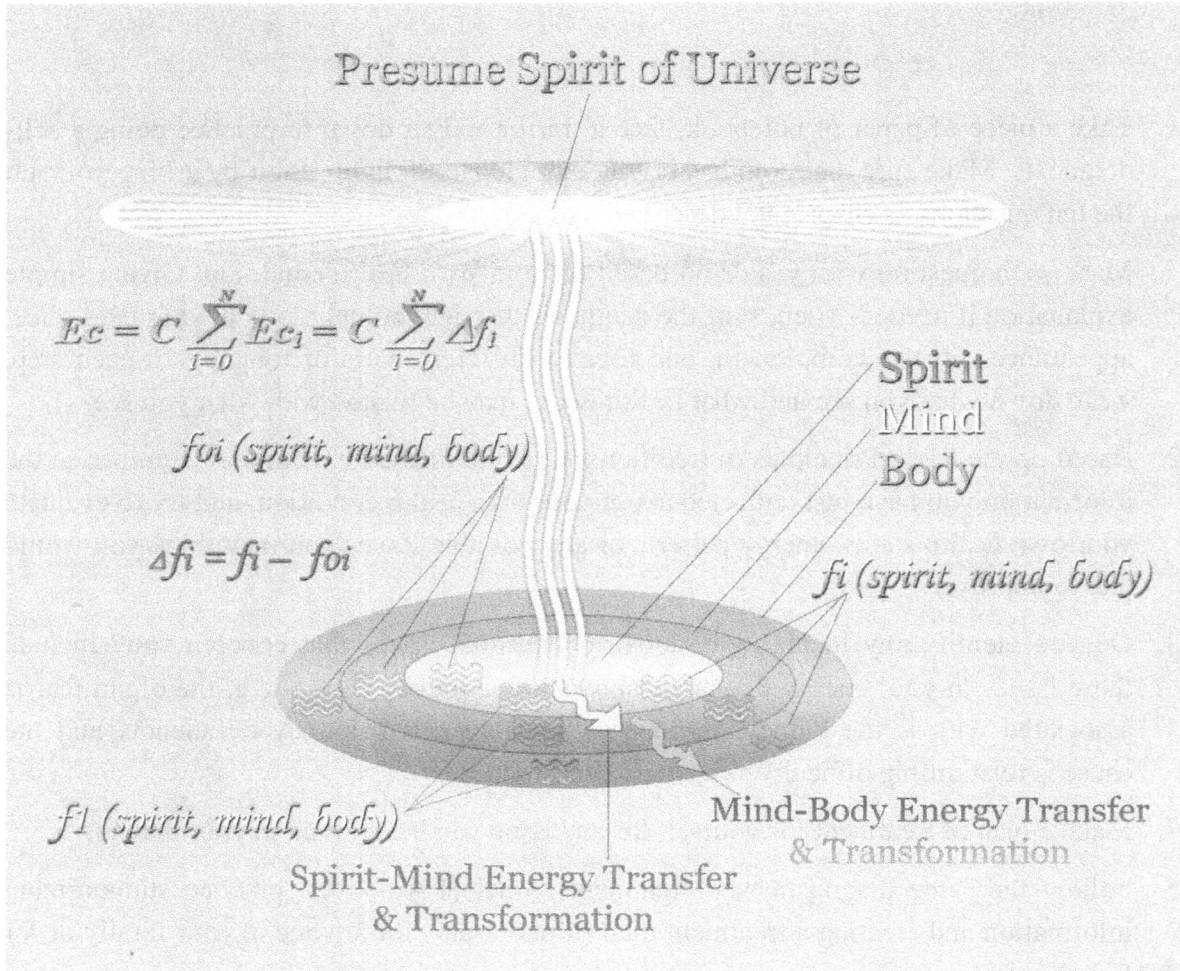

Presume Spirit of Universe

$$Ec = C \sum_{I=0}^{N} Ec_1 = C \sum_{I=0}^{N} \Delta f_1$$

f_{oi} (spirit, mind, body)

$$\Delta f_i = f_i - f_{oi}$$

Spirit
Mind
Body

f_i (spirit, mind, body)

f_1 (spirit, mind, body)

Mind-Body Energy Transfer & Transformation

Spirit-Mind Energy Transfer & Transformation

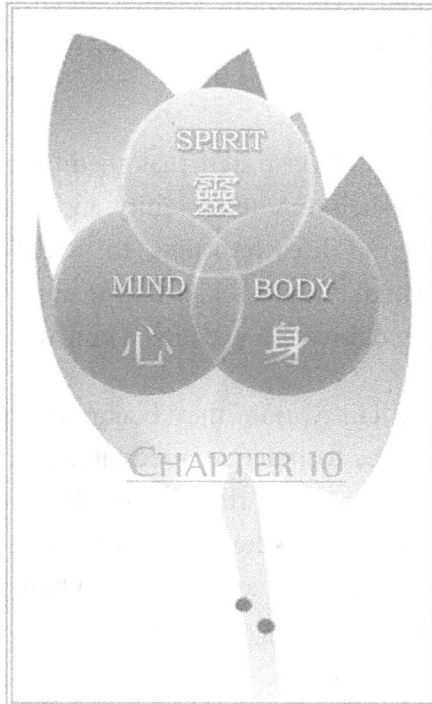

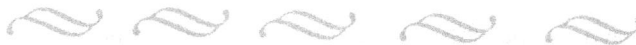

Meditation • Spiritual Realms: Mind-Body-Spirit Practice

In this chapter, I will take you to the joyful journey of meditation, the most fundamental and effective mind-body-spirit cultivation and MBM and healthology practice. We will also explore the wonderful spiritual realms in other dimensions beyond this material world and find out the answers to the following questions: What is the true health of the whole being? What is the true meaning and purpose of this life? And what is the eternal destination of our future life? Then, for true health and eternal destination, we will learn to practice higher energy life force, and cultivate the mind, body and spirit to a higher level.

We will not address any specific style of meditation such as Qigong, Taiji, Yoga, or other belief system associated meditations, but we do humbly and respectfully learn from those traditional practices and study meditation as a health practice and scientific field.

Meditation has a fairly long history. Its root travels back to ancient time, and parallels the same path and timeline as divine teaching for human enlightenment and civilization. At least in this human civilization, meditation culture began with the sage, Lao Tzu who taught humankind the Tao (Dao) and Buddha Shakyamuni taught the Fa, the way of enlightenment.

Some evidence, however, demonstrated that meditation cultivation practice came from a prehistoric civilization. In such remote antiquity, meditation was the way of a human being seeking the true meaning of life, returning to true Self, the origin of life, and connecting to the heaven or spiritual realm, as its lifetime purpose. This is called cultivation. And the person who practices the cultivation is called a cultivator.

As more people practiced cultivation, they began to organize together and set up a certain place, format and even rules to practice, meditate, chant, and even live together as group. This was how religion started in the Orient. It's why today people have the impression that only those monks and nuns or religious people practiced cultivation meditation and only in the temples or monasteries. Whenever mentioning meditation, people often easily associate it with a sort of religion, belief system, or those traditional monasteries, convents, monks and nuns.

Meditation, however, is actually not necessarily only practiced by monks or nuns in the temples or monasteries, but it indeed can be practiced by any human being. Meditation came to the human world originally without any religious format. It was simply known in our long history as the way toward spiritual enlightenment, human cultivation, longevity, health and wellness for the whole being, the body, mind and spirit.

Meditation itself is not any religion although various religions practice it in their temples or monasteries. In fact, today an increasing number of people practice meditation at home, community, public parks, or anywhere, in a free format and in their daily life.

At least over 5000 years ago during The Yellow Emperor's Era, people already knew and practiced meditation to calm their minds, stay still and quiet, balance their mind and body, and achieve inner peace and health. A typical example of a meditation practitioner is the well-known ancient longevity practitioner Peng Zu[13] who lived in the human world for over 800 hundred years. Based on the written record called "Pengzu Jing"

---

[13] **Peng Zu** (彭祖, Ancestor Peng) is an ancient longevity master in China. Based on many historical records, he lived over 800 years in the Yin Dynasty (殷朝 1900-1066 BC). Peng Zu was regarded as a saint in Taoism and longevity master. The longevity culture, meditation cultivation lifestyle and pursuit of eternity drugs in the Tao culture were deeply rooted in Peng Zu's cultivation life stories. He is well known in ancient and modern longevity culture as a symbol for long life, nutrition treatments, and long sex therapy treatments. It is said he married more than 100 wives and with them had hundreds of children, into the age of 800. He was regarded as the God of Longevity.

and other records in the history, at the ending period of Shang Yin (商殷末), Peng Zu was already 767 years old, but he was still healthy and strong, keeping his practice, and living his long life. He was excellent in cooking many kinds of longevity porridges (soups or gruels) and natural herbs to enrich his nutrition. He practiced meditation cultivation every day. Below is a very old description of his life and health practice:

He often sits there and meditates with slow breath, keeps his mind focused on Dantian, staying in a still upright position from morning until noon. Every time before he ends his practice, he gently rubs his eyes, massages every part of his body, his tongue licks his lips and he swallows his saliva, slowly breathes dozens of times. After that he takes a walk and has conversation with people while happily laughing. If he occasionally feels tired or uncomfortable physically, then he practices meditation and his breath exercise.

This, as described above, was the story as told many thousands of years ago when Peng Zu was already nearly 800 years old, without knowing science and technology as we have now at modern time.

At that time, he already knew the way to live long and stay healthy. There was no religious format he was associated with at that time. It was far earlier than the time Lao Tzu teaching the Dao and Shakyamuni teaching the Buddha Fa, and Jesus Christ teaching his enlightenment. In fact even during the times through which Lao Tzu and Shakyamuni lived their lives, Taoism or Buddhism were not yet "religions." Several hundreds of years later, after they left the human world, their disciples established these respective forms of religion.

Since then, meditation practice or cultivation methods were spread throughout the human world, with influences from different religions and belief systems, or in non-religious format. It is believed that originally these meditation cultivation forms mysteriously and divinely came to human world because the higher divines want human beings to be enlightened and to be able to return to the original life form in the spiritual dimension after this physical life. This is the original purpose of all cultivation practices. It's why, after a certain period of time in history, there were certainly high level masters coming forward to teach cultivation, such as Lao Tzu, Shakyamuni and Jesus Christ as we mentioned above.

Because meditation cultivation methods originally came from higher divines, they are very powerful and effective in improving the health of mind, body and spirit, crossing different dimensions. From ancient time, however, people already knew that meditation practice is an effective way for health of the whole being, the body, mind and spirit.

As a result, meditation has been practiced as a healing and health method for our entire civilized history, not only in the temples or monasteries, but also in the everyday society, family, healing places and health centers. In modern times, scientists, doctors, psychologists and holistic healthcare practitioners have widely researched and practiced meditation as a mind-body medicine practice, health practice or self-healing or self-improvement and development method. So many researches have been done and evidenced that meditation improves mental and physical health. One of the good examples is the research throughout many years by the Center for Investigating Healthy Minds at University of Wisconsin, founded by world-renowned neuroscientist Dr. Richard J. Davidson [54]. Some other scientists such as the group from Massachusetts General Hospital, Harvard Medical School, Boston, MA, found that meditation help improve brain structure and functions including gray matter, emotional state, memory, pain sensitivity, etc. [55-58].

Throughout a long history in the human world, however, these cultivation methods such as meditation practice have been gradually mixed with human thoughts, religious ideas and formats, impure messages and contaminated energy from lower spirits and material world. Some meditation forms, methods or procedures have nothing to do with the original purpose of meditation cultivation. Especially as the human world becomes more materialistic, people nowadays have so many attachments that it is not easy to empty the mind during meditation. Although some people try to meditate, their minds have so many thoughts evolving within the human realm, desires, and messages from daily life that they cannot really meditate with a quiet mind.

Many people today no longer even believe in meditation and spiritual cultivation as important lifetime practices at all. So, for many individuals, meditation practice is not really related with the original goal of spiritual enlightenment.

As well, many meditation practitioners no longer know or have ever heard about – much less studied and cultivated – the true meaning and purpose of meditation at all. For the majority of people today, the core truth and purpose of meditation is unfamiliar. This is especially so for those places influenced by atheism. Many people don't even believe in spiritual cultivation. They as well do not believe meditation has any benefit toward the health of body, mind and spirit. Some think spiritual belief and/or meditation cultivation is a form of superstition, and they are either drawn to it or turn off to it for that reason. The worst thing is that some cultivation practices and meditators are suppressed and persecuted – even during our modern times.

Today's materialistic world drives people more and more toward the loss of true Self, leaving their mindset far away from the original nature and looking outwards, ignoring truth, confused about the goodness and evil, being busy for the short term of material life pursuits and forgetting about the lifetime goal and the meaning of original life. As a result, health problems are caused at all levels, mentally, physically, and spiritually.

Due to all these reasons described above, understanding and learning the original and fundamental principle and practice of meditation is extremely important for either a mind-body medicine healthcare professional or any individual practicing mind-body self-healing and health.

In this chapter, instead of discussing any particular form of meditation or any religion or other belief system associated meditation forms, we will teach the original style of meditation cultivation that was rooted in the ancient cultivation practice for the mind, body and spirit as the most important part of mind-body medicine and health practice.

§10.2 General Principle, Form and Method of Meditation

The core principle of meditation is to cultivate your mind, body and spirit by letting go of human thoughts, desires, attachments, and purifying and elevating your life by assimilating with the universe's nature and resonating with the energy vibration of the universe while staying in a still position, calming the mind and body, and entering an empty, relaxed, meditated and energetic conscious state.

Extensively, meditation cultivation also includes practice in daily life to improve mind nature, spiritual quality and lifestyle. In our spirit-mind-body model discussed in the previous chapters, meditation cultivation is a practice that activates, cultivates and enhances the spiritual mind, switches on the energy generation system, and at the same time turns off the human mind, lets go of human attachments and ego mindset, increases the human mind threshold[14], and limits the energy consumption, achieving a higher level of mind-body-spirit, and its energy, health, longevity, and future destination life.

In the most fundamental style of sitting meditation, you choose a quiet location such as your bedroom, living room, reading room, back yard, or a park where you will have no interruption, no windy conditions, and a suitable temperature. Warm sunlight is fine, but not direct sunlight, especially if it is too hot. If inside a room, it is fine with or without a light on, depending on your preference or can be different from time to time, depending upon your mood or feeling.

The place where you meditate must have good quality fresh air and natural air circulation. Wear easy-to-relax-in, comfortable clothing and no shoes. Turn off your phones and any other alarm that may disturb you while you practice meditation. You can have a piece of meditation music or energy healing music playing continuously while you are

---

[14] Human Mind Threshold: the minimal amount of distractions or triggers from the material world which cause the mind to be moved, shaken, addicted, frustrated, attached to it, interrupted, contaminated, and energy consumed.

meditating. Adjust the music in a comfortable volume, and let it go on without stopping throughout your meditation. A regular music CD is not recommended because it is not designed for a continuous peaceful meditation not only because of the musical style, expression and energy pattern, but also each track of such a regular music CD is usually only a few minutes long, so it will keep changing from one track to another, aimed at different musical moods and sound flow, disturbing your meditation when the track changes.

Relax your mind and body to get ready to enjoy your meditation. If you have a meditation cushion, you can sit on it, otherwise a carpeted floor or firm bed is fine. The cross-legged double lotus position is a typical traditional meditation posture and recommended for you as the best sitting meditation position. In the position of cross-legged sitting, for ladies, first you bring your right foot up and place on your left thigh, then your left foot set up to your right thigh. For gentlemen, just do the opposite; your left foot is first placed above the right thigh, and then the right foot sets above your left thigh. Your overlapped/conjoined hands (palms) set around your lower abdomen area or placed above your crossed lower legs. The hands form a circle by conjoining your thumb tips together. For ladies, your right hand is on top above your left palm, and for gentlemen you do the opposite. Sit upright with your spine and neck straight, but naturally relaxed.

Relax your shoulders and naturally drop them down, but never hold them up or tightly up while you are meditating. Gently close your eyes and your mouth, leave a space between upper and lower teeth, the tip of your tongue naturally touches your upper (hard) palate, and bring a peaceful smile to your face with your mind feeling compassionate, love, peaceful, truthful, righteous, and positive. Then, gradually get into a deep stillness. At the beginning if you are not relaxed well, use your mind to check through all parts of your mind and body to make sure you completely relaxed, but not too loose, so your conscious mind stays clear, empty, relaxed and energized.

In addition to the sitting position, you also can stand in a still posture to meditate. You stand with feet at shoulder width, legs slightly bended at a comfortable angle, your back upright straight, arms relaxed naturally forming a circle in the front of your body, hands overlapped and placed at the Dantian (main location of Qi) area, about 2 inches below the belly. For women your right hand is above left hand, while men do the opposite. Same as within the sitting meditation described above, peacefully close your eyes and mouth, tip of your tongue touches the upper palate, empty your mind, and stay still to meditate. Relax your entire body, but not too loose, and keep your mind quiet, still, peaceful, empty, free of any thought – note, however, that your consciousness is aware that you are meditating.

This is the simplest posture for the standing meditation that can be practiced as an alternative to the sitting meditation. You can even vary positions if you like. For example, you may practice sitting meditation during the evening and then try your standing meditation in the morning.

During meditation, your mind is empty, has no other thought or negative emotions, stays inward instead of outward, and keeps a positive mood, but not excited. Your conscious mind and subconscious mind have no wandering or random thinking, no attachment and desire or intention, no narrowed mind and stubbornness, just remaining open minded and broad hearted, so that you are being one with the universe, surrounded by the universe's energy, and getting deeper and deeper into a meditation state.

At the beginning, you may check through your mind and body to make sure everything is relaxed and quiet, and then you gradually get into stillness, a deep meditation state, so that you almost unaware of your surroundings, but your conscious mind is still aware that you are meditating. Sometimes, you may notice a bright light right front of your third eye (as it is referred to, the point between eyebrows and connecting to the pineal gland). It is a good thing and may mean you are gaining good energy and spiritually energized. Do not attach on it too much; simply let it progress naturally.

§10.3 Meditation State: Beautiful & Joyful Spiritual Dimensions

There is no better joyful experience than a deep meditation that truly gives you a meaningful, inspiring and fantastic quality time, making you feel that you have gone back to your real home extremely peaceful and lovely – this is your permanent home that belongs to your Self forever. No matter what you have in this material world including fame, material interest and human sentiments, they are all outside of you and never truly belong to you nor stay with you, but the energy and spiritual power cultivated during your meditation are inside you, belong to your own life, stay with you this moment, every moment and forever. This is absolutely true, and not an overstatement.

As you go deeper and deeper in your meditation, your physical body is sitting there and relaxed, but you feel all parts of your body have disappeared, all surroundings have disappeared, space has disappeared, time has disappeared, thoughts have disappeared, and there is only a very little consciousness, which knows you are meditating … all becomes one, and you stay with the whole, while in the front of you and surrounding you is an unshaped light-space that is so peaceful, soft, gentle, friendly, lovely, warm, safe, trustworthy, very transparent, immersive, totally new and mysterious to you, extremely beautiful, colorful, lightening, stable, constantly there forever into infinity – with no intentional consciousness, no thinking – total empty – and you are witnessing colorful lights, images, and magnificence the likes of which you have never experienced in the physical world.

Stay still into the infinity. In fact, this is actually your own spirit you are experiencing, at your own home ... forever.

If you meditate with energy music (see later chapters), the musical vibrations bring you more colorful lights, flowers, and never seen images. Those colors are never seen in this physical world. They are so fresh, real, clear, immersive (multidimensional), impressive, striking, transparent, very friendly belonging to only you and connecting to your spirit, making you want to stay with them forever and never want to leave them.

You probably have heard people talking about heavenly out-of-body experience, near death experience, deep trance experience, past life regression, entering other dimensions beyond this physical world, and so on. These are all real occurrences in other dimensions which your soul can enter and directly experience during your meditation.

As a meditation cultivator and spiritual healing practitioner, I myself have had similar experiences during meditation every day. These are amazing, fantastic experiences that give me so many blessings, happiness and strength mentally, spiritually and physically. I have interviewed some dear friends who had near death experiences (NDE), including their senior leaders and members in their San Diego local group of the International Association for Near-Death Studies (ISNDS). We will discuss the topic of NDE in a separate chapter. As a quick point, however, here I would like to mention that many peaceful happy experiences during meditation are pretty similar to the experiences of the NDE people. The only difference, however, is that meditation process still has slightly conscious feelings involved while NDE totally has no main conscious mind experience involved. This implies that meditation allows the soul or spirit of the meditator to enter spiritual dimensions and have an out of body experience similar to NDE.

Also, differences between meditation experience and NDE depend upon each individual and their cultivation level, Virtue and belief. This may be why NDE, in general, can be more dramatic, stronger and richer. The most recent Newsweek Magazine's cover story told by Dr. Eben Alexander, a neurosurgeon who taught at Harvard Medical School and other universities. Alexander explored the secret of spiritual realms, and provides experiential proof of the existence of a heaven [59-60]. "Toward the beginning of my adventure, I was in a place of clouds. Big, puffy, pink-white ones that showed up sharply against the deep blue-black sky." Dr. Alexander described his NDE. "Higher than the clouds—immeasurably higher—flocks of transparent, shimmering beings arced across the sky, leaving long, streamer-like lines behind them." He saw and experienced these wonderful beings and described how they appeared: "Birds? Angels? These words registered later, when I was writing down my recollections. But neither of these words do justice to the beings themselves, which were quite simply different from anything I have known on this planet. They were more advanced. Higher forms." He even heard "a sound, huge and booming like a glorious chant, came down from above, and I wondered if the winged beings were producing it. Again, thinking about it later, it occurred to me that the joy of these creatures, as they soared along, was such that they had to make this noise – that if the joy didn't come out of them this way then they would simply not otherwise be able to contain it. The sound was palpable and almost material, like a rain that you can feel on your skin but doesn't get you wet." Dr. Alexander traveled through the heavens, surrounded by "millions of butterflies," with a woman. This woman even gave him three clear messages: "You are loved and cherished, dearly, forever," and "You have nothing to fear," and "There is nothing you can do wrong." [59-60].

The NDE described by Dr. Alexander and by other NDE people give us a similar message: there is a much more beautiful life after this physical life in other dimension(s) where one can reach, only the physical brain is shut down or nearly shut down. It's why during meditation if we stop conscious and subconscious activities in the brain, our soul or spirit can enter such high dimension(s) and experience the heavenly kingdom as occurs for those within a near death experience.

If there are so many human thoughts and desires in the mind during meditation, however, there is no way to reach the higher level dimensions. It's why letting go of human attachments and ego through cultivation in meditation and daily life is very important for this life and future life. Only good cultivation practice such as a deep meditation can allow you to enter such higher dimensions and give you these experiences. Through such practice and experience at other dimension(s), you actually travel different levels of the spiritual realms crossing all higher dimensions.

As you progress with your practice, you can enrich your experience, reach different levels of spiritual cultivation energy, and achieve an energetically higher level of spiritual life and future life, the destination of your current life.

These experiences are not just experiences. Indeed, they are the processes of your permanent life journey from the true health of this life to the eternal destination. They are meaningful teaching lessons and experiences that teach us about the real purpose of this life and how to accomplish the purpose. In fact the mind-body-spirit cultivation process is the actual path by which you can reach the final destination to the heavenly kingdom: you are taking action to make the purpose comes true. From this understanding, we can say spiritual cultivation, such as meditation guided by the highest law of universe, is actually a preparation and exercise for the future life after this life. Therefore it is the most important task that we have to take good care of, on a daily basis.

At the beginning of each practice, if you may have some thoughts in your mind or subconscious mind and cannot be quiet to meditate, you can use your mind to send the message throughout yourself to quietly calm. Say: "Relax my mind and body, and let go of all attachments and human thoughts. I am so relaxed and empty that I am completely disappeared from this physical world." Say it gently and even a few times if necessary. Check through all parts of your body to relax completely. You can use your mental eye to look at the front area of your third eye, focus on it and stay still and quiet. You may see the peaceful lights right front of your third eye. Enjoy the peaceful stillness while getting deeper and deeper.

Physiologically, biologically and genetically in such an ideal meditation state all cells, molecules, and particles inside you are transformed to another energetic dimension out of the physical realm and recharged with new fresh energy, cleansing and repairing all the contaminations and damages over the microenvironments of the organs, cells, nerves, blood vessels, hormones, cellular membranes and contents, ion channels, immune cells, and DNA molecules, etc. so that your life is rejuvenated and locked into a younger age or at an even better state than when you were in your younger age. You will get into a totally new dimension, very beautiful and joyful spiritual kingdom. You really want to stay there forever and don't want to come back. But you still have a clear consciousness that tells you that after this trip you still need to go back to the physical world where you can continue your cultivation and achieve the consummation. Thus, you finally do come back to this life time-space with much freshened energy.

If you are a beginner of meditation, you may not immediately achieve such an ideal meditation state, but it is fine to take time to practice and progress gradually. Each person may have different experiences in meditation. However, with no intentional pursuit in meditation, yet with the persistence to keep up your practice, no matter what you have experienced in meditation, you will progress in your practice, and you will have those aforementioned benefits as well as those described in the following section.

Meditation has many unexpected benefits. Knowing the benefits or just reading the benefits listed below will help you improve your meditation with great progress and will also encourage you to meditate daily persistently. The following is a summarized list that describes the major proven benefits of meditation cultivation. But there are many more benefits for sure, yet a complete list would go on too long for the purposes of this book. You will discover more benefits of your meditation as you experience it more over times. As you read the following benefits, your mind will move forward with me to encourage you to practice meditation cultivation every day and improve your health and all aspects of your life. Let's take a look.

1. Spiritual Benefits and Overall Life Improvement: Meditation cultivation transforms one's fundamental life path and quality to higher levels, improves the whole being of mind, body and spirit, eliminates bad Karmas, builds up good Virtues, brings good luck and bright future to your life. This is the first and ultimate benefit. Others include enhancing: physical or physiological health, mental or psychological health, daily performance, efficiency, wisdom, creativity, relationships, friendships, beauty, the deceleration of aging, and promotion of longevity. There are many benefits that meditation cultivation brings you, your family, your business or work. Additionally, you will probably discover even more benefits through your own practice.

2. Personality, Character, Mindfulness and Spirituality: Meditation helps you develop a peaceful mind and a harmonious, happy and meaningful life, brings you self-awareness of the purpose and meaning of your life, helps you develop self-actualization and self-valuation, grows your compassion, love, kindness, righteousness, truthfulness, forgiveness, patience, wisdom, creativity, talents, ability of understanding yourself and others, broadens your heart, and helps you develop acceptance and positive attitudes for changing your life and helping others, brings you inner peace, inward mindset, and synchronicity with society, family, nature and the universe, gives you the wonderful experience of Oneness with the universe, and helps you develop pure spirituality and deeper relationship with the super power towards enlightenment.

3. Energy, Healing and Health: Meditation cultivation opens all your energy channels (meridians), circulates Qi/energy and blood throughout your body and mind, and balances Yin And Yang of your whole being to naturally heal existing health problems, prevent future diseases and improve your health quality, strength, beauty and longevity. Almost all kinds of physical and mental chronic health issues or diseases can be healed, improved or prevented through meditation from simple headaches, migraines, stomachache, common cold, fatigue, stress, and insomnia, to depression, anxiety, high blood pressure, high blood sugar, high cholesterol, weight problems, major organ problems – e.g., heart, lungs, kidneys, liver, stomach – allergies, arthritis, asthma, chronic pain, cancers, bad addictions – e.g., drug, smoke, alcohol – family and social relationship problems.

4. Immune System: Meditation practice naturally and effectively strengthens your immune system, physical and mental strength, vital energy and vigor. There isn't any better way to strengthen your vital energy and vigor than with meditation. It brings you the benefits immediately, effectively and naturally, without side effects, cost, or need of any equipment, but with more conveniences such as time and location. A good meditator has a strong immune system so that he or she never easily gets sick, not even a single common cold as the season changes.

5. Health Benefits on Cardiovascular and Respiratory Systems: Meditation practice deepens your breath, improves oxygen take-up, lowers oxygen consumption, decreases respiratory rate, balances sympathetic and parasympathetic nervous systems, drops down cholesterol levels, lowers risk of cardiovascular diseases, slows your heart rate and improves your heart functions.

6. Nervous Systems/Brain Chemicals/Deep Relaxation: Meditation takes you to the deeper level of physical and mental relaxation, calms and cleans your mind, brain and nervous systems, balances the sympathetic and parasympathetic nervous systems, regulates and balances brain chemicals, betters your sleeping quality and daily performance. Meditation reduces anxiety attacks by lowering the levels of blood lactate. Researches indicate that meditation can improve brain functions and help heal brain chemical imbalance related diseases such as ADD, ADHD, and autism. It reduces the tensions of your muscles, joints and all parts of your body and mind, so you remain in the peaceful, joyful, energetic and positive state physically and mentally.

7. Health Benefits on Hormone/Endocrine System and Sexuality: Meditation balances and strengthens your hormone or endocrine systems, heals and prevents hormonal diseases, improves and prevents female problems – e.g. pre-menstrual symptoms, breast tumors, infertility – and male problems – e.g. impotence, premature ejaculation and improves both male and female sexuality, sexual health, performance, and loving relationships.

8. Prevention of Virus Infection: Meditation reduces the risk of infections from viruses and virus activities that affect your health. The practice also prevents virus-caused diseases, including influenza, avian influenza, plagues, or other kinds of infectious diseases. Not only does meditation strengthen your immunity so that it can fight off the bad viruses in your body, but it also improves your spiritual and mental awareness, helps you let go of attachments, so you will no longer attach to those unhealthy foods, eating habits, living schedules, desires, addictions, negative thoughts and emotions, relationships, and so on – all of which lead you to the risks of poisoning your whole being and to negative karmic factors in your life.

9. Beauty, Fitness and Longevity: Meditation is the best and most effective natural way to transform your life and beauty, improve your skin, improve vitality, appearance, fitness, attractiveness, communication skills and expression, slow down your aging process naturally so you can feel forever youthful, as well as improve your strength and engender a happy longevity. There is really no better way to truly and fundamentally transform your life to such an unexpected high level, no matter with what chemical, mechanical, genetic, cosmetic or other artificial products or advanced technologies you might have already tried.

All those artificial ways only change the surface of your body, but do not really improve your original life force, vital energy and functions, so such beauty is fake, superficial and temporary. Also in most cases those ways are poisoning, contaminating and damaging to your body and mind. Meditation cultivation directly works on your original life mechanism, increases your vital energy, unblocks the blockages of energy flow, cleanses the poisons and toxins, reduces free radicals and limits tissue damage.

Meditation makes your own cells, tissues and organs as well as mind and soul all work together to rejuvenate and transform your entire being so it is refreshed and new. You should see your Self become even younger, more beautiful, and energetic each day as you practice meditation cultivation and begin to let go of attachments to bad lifestyle habits, whether they are staying up late night, eating unhealthy foods, or participating in high risk social behaviors as well as meaningless but time and life energy-consuming activities and entertainments.

10. Pain Improvement and Management: Meditation calms down the mind and body, reduces the internal heat, infection and inflammations, and eases chronic pains such as fibromyalgia, low back pain, and a whole list of others. Some researches indicate that meditation increases the thickness of certain brain regions that are involved in regulating pain. In fact clinical experience has proven that meditation very effectively heals pain [61].

11. Mental Strength, Intelligence and Creativity: Meditation is the best way to improve your mental strength and health, inspire your intelligence, wisdom, intuition, talents, artistic and musical talents and skills, creativity and productivity, improve your learning ability and memory, help develop your imagination and visualization abilities, enhance your confidence and emotional stability, improve your brainwave coherence, focus and concentration, and optimize your daily performance and achievement.

12. Communication and Relationship: Research shows meditation improves the functions of both brain hemispheres, as well as enhances communication and language skills. Through meditation practice, you will improve your communication skills, and develop harmonious relationships with your partner, family, friends, people at work, and community members.

13. Performance of Business, Work and Life: As meditation empowers your mindfulness, spirituality, vital energy and best health, your entire person is completely transformed and you become more capable, more intelligent, creative, flexible, not stubborn, broadminded, inspired and more easily get along with people. Meditation will improve your work, business, and social skills. This is because you begin to simplify complications of all issues in this life as you optimize your plan, design, techniques, management, execution and performance of work, both in business and within your personal life. Your perspective on success becomes more about the quality, beauty, and joy that emanates from your life, work, living style and daily cultivation practice.

§10.5 Why Mind Can't Be Quiet During Meditation

The key issue in meditation is to empty the mind and stay quiet and still of consciousness and subconsciousness. For many people, however, this is not an easy thing to do. Often we hear people complain that they have hard time meditating. It is because their minds are always busy with all kinds of thoughts or random messages that make them unable to quiet the mind and meditate. Because of the busy mind, sometimes they get tired after a meditation. Obviously for these individuals, the meditation quality needs to improve.

The main reason why the mind cannot be quiet is because of too many attachments in daily life. The only solution for this problem is to work on your own mind inwardly, but not outwardly. There is no other solution. In fact, the purpose of meditation is to improve the stillness of the mind and let go of human attachments and desires so that you can connect to the higher spiritual dimension and obtain the higher energy that can transform your body, mind and spirit to a higher level.

If your mind is full of all human things, then you are disconnected with the higher dimension, so your meditation cannot progress – or you will be wasting your time if you try. Of course for beginners, it is normal that you have thoughts in mind and cannot get into a deeper state of meditation. It is also why you need to cultivate mind nature during daily life in addition to persistent daily practice of meditation and gradually improve the purity of your mind with clear self-regulation of conscious activities, and subconscious shutdown.

Why do we attach so much to all things in this life such as material interests, fame or power, and human sentiments? It is simply because the meditator forgets the true purpose of this life or has yet to discover what the true purpose of this life is. To such people all things in their daily material life, human relationships and sentiments become the first priority in their minds, so much so that they have formed an uncontrollable habit within the mind to constantly think about them. This happens because as day-to-day life progresses, such individuals have kept all these "human things" in their conscious mind and remain in constant pursuit of them. As a result, their subconscious mind stores this information in memory, and thus plays back its messages over and over all the time. As a result, even during their meditation, such a person's head will keep running all of these things (attachments) unstoppably and uncontrollably.

Some meditators may be able to quiet their minds during meditation, but after meditation they go back to the human life in the same way and attach to human daily issues as a non-meditation practitioner does. So in such cases, their meditation, likewise, cannot progress that much because their mind nature and spiritual quality have not been improved.

As we discussed in previous chapters, it doesn't matter whether you are involved in a religion or other belief system, the true purpose of this life is to cultivate your own life and have a transformational journey that takes you to the energy state from whence you initially came, the origin of your life, your being's highest energetic spiritual level.

Of course, no one can change others unless the individual wants to cultivate him/her Self and better the whole being of their life. A person has the right to not to change. But the result is that they will not be able to accomplish the transformation as described above, and their life will drop down to the lower energy level, and have health issues, troubles, ill luck and difficulties followed by a death – that is not understood or worse, misunderstood – in this life and future lives. This applies to all human beings no matter what social, economic and/or educational level they are living in. For an ordinary individual person, what will happen in this life is not under his or her control of, but is an unpredictable life path that has been already arranged upon their cultivated Virtue and self-created Karma in the past lives and this life. For a successful mind-body-spirit cultivator, however, your destination of this life and future life is certain – having a high quality of life journey of this life followed by returning the origin of your life, the highest energetic spiritual kingdom.

Even for a plant or flower, without water and nutrient, eventually they will become dry and die. It is a natural law. Human beings are the same. Without mind-body-spirit cultivation, we will have conflicts with the universe's law and will have difficulties in our life or will even be eliminated by the universe, by way of sickness, diseases and death. Medicine, drugs, money or better material conditions may or may not help you on the surface of this life, but they cannot change your entire life path, cannot better the whole being, and cannot transform the fundamental life to a better path in all aspects including health and luck.

People want to be healthy, want to be looking beautiful, and want to have good lucks in life, but their life path, inborn nature, and quality and ability of being, as a whole of mind-body-spirit, may not really have such Virtue and essence to give them those good things.

Therefore, life cultivation is the number one important thing to do in this life. It must be done daily with clear awareness, righteous mind, strong perseverance and serious effort as first priority on top of anything else. It will not only help improve your health concerns in general, but will also transform your entire life, the whole being, to a better life path and higher energetic level. If keeping this in mind as your first priority, you will stave off many damaging daily life issues such as destructive thoughts, emotions, attachments, desires, struggles, conflicts, worries, as you are meditating and then your mind will begin to perform that way more often in your daily activities until that mindset becomes your normal daily state. As a result, you will naturally simplify your life, avoid meaningless and stressful things, build a healthy lifestyle and organized cultivator's living schedule, and stay in a clearheaded and energetic spiritual state all the time.

This is the most basic core principle and purpose of why we practice cultivation meditation. Understanding this will also help us further discuss how to improve meditation quality in the following sections.

§10.6 Improve Meditation Quality and Become a True Cultivator

We do often see the fact that many meditation practitioners have practiced for years already, but they have not really improved their lives that much in terms of physical and mental health, fitness, aging, beauty, emotional strength, lifestyle, personality, mind nature, thought, relationships, family issues, working efficiency, study, and wisdom. Why is that?

This is a big issue we need to consider and for which we need to find a solution. Otherwise no matter how much you meditate, you will just waste your time and not really cultivate at all. And additionally, it is not good for other people to look at you as an example of what a meditation practitioner is supposed to be.

A good meditation cultivator should be very healthy mentally, physically and spiritually, should stay young, look beautiful, behave with truthfulness, kindness, compassion, tolerance, forgiveness and peace, and think, work and study with a clear head, good wisdom, high efficiency, simple solutions, easy procedures and a smooth performance, effective action and guaranteed result. These good benefits of meditation, however, cannot be obtained by pursuit or desire. But they can be achieved by good cultivation practice through right principle and form, as well as through perseverance and persistent solid efforts.

The following is a self-checklist that helps you improve your meditation quality. Each topic has a question so you can evaluate your own situation. Each is immediately followed by a discussion on the topic.

1. Meditation: First Priority for Life-Saving Transformation

Do you truly understand why you need to practice cultivation meditation, truly consider the practice as the most important issue in your life and truly practice it as daily routine at a preserved time no matter what circumstances you are dealing with?

As we discussed above, it is crucial to understand how important the cultivation is and why we need to cultivate our mind, body and spirit. This is not just a theory, logic or knowledge that you may or may not need to know, or you can just know it but you can leave it there and do nothing about it or with it.

No, it is not something like that. This is must be truly understood inside your own soul as an awakened being who has to know the true meaning of this life and at the same time you need to put solid effort into and take your own responsibility for its practice. As we addressed in previous chapters, this life is just a short period of your entire life that originally came from the universe a long time ago, and will have endless eternal time to go into the future.

Where to go, how to go, and whether you are able to go after this life, and how it will be in this life, including health conditions, life quality and solutions for all problems in this life, all these are depending on the quality of your whole being (mind-body-spirit) and at what level you have cultivated to.

Therefore, this issue is above all other issues in this life. Understanding and practicing this concept is not for anyone else, but it is for your own Self. Every individual has the same issue about his/her own life presently and for the future. It is not something on the surface for just looking good or showing off, nor is it a belief or religion, or just an optional choice of lifestyle or habit, nor something we can put aside and delay for later. Indeed it is an actual, absolutely necessary, first priority and indispensable issue we have to take care of throughout this entire life. Otherwise many problems will arise sequentially starting with health problems and then proceeding to a host of other issues.

Through meditation cultivation, many problems in this life, as well as within your future life, are resolved because meditation cultivation improves your entire life path from the root and transforms your fundamental life quality.

Therefore, meditation cultivation is a first priority and life-saving practice. If you want a better quality of life, then you have to have a better quality of cultivation meditation practice. Only when you truly understand this and take responsibility for the practice, as your own task will you improve your meditation quality.

2. Cultivate Entire Being in Daily Life

Do you just rest and relax yourself by your meditation, but not really cultivate your whole being, mind, body and spirit, and improve mind nature, mentality, character, morality and behavior as a cultivator in daily life?

Some meditators simply rest themselves during the meditation and enjoy it as a way to relax and calm down, but do not really understand the true meaning of this life and why they need to meditate and cultivate, and do not put effort toward the improving the internal self so they still stay in the original ordinary human lifestyle and thinking mode, pursuing ordinary human desires and carrying a lot of attachments in their daily life. Such meditators do not look inside themselves and into their entire life, and do not let go of human attachments to improve their mind, attitude, thought, emotion, lifestyle, habit, behavior, manner, food, and living schedule. So the way they think and behave, the way they live, eat, sleep, speak, dress, look, work, treat themselves and others, deal with their life issues and complications, the kinds of people with whom they involve, the activities with which they involve, and so on, all these remain unchanged. Such meditators do not want to change as a mind-body-spirit cultivator or ever think about changing and improving. This means those meditators are not really cultivated at all. To them, meditation itself is just a form, in the still position, to rest the mind and body, but is nothing about improving and transforming their entire being.

To improve the quality of meditation, the meditator needs to look into his/her own mind and entire life issues for positive changes from surface things such as daily living schedule, eating habit, manner and temper, dress style and colors, to deep issues such as personality, belief, value system, purpose of life, mind nature (such as compassion, kindness, truthfulness, forgiveness), behavior, energy vibrations in daily life, letting go of selfishness, desires, attachments, and upgrading standards of good and bad, beauty and ugliness as a cultivator, cultivating mind-body-spirit by following the universal law and energy principle. Looking at oneself and changing oneself is not easy because human beings often look at their own lives as okay or at themselves as a perfect person, and it is hard to see the problems. As a cultivator, the standards for good and bad, beauty and ugly are much higher and different from ordinary people. To become a true cultivator, your mind must turn inwardly, looking inside yourself for the improvement of all the details of your life, instead of looking outward toward others or your surroundings.

In the daily life you cultivate great characteristics such as compassion, love, kindness, opened mind, forgiveness, tolerance, positive and righteous thought, giving, sharing, and caring for others and the world, so you deeply connect with the spirit of the universe. With such mind natures, you do not easily accrue negative messages and distractions in your mind during meditation and daily life. In the event you do discover negative thoughts, you can eliminate them during your meditation practice and everyday living.

Meditation cultivation is not just a way to relax, rest, reduce stress, and gain health, but most importantly it allows you to connect to the higher spirit of the universe and resonate with the spiritual nature and energy vibrations of the universe, so that you can eliminate bad Karma, negative messages, darkness, sick information and bad thoughts in your mind, body and spirit, and transform human life to a higher level.

When you meditate, especially at the beginning, you remind yourself: I am a true cultivator, having a high goal to transform my entire being to a higher level, sitting here to purify my body, mind and spirit, all darkness and negativities inside myself at all dimensions are eliminated, so that the pure and shining energies from the universe fill my entire being. You let go of all attachments, desires, worries, stubbornness, narrowed thoughts, selfishness, other negative emotions, and fill your whole being with great compassion, love, truthfulness, and forgiveness. And then you stay in such stillness throughout your entire meditation process.

3. Meditate in Correct Form and with Smiling Face

Do you really practice the cultivation meditation in a correct form during the entire process or are you just resting in a loose style so that there really isn't that much meditation energy building, transferring and transforming?

As we know that meditation is not just a form to rest and relax, but it involves spiritual divine energy in the higher dimensions, so a certain precise form in the meditation practice is very important in order to generate the powerful energy at all levels of your whole being crossing the body, mind and spirit.

The spirit leads the mind, and then both mind and spirit lead the body. You should always keep in mind that cultivation meditation is a serious life transformation practice involving high divine energy source, so your spirit is at a high level and in an alert, relaxing, peaceful, compassionate, righteous, and energetic mode to guide your mind and body to practice the meditation in the correct form precisely. You should sit upright with spine straight up, crossed legs, and your entire body and mind relaxed, but not loosening. You do not fall asleep while meditating, so your consciousness stays aware that you are meditating and cultivating.

Meditating with a smiling face is a very effective way to improve meditation quality because smiling can influence your mind to be more peaceful and positive. Body and Mind are one, and they influence each other. When your facial expression is peaceful, happy and positive, your mind follows it in the same way, so that your mind will bring more peaceful energy back to your body. Try peacefully smiling all the time during your meditation, and you will see how it helps you improve meditation quality, generate great energy of peace, love and compassion, and bring you beautiful skin, rosy face and attractive expression. And then you will hear from people praising you, as you will be smiling all the time during your daily life.

4. Perseverance to Secure Your Persistent Daily Practice

Do you secure your meditation time daily in the morning and night and persistently practice it long enough (1 hour at least) each time or are you just doing it in your spare time occasionally?

Modern life is very energy driven, and there are so many disturbances, distractions, contaminations and toxins to the mind and body, causing health problems. Daily meditation practice with extensive cultivation practice in daily life is very much needed for everyone in our modern society. If you just wait until you have spare time to meditate, then you will probably never have time to do it. If you wait until you get all things done before you meditate, then you will never get a chance to do so. As the first priority in this life, you need to have a strong determination in your mind to schedule and secure the time for your meditation every morning and night. Your scheduled meditation time cannot be moved by anything, anyone, or any reason, or for any circumstance. You also need strong perseverance to actually put effort toward doing it every day on time as scheduled. This is the way a good meditation practitioner is supposed to practice and the only way you can have guaranteed good quality beneficial meditation.

When it's time to practice you just count "1-2-3!" Then you start it without wondering.

5. Live in Meditation Lifestyle

Do you live with a simple and healthy cultivation mindset and in such a lifestyle as to have a peaceful, relaxing, spiritual, energetic, and simplified daily life or you are usually very busy all the time with all things surrounding you, many and all kinds of people surrounding you, fully scheduled activities, and have no time for yourself to stay with your own spirit, or have no, or rarely have, quiet time to meditate?

Human beings are originally rooted in the higher spirit of the universe that supplies the pure energy source from the higher spiritual dimension down to the lower physical dimension for our physical and mental health needs. This energy pathway is mediated through human mind that bridges the physical being to the spiritual energy source. The main conscious mind, your true Self, must be involved in this energy networking process, crossing the high to the low energy dimensions.

In our daily life, however, all the activities keep our mind focusing on all kinds of overwhelming everyday issues at low dimensions. As a result, therefore, our mind is often in the energy output (consumption) mode, instead of energy input (generation) mode. This is why that people get tired, sick and age, and have an array of other troubles and difficulties in this life. And this is why we practice cultivation meditation to connect the true Self to the spiritual origin and refresh, purify, energize, rejuvenate, and cultivate the whole being, integrating all components (mind, body, spirit) into one whole.

Meditation cultivation practice (including meditative movement such as Qigong, Taiji, Yoga with spiritual discipline) is a practice for greater self-awareness and spiritual connection with the true spirit, the higher spirit in order to assimilate the whole being (body, mind and spirit) with the original life force, the universe's divine power. Therefore, every human being needs a certain amount of time each day to stay with his/her own Self internally, without any external interruption and distraction, allowing the true Self to communicate with the higher spirit, bring the higher energy to link the body, mind and spirit together for inner cleansing, repairing, detoxification, integrating, alignment, energizing, and cultivation. From this meaning, meditation is a natural life process of self-repairing, self-recharging and self-rejuvenating which is absolutely needed for the continuation of life functions.

In the material realm especially during these modern times, however, people are so busy for their material life and too many desires-driven activities that the mind is involved in many things and complications externally, making the true Self tightly bound to the physical world and disconnected with the universe's spiritual energy source. As a result all the life components (mind, body, spirit) stay apart separately without repairing, recharging and integrating, resulting in low energy, inner conflicts, fast aging, and health problems. This makes meditation even more difficult because the mind is full of all human thoughts and attachments, and the body is driven by all the desires of being busy all the time. To persistently practice meditation, you have to simplify your thoughts, lifestyle, relationships, friendships, family activities, social activities, working procedures, and all issues in daily life, so that you can save more time for your spiritual reading, learning, healing, meditation, exercise, health improvement, personal development, and cultivation practice.

As you let go of more attachments and human thoughts, you will find the way to simplify your life. As you practice more meditation cultivation, energy, health, wisdom, working efficiency, and capability to manage your work and deal with your life – all will be improved. This will then further motivate you to have more time to practice better.

As your meditation quality improves, all things in daily life become simple and easy to you, and you will no longer need so many hours to sleep but you have much more energy and better life quality. This forms a positive feedback circle, and establishes the true cultivator's lifestyle.

6. Quiet Conscious and Subconscious During Meditation

Do you meditate with completely quiet mind and have no any unconscious and conscious activities in your mind, or do you have uncontrollable random thoughts, intentional or unintentional thinking, negative emotions, struggling conflicts, troubles, problems or stressful issues in your life that bother your mind during your meditation?

If your answer to the later part is yes, then your meditation is obviously not right. You need to stop all the thoughts during your meditation no matter whether they are conscious or unconscious. To connect and synchronize your original true Self with the universe's nature during your meditation, you need to let go of your human thoughts. This is the way your meditation is supposed to be, so that you can truly receive the benefits of meditation as we described in the previous section.

Look deeply into your mind inwardly, and find out what are the attachments, desires, addictions, human notions, and habits that you have formed in this life in this material world, and let them go, so that your mind can stay peaceful and quiet to meditate well.

Sometimes you may find that your subconsciousness runs a circular series of mental activities over and over, and those thoughts have no actual meaning or you did not intentionally think of them at all, but they just come to your head uncontrollably. To stop these subconscious activities in your head, your conscious mind must stand out, stay strong and clear to tell your subconsciousness to stop the thinking, be quiet, and then your whole being will stay quiet, empty, still, and peaceful. This way you can get into the deep meditation state. If sometimes your subconscious thought comes back to you again, then you can use your mental eye to look at the front part of your third eye area, let your attention focus there and stay still and quiet. You may see the peaceful lights right in front of your third eye and enjoy the calming stillness while you get deeper and deeper in meditation.

7. No Excuses to Skip Your Practice

Do you often feel tired, busy and lazy or for other reasons or excuses such as having no time to skip daily meditation and cultivation practice?

We often hear people give so many excuses that require them to skip meditation and energy practice day after day. Although in the previous sections we have already pointed out some common excuses with which people often skip their daily practice, here we address a few more common excuses that prevent you from establishing a routine lifestyle with daily meditation practice. We will give a brief explanation to help you keep your practice consistent and persistent.

Excuses, for example: "I am too tired after work, so I have to lie down to sleep and cannot meditate."

If this is the case occasionally, but not one that often happens to you, when it does occur, it is fine you just go ahead and sleep, and get good rest. After that you can meditate. However if you often feel tired and always skip your meditation practice or only can do so for a very short time during which you get tired and fall asleep, then it means you are still not a meditation practitioner at all or your meditation did not energize you at all or you have not established a meditation practitioner's lifestyle. You still live in a non-practitioner's lifestyle and still use the non-practitioner's way to rest yourself. Every non-practitioner sleeps every night and tries for an even 8 hours, 9 hours or even 10 hours, but these individuals can still get tired or even sick. By regular daily sleep you won't really have a high quality rest or ever get enough rest because simple sleep is not comparable with a deep meditation or Qigong movement exercise that can completely refresh you, and energize you dramatically with tremendous energy gains.

In fact the truth is just the opposite compared to what you think when thinking in a non-meditator's way: because you often get tired and want to sleep and rest, it means regular sleep did not do enough to energize you, or your sleeping quality is not good enough, or your daily work or activities overloaded you and made you tired. For such a case, you need more meditation to gain higher energy and better sleep quality. In fact as you put more effort and time into meditating daily, you will no longer need so many hours of sleep, but you will have much better energy in your daily performance.

I am not saying you will replace all your sleeping time with meditation, but please keep in your mind that meditation will give you much better quality rest, more energy and unexpected transformational benefits than regular sleep.

For example, if you have 9 hours for resting time, it is better that you take 7 hours for good quality sleep and then do 2 hours deep meditation and energy movement exercise instead of just sleeping 9 hours. Of course, the order can be arranged as you prefer, for example, you can meditate 1 hour first, then sleep 7 hours, and after waking up, meditate or practice energy movement for 1 hour.

As a result you will have more energy to deal with your daytime work and activities, and after work you will not feel tired. Also as a meditation cultivator, when you are more progressed, you will simplify your life and reduce many meaningless activities, so you won't be as busy as before. This way you will have more time to meditate, better quality of sleep, and involve yourself in activities that are more meaningful and energy producing rather than energy draining. All of this will form into a positive feedback circle; and you will be experiencing a true meditation cultivator's lifestyle.

Someone may say, "I have no time for meditation because my work is very busy, fully scheduled every day, and on the weekend I have so many things to do such as meeting friends, going to birthday parties, shopping, moving, dancing, and so forth."

As we addressed previously, you need to know what is the most important thing to do in this life. Read this book and you will understand why you should take cultivating your mind, body and spirit seriously and as your first priority thing in this life. You should reduce many activities and give yourself more personal time to improve your health, inner peace, spirituality, strength, beauty, youthful zest, longevity, talents, wisdom, good quality time within the arts, music, meditation, reading, spiritual leaning and practice for your own vital energy, high quality beautiful confident life and meaningful living, instead of focusing on too many outward activities.

8. Extensive Meditation Cultivation State During Entire Day

Do you still feel stressful, tired, inefficient, and not really benefited from your practice even though you have kept practicing meditation and cultivation?

Even if you practice meditation and energy movements for a long enough timeframe (e.g., 2 hours) everyday, you may find that when going back daily work and life activities you still feel stressful, tired, inefficient, emotionally unstable (such as anxious, worried, depressed, etc.), ungrounded, or sometimes you may still catch a cold or develop some other health problems. The reason for this is because: as soon as you have done your practice, your meditation cultivation state turned off and your mind went back to the low energy state (energy consuming state) with human attachments to material life and desires. You need to extent your meditation cultivation state after the practice, during your entire day. To do so, your higher Self should lead your entire mind-body-spirit and keep telling you to let go of human attachments and desires during your daily work and life activities. Let it resume you to a peaceful, relaxing, alert, simple, quiet, broad-hearted, clear-headed meditative mindset and help you sustain it for all your daily undertakings. When your higher Self keeps your entire being of mind-body-spirit staying in the cultivator's mentality, energy state, thinking mode, and behaving status naturally and spontaneously, you will stay connected with the higher spirit and energy source, and will not fall into an ordinary human state – energy burning state – so that you will constantly generate good energy and perform energetically and effortlessly.

9. Checklist For You to Change

In order for you to testify by yourself whether you are a true mind-body-spirit cultivator, the following is a checklist that you can go through often to remind yourself to keep a good cultivation lifestyle:

(1). How many hours do you practice meditation and energy movement exercise a day?

(2). How many hours do you read your spiritual cultivation teaching book a day?

(3). How long do you exercise a day – walk, workout, etc. in the healthy way?

(4). How much time do you spend with your close one – wife or husband, girlfriend or boyfriend, and/or children? Do you often meditate with them? Do you have close talk with them spiritually?

(5). How much time do you have outdoor activities to get in contact with nature?

(6). For how much time do you participate in health related activities, lectures, seminars, workshops, and holistic health activities?

(7). Do you spend some time reading and studying about your health of mind, body and spirit, and about healthy lifestyle, diet, food, nutrition, supplement, and traditional methods for achieving healthy and long living?

(8). Do you sleep early and wake up early every day and have enough sleep and meditation practice every night and every morning?

(9). Do you pay attention to your nutritional diet and eat healthy? Do you eat too much or too little? Do you eat on time and regularly, especially for breakfast and lunch, and for dinner not too late and not too much?

(10). Do you spend some time on the arts, news, science, humanity, important issues and concerns about the society, environment, social justice, human rights, freedom within the nation and worldwide?

(11). How many hours do you currently spend a week for shopping? Is it too much? Can you cut it short?

(12). How many hours do you currently spend a week for partying, meeting friends or dining out? Is it too much and can you shorten it?

(13). How many hours do you currently spend a week on the Internet surfing, YouTube and Netflix videos? Is it too much and can you shorten it?

(14). How much time do you currently spend a day for checking, reading and writing emails that are not related with your work or are mostly from all kinds of people not related too much to your work, necessary issues and your personal cultivation? Is it too much and can you shorten it?

(15). How much time do you currently spend a day or week for telephone conversations or phone texts that are not really needed? Do you think you can skip some phone calls, texts or talk as short as possible, so you can have more meaningful and quality time for your health practice, personal grow and cultivation?

§10.7 How Meditation Heals – Mind • Body • Spirit Are One

From the perspective of biology-based modern medicine, it is hard to understand how spiritual and mental practice can achieve physical health or even heal disease. For people of today who are educated by modern science or for those people who used to rely on chemical medication to deal with diseases, it is difficult to understand how meditation without physical, chemical, medical and genetic approaches can improve physical health or even heal the physical body. In this section we will look closer at this issue.

§10.7.1 Change Old Thought and Do Not Rely On Drugs

We often hear people talking about what to take, what to eat, and what to drink to heal or feel better. People used to think that we have to take something such as a pill of medication into the body; otherwise we won't get better or heal the problem. Of course essential nutrition is needed (we will discuss this in the later chapter). It's hard for ordinary people to believe how one just sits there, meditates and quiets the mind, and then the sickness or discomfort is gone.

For you as a meditator, however, you should not only believe it, but also understand it. If you want to improve your meditation quality and achieve the benefits from the practice, you need to truly understand how the spiritual and mental energy heals the whole person including the physical body. As a practice for now, please read the following content while you stay in a meditated state, and let your mind work through your body, so all parts of you will be purified, refreshed and rejuvenated. How much you believe will determine how many benefits you will gain. No more relying on medication. Healing starts from changing old thought.

§10.7.2 Mind and Body and Spirit Are One

Matter and Spirit are one. Body and Mind are one. They are energy forms at different dimensions and influence each other. The spirit has the highest energy in the spiritual dimensions that can lead to health and strength of the mind and body. The mind has higher energy than the body, so it can lead the way toward physical health and strength. The body is the vehicle of the mind and spirit, so physical health can influence the mental and spiritual health and strength. Mental and spiritual energy from the higher dimensions always plays the leading role in physical health and strength, while physical condition can be reflected on mental and spiritual wellness. Purified mind and spirit and their synchronicity with the universe's nature have the power to re-harmonize, rejuvenate and heal the body. As a meditation practitioner or health professional, we should truly understand and believe in this relationship in order to improve meditation quality, healing results and cultivation progression.

§10.7.3 Structures and Functions of the Physical Body

Let's see how the physical body itself works. The human body is composed of cells which contain cellular contents, biochemical compounds, molecules and atoms, nucleic acids, proteins, lipids, carbohydrates, water, etc. The cell is the basic unit that constitutes the structure and function of the body. The cells with similar shape and related functions combine together through stromal cells (connective tissue cells) and constitute the tissue. Several tissues jointly combined perform a specific function, have certain morphological characteristics and constitute an organ. The certain functional organs together accomplish a certain continuity of physiological functions, and form a system. The human body consists of nine systems: motion system, digestive system, respiratory system, urinary system, reproductive system, endocrine system, nervous system, circulatory system, and immune system. These physiological systems work together organically as a living body. For example, your heart is pumping blood, lungs are breathing for oxygen, stomach and intestines are digesting food and absorbing nutrition, liver is generating blood cells, and kidneys are filtering out wastes, and circulating fluid, and muscles, joints and bones are working together to generate force and handle labor works and body movement, immune system is defending the body from diseases, and nerves are receiving and sending signals to communicate with all organs and tissues for the entire body's functioning.

The central nervous system, the brain, as the supreme headquarters of the physical body, directs all other eight systems to perform the physiological functions. At the same time while they execute commands from the brain and perform their tasks, these systems give feedback to the central nervous system, and allow the brain to make appropriate adjustments in neurological signals, balancing functions for all systems.

For instance, all kinds of hormone secretion cycling, blood sugar level controlling, nutrition and transportation, all these physiological functions, are precisely performed by the mutual cooperation and communications within all the nine systems and their associated organs, tissues, cells, cellular compounds or chemical molecules and atoms, under the supervision and management of neuron networks.

Above is just a brief review on the physical body's structures and functions from the conceptual point of view of modern physiology. We see that the physical body itself is like a mechanical unit that works through several solid body parts, their cooperation and task performance. It's why when the body is sick, modern medicine tries to find out what is missing in the body parts, what procedure is wrong, and then add some chemical compounds (medication or drugs) to react with the body in attempt to make it function well again. Does this way work? Yes or No.

The problem is the body is a very complicated system with all kinds of living components and chemicals, so that it is very hard to balance them to the original level and healthy state as it is originally supposed to be.

Drugs or medications react with the cells, molecules and chemicals inside the body, so that they may fix some problem but also, and often, they damage other parts of the body or cause further imbalances. For example, antibiotics kill bacteria that caused the infection or inflammation, but they also damage some healthy cells or necessary bacteria, or cause other bacteria to grow abnormally. As a result this causes other health problems. As an example, many patients who receive antibiotics treatment in the hospital can get antibiotic-associated diarrhea (AAD), which can lead to pseudomembranous colitis, clostridium difficile colitis, a severe inflammation of the colon that sometimes can even cause loss of life [62-64].

§10.7.4 Brain Is Not Your Whole Being • Spirit-Mind Is Boss

The modern medicine considers the brain itself as the physical unit of the mind or the mental organ. This is why some people think psychology or mental health science itself is almost equivalent to brain science or neuron science. People even think the brain has everything necessary to work with the entire being, and that it is the highest ultimate supervision system of the entire person. It's why some brain scientists try to work with brain chemicals and think those brain chemicals control all functions of the body. In fact from the understanding of mind-body-spirit medicine, however, we know the mind and spirit exist outside of the brain and body without physical form, size or shape, and both influence all functions and performances of the physical being. The brain is just the container or storage of memories in this lifetime, a neurological information processing unit, and an antenna and information transmission station between the individual physical being and the higher spiritual divine, intermediated through the mind. The mind is an intelligent, emotional, affective, intuitional, and inspirational mental unit intermediated between the brain (body) and spirit for conscious, unconscious, emotional, intelligent and energetic information processing, transmission and performance of mental or psychological functions.

§10.7.5 High Energy & Meridians in Spirit-Mind-Body

Therefore, above the level of physical body including brain, the mind and spirit (from higher levels) can cross multiple dimensions of physical, mental and spiritual worlds to interact with multi-dimensional energy vibrations and help the physical body function smoothly and live in a healthy condition.

As an opposite example, when there are no mental and spiritual inputs and activities, only physical input and activity, as some (actually many) individuals have come to believe and understand that the body lives with such materials needed for its survival, the physical body will – in fact – die.

Such a test was done during the WWII. In the test children were provided with foods and drinks on time each day, but had no human or animal contact under isolated conditions. As a result, however, the babies were all dead within months. Although such a test is totally inhumane and, of course, never ever recommended – in fact, we condemn it – the result is marked in history and indeed demonstrated how the mental and spiritual life is absolutely needed for the survival of physical being. This was an extreme situation. In everyday society, however, we still often see many patients with mental disorders contract physical health problems, indicating that the mind and spirit can directly determine, influence, and involve physical health. From another historical perspective, history is filled with examples of individuals who have overcome the most brutal of physical conditions and depravations entirely on the power of their mind (mindset) and spirit.

Without mind and spirit, the body is like a piece of dead meat. The mental and spiritual energy is a powerful life force with great compassionate living spirit and wisdom that travels your body and mind, especially during meditation and everyday cultivation practice, to heal diseases and make your body and mind healthy, beautiful and long living.

These higher energy vibrations, spiritual messages, and high divine powers are activated and delivered to your mind and body when you meditate, cultivate and assimilate with the positive spiritual characters such as compassion, love, kindness, forgiveness, truthfulness, and tolerance, and at the same time let go of human mind, attachments and negative emotions. The process of meditation cultivation is just such a way for you to work on your whole being through your mind and spirit communicating with the higher energy vibrations.

Meditation (especially with energy healing music) gives your body and mind an energy shower to purify, cleanse, energize, refresh, reorganize, realign, change, correct, improve, and optimize their functions, health and strength. Once the spirit and mind resonate with the universe's original vibration, all energy channels (meridians) within body-mind-spirit will be opened, and the energy will flow and circulate all over the body and mind. As a result the whole being is re-harmonized, synchronized, and rejuvenated. The physiological body and its all components such as physiological systems, organs, tissues, cells, biochemical molecules and atoms are balanced to the original healthy state. Compared to complicated and cost-ineffective drug-based medicine practice, this way is much more transformational, effective, safe, comprehensive, fast, result-lasting, direct, natural, and has no negative side effects, therefore the smartest and simplest way to achieve mind-body-spirit health.

When you sit there and meditate, in fact inside your body, all cells and molecules are receiving the healthy and powerful energy messages to heal, rejuvenate and transform. If we had an instrument that could truly and dynamically visualize the changes inside our body during the meditation, we all would be surprised by the steady plethora of magnificent transformations. In fact some of our experiments and some other scientists' researches have already sketched out this kind of spectacular imagery from different angles.

§10.7.6 Spiritual & Mental Energies Work Intelligently

So far, we discussed that meditation cultivation works on the physical body through connecting to the higher energy source in the dimensions of mind and spirit while letting go of human mind, attachments, desires, negative emotions, and narrowed mindset which prevent you from communicating with the higher divines and your own true Self. Through the meditation practice and daily cultivation, the high energy featured with an intelligent living spirit automatically and intelligently works on your entire body and mind to transform you to the higher level of life.

As a meditation practitioner, we often experience the powerful energy generated during meditation cultivation. This energy is surrounding the entire body and mind, and spread all over inside the body and mind. Sometimes it massages some parts of your body, and sometimes it travels everywhere throughout your body and mind. Sometimes you may sense the energy is warm and other times it is nice and cooling and cleansing, depending on your body condition at the time. In fact it feels differently in this way because it balances the energy state of your body and mind, depending on what you need. For example, if you have a yang type of body and often feel your body has extra heat, then during meditation you will feel calm and cooling comfort. While if your body is a cold type, and you feel cold, especially cold hands and feet, then during meditation you will feel comfortable warmth over your body. As a result, you are balanced and you don't feel hot or cold, just perfectly comfortable.

Similarly regarding the mental feelings, if you are too excited or anxious (excessive yang), then during the meditation you will gradually calm down and feel peaceful (yin energy). While if you feel depressed and unhappy (excessive yin), then the meditation will make you feel happier and positive (yang).

The meditation energy is a living spirit that knows what kind of energy you need and where to go in your body and mind. For any unhealthy or imbalanced condition you have, the energy automatically finds it out and corrects it. As a result, you get healed and rejuvenated. For example if someone has a hyperthyroid condition, then the healing meditation energy automatically slows down the metabolism, while if the meditator has a hypothyroid condition, then the energy will automatically enhance the metabolism to the healthy level. If a young female meditator has too active hormonal production that develops some problems, then during meditation the energy will automatically balance her hormone level and improve the problems. However through mediation and daily cultivation practice, a female meditator at her menopause age can rejuvenate her hormone system and keep younger hormone production level, slowing down her aging process, and maintaining a young look and overall health.

This healing is totally different from treatment at the human level such as drug-based medicine uses. The god-made life mechanism is repaired and reactivated by the meditation energy, so that the mechanism works to automatically and intelligently heal the problem in terms of whatever it needs. There is no need to know logically and exactly how it works because the meditation energy works on the entire body-mind-spirit at the same time in the holistic way, but not specifically targeting where or what. Whatever imbalance or incorrect health condition you have, it re-boots your entire being back to its original balanced state and thereby corrects the problem. If your blood pressure is high, for instance, then it reboots it to normal, while if it is low, then it brings that back to normal. The smart and powerful cultivation energy makes alignments and adjustments wherever necessary.

Rather than saying the meditation energy heals the problem, we may better say it heals/fixes the original life mechanism and then the mechanism works again to heal the body.

Sometimes you will feel or may even see the energy as bright light that surrounds you, flows into your body, fills all your cells, purifies and energizes you. The light replaces darkness within your body and mind and your surrounding environments, making your entire world transparent. In a good meditation practice, you can experience the energy flowing into you like an "energy shower" or like a warm and comfortable sunlight shining on you. Each meditator may have a different experience, or the same person may have a different experience each time he or she meditates. No matter, if the meditation is of certain quality then all are good for you and will improve your health and transform you to a higher level of life. As long as you keep practicing in the right way, you will receive the benefits we have described in the previous section. Sometimes the great healing results can be much more than what you expected.

§10.8 Meditation Strengthens Your Own Healing Power

Besides the powerful spiritual "energy shower" that heals you and rejuvenates you during your meditation, meditation energy also enhances and strengthens your immune system and all other physiological functions to bring you direct and long-term health benefits physiologically and psychologically. As we discussed in last section, our physical body has nine physiological systems, and among them, the immune system performs the task of safeguarding the body and preventing diseases or harmful attacks that may cause the body to be sick. The immune system recognizes the body's own cells, identifies foreign materials or anything unfamiliar such as bacteria, viruses and parasites, and then destroys them to protect the body from sickness or disease.

A strong immune system also defends you against other external harmful attacks, such as poisoning foods, stress, and emotional disturbance that can cause your body to become sick and weak. From the common cold to difficult diseases such as all kinds of infections, inflammations, heart failure, kidney failure, cancers, hormone imbalance, and so forth, all these health problems can be prevented and healed if our own immune system is healthy and strong. Meditation cultivation very effectively and directly strengthens your immune system. It's why a good meditator does not easily get sick or even catch a common cold and may, in fact, not get sick for many years on end, no matter how young or old they are.

Besides immune system defenses, your body, in fact, employs other physiological systems that are also created with a self-protection mechanism. We all have the experience that after the body has a good rest, some health problems or discomforts are gone automatically. It is because the body does heal itself naturally. It is the natural law. The key is the body must be strong, operating with a balanced and healthy condition – e.g. a strong heart, lungs, liver, kidney, stomach, gallbladder, bladder, hormone system, and nervous system, all parts of the body, and a strong and healthy mind and spirit, as well as a strong immune system.

As shown in Fig. 10.8, along the axis of health level, if we set the reference point, origin, as the minimal health level (health critical point or sick warning point) for a person's physical and mental condition as $Ho = 0$, and maximum health level as $Hmax = 100$, then the ideal health condition H value should be over $H = 80$ or higher. Many people nowadays keep a busy life and do not take good care of their health, so their health level is around the critical point (minimal level) $H = Ho = 0$. Therefore whenever even the slightest bit of negative factors "intrude" on the individual, they can tip the scale fast and the person becomes sick fairly easily (**H** < 0).

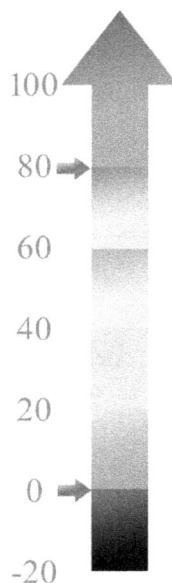

Fig. 10.8. Health Level Scale as a conceptual measure shows a recommended health condition at the value of H ≥ 80, and a warning value (health critical point) as around the origin point at zero (H = 0), and the sick point under zero (H < 0). Along the axis of health level, the reference point, origin, zero point is the minimal health level for a person's physical and mental condition (Ho = 0). The maximum health level is Hmax = 100. The recommended ideal health condition should be over the value of H ≥ 80 for a good meditation cultivator. If one's health level is around the critical point (lowest health level) Ho = 0, then even slight negative factors can cause sickness (H < 0).

A good meditation practitioner should improve their health level to above 80 or near 100. We often see people nowadays, including our patients, always waiting until they feel very sick to see a doctor. Only when feeling sick do they start caring about their health. They are not thinking preventatively and putting the effort into health improvement when they need it most – before sickness arrives. As long as they are still functioning, they still keep insisting that what they "do," their job, their recreation, whatever they are busily "doing" is what really matters – seems health, at that point, is the most unimportant thing in their life. Then, after having some sessions and getting "better" to the point to where they are a little bit above the health-sick critical point **H** = **Ho** = 0, they go right back their life of putting the most importance on their daily "things" and physical attachments. They suddenly don't want to put any more effort into healing completely or strengthening to the optimal level. In fact this is another reason why people do not persistently practice their meditation cultivation.

Your own body was originally created as a perfect self-defense system. The best doctor, your most powerful medicine, is your own body. The immune system and all other systems with your healthy mind and spirit together can prevent and heal all kinds of diseases and discomforts. Therefore, all you need to do is to strengthen your own body, mind and spirit. Cultivation meditation is the best and effective way for such a benefit. You will see how you become much healthier, stronger, younger and more beautiful as you progress your meditation cultivation persistently day after day and year after year.

Sometimes we hear from people who practice meditation but do not progress as expected or have not received progressive benefits in their health. There are many reasons as to why this may be. But one of the more common and predictable reasons they convey is that they have not motivated themselves for daily practice. There are many possible reasons for this, too, as we discussed in the previous section. One I wish to emphasize, however, is that some individuals do not really understand why the meditation can improve their health condition in a positive way. In fact, the meditation healing power and health benefit is gained through the meditator's own system – the mind-body-spirit has that power originally. Understanding this point is very important because that understanding will help you become more trusting in your practice, and you will motivate yourself for your meditation cultivation with a much more positive attitude, strong confidence, extraordinary perseverance, and a persistent schedule.

§10.9 Balance Spirituality, Daily Living & Practice

Although we know that if the mind is cultivated, the body should also become healthy, sometimes we do see that some spiritual cultivators are not in a good health, especially physical health or longevity health, and sometimes they go so far as to not even take good care of their health. Why is this?

Besides all other possible reasons individually, one of the reasons is that these practitioners have an understanding: spiritual practice is purely spiritual and should not attach on physical health or healing diseases, so they do not eat healthily and regularly, do not balance nutrition, do not have a healthy living schedule, do not have contact with nature, and especially do not regularly practice meditation and energy exercise, although they do read their spiritual teaching book, actively go to their spiritual group to attend activities, do volunteer works, or group readings. We fully understand them and respect their belief, but we would like to make a friendly suggestion that a spiritual practitioner should take good care of their health.

These things (concepts/practices) are all related. Spiritual growth helps improve physical health, while physical health also helps one grow spiritually. Longevity health will allow you to have more time and strength in this life to cultivate and ensure your final consummation towards your spiritual goal.

Of course your mind does not attach on your physical health as an attachment. However the key is to understand improving physical health and longevity itself is also the part of your efforts that favors spiritual cultivation and its final goal achievement. You need to balance your spiritual cultivation and health practice simultaneously as one thing, but not go to either extreme because they are all important parts of your cultivation.

We suggest that a meditation cultivator also balance nutrition, eat healthy, have some exercises, and live in a healthy lifestyle and daily schedule, energetic and relaxing entertainments and family times, so you offer a good example as a cultivator: being in good health mentally, physically and spiritually.

§10.10 Health, Beauty & Longevity Motivate Your Cultivation

Health, beauty and longevity are not the ultimate goal of spiritual cultivation, but they are good side-benefits, reminders, encouragement, motivation, and natural results of spiritual cultivation.

We believe that sickness, discomfort, or difficulty in this life has its spiritual meaning. It could be a good lesson and reminder for us to practice cultivation. Human beings have Karma that leads to sickness or difficulties in this life. Therefore sickness or some difficulties in this life can urge us to cultivate more seriously and urgently, in order to eliminate Karma. Otherwise, if we never get sick or never have difficulty in this life, then cultivation may never be treated as an important pursuit in this life.

We human beings have so many attachments in this material world. It is not easy for human beings to resist the temptations of material interests. If we do not have a clear spiritual awareness and strong perseverance for such pure spiritual goal, our desires often drive us to fully attaching on all kinds of attachments or daily things in this physical world, including fame, interests, power, money, human sentiments/emotions, families, relatives, relationships, work, business, and so on. As a result, sometimes we overload in this life for material interests and do not think spiritual practice is important or do not think our future destination after this physical life is of any urgent concern. Some people don't even believe there is actually such a spiritual life destination in the future at all. Some people may even have an excuse that there is no such evidence to demonstrate that there is such a future spiritual destination. In other words, in our modern times, people would rather rigidly believe in science on the surface, so they do not believe there is a spiritual world after this physical life unless they see so-called scientific evidence.

In fact, the spiritual world and its blessing power will never appear to and benefit those people who do not believe in it. Whether believing in it is just the very first gate or front entrance of the spiritual world, if one does not believe in the spiritual world, its power, energy and magnificence, then he/she will hardly achieve progress in meditation cultivation or even want to do so at all.

This is one of the most common reasons why modern day people can easily get sick, but not so easily get themselves healed. That is to say, people attach on the physical world or material life, but don't really believe in life's spiritual aspects, therefore cultivation practice or meditation is not taken as high priority in daily life. So sometimes we can say sickness and difficulty in this life can be a good lesson and reminder to help people think deeper about life, and wake up for the cultivation practice.

On other hand, if a good meditation cultivator can achieve wonderful health, beauty and longevity through meditation cultivation practice, then it will greatly encourage him/her to progress in cultivation. As you practice cultivation day after day and year after year, you see your health improved more and more, you become stronger physically and mentally, and you become more and more beautiful in appearance, and become clearer headed, efficient and intelligent in daily performance, and you can contribute more and more in your family and society, and in many ways. These benefits are real and will encourage you to practice meditation cultivation more and more. At the same time, you should remember to set a good example as a spiritual cultivator and meditator for people surrounding you.

Meditation is the most beautiful and joyful practice and also a smart choice for you in this life. As you progress persistently every day and never skip even one morning or one evening, you will see your positive changes in many ways unexpectedly and surprisingly. Let your health, beauty and longevity improvement motivate you to further progressing in meditation practice every day.

§10.11 Why Sometimes Meditation Works But Sometimes Not

Belief and Understanding

People often ask why spiritual medicine, mind-body medicine, or mind-body-spirit self-improvement practice – e.g. meditation, Qigong, Taiji, Yoga, hypnosis, music healing, etc., sometimes works and at other times does not, or works for some people and does not for other people. If you understand the previous sections and chapters as well as the fish-water model to explain how mind-body medicine works, then you probably already have the answer for this question.

Some patients, who come to a mind-body medicine doctor, do not understand or even do not believe there is such a spiritual, mental and emotional energy beyond the physical being, and do not believe such energy can have the power to heal, transform and rejuvenate life. Because their mind is not open to receive such energy, the doctor cannot heal the individual.

The healing process in mind-body medicine must be through the person's mind, spirit, emotions, belief system or value system, everyday life performance and lifestyle. In other words, the healing power of mind-body medicine relies on the energy that comes from the high divine source, through the mind and spirit of the person; his/her own Self and then, the doctor works with his/her daily cultivation practice and life experience.

If the person does not believe in the process and/or discipline, that means he/she refuses the spiritual energy, divine power and healing energy, and therefore there is no way he/she can receive the healing energy nor can the person gather the benefits from it. If a person does not understand the principle of this healing art and health practice, then the energy cannot transfer and transform for that person, and he/she will also not practice it correctly (see more details in the following sections), and so, as such, the process will not work for that individual.

In addition, if the person does not directly practice the cultivation of energy, then the energy will not work with the person at all. Belief, understanding and practice are necessary requirements for the mind-body healing and health practice to work effectively with the subject.

Of course, sometimes, a powerful master may heal the person without effort from the person or even without awareness from the person. But there is usually a certain reason for that. In fact in such a case, the person must have exceptional good Virtue in this life or past lives, so there is good faith within the person. In other words, the individual may already have an inborn spirit connecting with the higher healing source, so even though he or she does not really understand the healing process, nor is the mind directly involved, the person can still be healed. This is a very special case. Yet, even when it is the case, the person still needs self-cultivation practice to maintain the healing result afterward.

Modern science, the entire education system from elementary school to graduate school, and all modern living activities, material life experience, etc. guide most people today toward more materialism, superficial and non-spiritual desires and goals. Even for some believers, cultivators, or meditators of spiritual practice, thinking in the physical way and ignoring invisible spiritual dimensions, energies and powers has already become their typical, "normal" thinking mode. And of course, this mindset is not healthy in that it cuts the person off from their higher level of energies which they will need to progress and evolve in this life as healthy, happy, purposeful beings. A physical-level mindset also makes the practice for either the healthcare practitioner or self-improvement and self-healing cultivator much less effective.

The spirituality and belief of the person are extremely important in mind-body medicine healing and health. This is actually the concept called *Wu Xing* as we mentioned early. If the person is open minded, believes in the spiritual or divine power, has great imagination, intuition, sense, and understands the idea and principle of mind-body medicine and spiritual cultivation practice, then it will help the healing work or self-healing and health practice achieve a good result. If the person, however, has a narrowed mind, does not believe in such practice or is doubting, skeptical, wondering, or even refuses these spiritual concepts, then it will be hard for the person to be healed or to improve his/her health condition by this method.

Practice Must Involve True Self - Mind and Soul

There is another important reason why sometimes the spiritual healing process does not work for some people. These individuals only involve themselves in the physical practice or the physical form of the mind-body-spirit techniques which they try. They mistakenly see them and treat them like sports or other forms of physical training. For example, some individuals do meditation like a daily relaxation activity – perhaps, you may remember when your teacher in the early days of school would tell students to lay their head down on the desk and "rest." When meditation is treated this way, the individual never really practices mind cultivation or introspection or works to improve the mind, emotions, character, lifestyle, or to let go of attachments, addiction, unhealthy habits, etc. as part of the meditation, thereby activating the transference and transformation of energy into their life.

Some people meditate or practice energy exercises such as Qigong, Taiji, or Yoga, receive treatments of hypnotherapy, music healing, or other mind-body medicine practice, but their minds keep wandering and thinking and are filled with a lot of noise, attachments, desires, emotions, anger, complaints, and random thoughts, and as a result they are never really able to relax, calm and empty their minds, and never get into deep dimensions and experience the energy to heal, rejuvenate or energize. Therefore they never acquire the benefits of whatever they do in the mind-body practice.

Sometimes the doctor uses hypnosis on the patient, but the patient's mind keeps busy, wandering, is filled with a lot of attachments, desires, thoughts, emotions and confusions and therefore, the hypnotherapy has little benefit.

If one just wants to get better health but does not improve their mind nature and let go of negative emotions, attachments, stubbornness – just keeps clinging to old unhealthy habits and shortcomings, does not want to change for improvement or refuses suggestions to change, does not cultivate his/her Self inwardly, does not look into their own mind, character, emotions, lifestyle, relationships, does not purify and upgrade spiritually and explore true Self, does not improve the whole being, but just does the physical form of the meditation, Qigong, Taiji, Yoga, music healing, hypnosis, or whatever the healing or health practice, then the cause(s) of the health problem(s) will still remain unchanged and the health condition will not be improved.

Sometimes people only want the doctor to help heal the problem, but don't understand that the healing process must go through the person him/her Self at the mental and spiritual levels and involve their daily lifestyle, activities and self-improvement practice. This is why mind-body health practice or treatment does not work for those people.

Consistently Practice Self-Healing as First Priority

If you receive the healing treatment of mind-body medicine or your doctor teaches you a self-healing practice and lets you do it at home, you should keep focusing on the practice consistently. Some patients expect mind-body holistic healing treatment to work like magic that is immediate and without any effort. Although it is true that sometimes the healing works dramatically and you see the result right away, you may not see results immediately. It depends upon the case. For most chronic conditions, no matter if the treatment works right away or takes some time, you will need to following up with your doctor's instructions, and especially keep practicing your self-healing activities daily.

Modern lifestyle is busy, stressful, overwhelming, energy consuming, desire-driven, taking one's true soul and mind away, and indeed unhealthy. All activities in this lifetime including work, family, desires, attachments, entertainments, relationships, and so on will take the entire person away from the true Self and make the person work and behave like a machine without freedom of mind and spirit.

Body, mind and spirit are one. All of them must stay together as one unified whole being in order to be healthy. Many people today have lost the entity of Self, the true soul, because the majority or all of their activities are outward, not inward. Therefore, mind-body-spirit cultivation practice becomes especially important and extremely necessary.

Some people know meditation or energy practice is important for their health, but most still cannot keep practicing it daily. You may often think after you get done with your work or after your scheduled activities are completed that you can have the time to do your meditation, energy practice or exercise. In reality, however, actually you will realize that you never finish your work or scheduled activities, and you always have something to do – probably one thing after another – thus you find you conclude that there is little or no time to practice your Self healing improvement meditation. Your intention is to practice often, but you actually often skip practicing because of every busy day with a full schedule.

In fact most people today are tightly bound to their daily work, entertainments, family activities, relationships, all these daily things that fully occupy their time and mind the whole day and every day, making it hard for them to detach from these and keeping their daily health practice random at best or stopping it completely at worst.

Every time you skip, you may think: "tomorrow I will get back into it," and then tomorrow you skip it again. This is always a difficult problem for you until you fundamentally realize what your purpose of this life is and what the most important thing is in your life. Interestingly, taking care of this primary need, empowers you to properly attend to all other important things connected to your life more fluidly and more satisfyingly, and allows you to more mindfully interact with them and grow them. At the end of each day, you will find you are more energized, fulfilled, and happier and have contributed goodness to your own progress, those around you and the bigger picture.

Sometimes people get sick and suffer from certain health problems. This is, of course, not a good thing in our life, but it may become a warning for us to take care of our health seriously. As a mind-body doctor and cultivation practitioner myself, I often see that some of my patients seriously practice meditation and cultivation practice more so when they get sick. As a result they get healed and become even healthier, gain more energy and better efficiency and improve their quality of work and life. They realize that cultivation practice for their body, mind, and spirit actually did not waste their time or make their schedule busy, but just the opposite; it gave them more time, energy, ideas, motivations, interests, passions and wisdom to live and work by and much more efficiency, quality, achievement and happiness.

From this, it appears their sickness woke them up to something good they could do for themselves for the rest of their life. The healing became a turning point in their life journey and steered them towards a healthier lifestyle and spiritual enlightenment.

Of course, the best way is not waiting to get sick before you start practicing healthier living and cultivation.

As you read this book, it will help you make the decision to practice your health training daily, so that you can begin to prevent sickness and aging and keep yourself healthy, strong, beautiful and young. This is what this book is written for and what this book promises you will be able to do.

Letting Go of Attachments Is the Key

Human beings have so many attachments and desires that revolve around all the details of their daily lives, such as families, job, career, study, money, power, fame, emotions, sentiments, love, relationships, entertainments, computers, habits, addictions, on and on. The operative word here is "attachments." We are not against these daily life issues as basic needs for human life. But we mean to emphasize that these (as "attachments") will cause problems in your life and health. These, as daily attachments, drive your soul and mind away from your true Self, make you unclear about your goal of living a meaningful life, keep you busy all the time, so you have no time to care for your health and true soul, cannot have a clear mind to live in a regular healthy lifestyle and schedule of health practice, mind-body cultivation, meditation, exercise, food, sleep, work, and rest.

Some people including youth, middle aged adults or elders may never seriously think about what is the true meaning or purpose of this life, and how to live with the true health of the body, mind, and spirit. Younger generations or teenagers may never hear parents or teachers talking about these serious and fundamental issues of life nor teach them the way to practice their mind, body and spirit for health and spiritual growth – despite the fact that they will amass a lot of information about science and technologies in their education. Many life activities today are aimed at accruing or living a "better life," but not many are aimed at growing as a human being with mind and spirit. I am not suggesting that we human beings should do nothing in or with this physical, material life. Actually I am talking about how we set a right relationship between establishing a healthy meaningful lifestyle for body-mind-spirit growth and basic physical life needs. An attachment driven by desire in the physical life is sort of like a drug that can turn you into an addict and is hard to let go of. If there is no higher guide in your clear conscious mind to steer you toward a healthy and energetic life, these attachments can make you lose perspective and direction fast and catch you in a maze where your whole being, body, mind and spirit, can easily disconnect and get sick.

The more you attach on the daily things, and the more you do not practice daily health, energy and spirituality, then more of your energy diminishes, and the more you will live and work in a low efficiency, low quality and with more troubles and hardships – and the more you will not have time for health improvement, spiritual cultivation and energy practice. This forms a damaging feedback circle that will cause you sickness, fatigue, discomfort, aging, hardships and difficulties in many ways throughout your life.

To end this harmful feedback circle, you need to make yourself determined to put health practice and personal cultivation on the top of your priority list. Once you make your mind up and set a time to practice mind-body-spirit daily, you will gain great energy physically, mentally and spiritually. As a result, you will get into a positive feedback loop.

You will stay clear headed, energized and enlightened with great wisdom and divine power, and connected with the boundless great energy sources, you will have much more energy, efficiency, and wisdom to work, learn, live and achieve the best quality and most meaningful life possible.

Full Practice for Total Transformation and Rejuvenation

Some people do not practice cultivation or meditation with a focused mind, but, instead, allow many interruptions, disturbances, or interferences when practicing. For example, while meditating, some individuals think about work, family, kids, parents, girlfriend, boyfriend, husband, wife, sister, brother, friends, business, income, housing, shopping, cooking, food, job, and entertainments, a long list goes on. Some stop in the middle of the practice and do something else and may come back later or never come back again, so the practice, at least for the time, could not be completed. This is not a good way to approach spiritual cultivation practice or health energy practice because you need to go deep enough and get into other dimensions without interruption, otherwise you will start over from the beginning when you stop and come back again.

Some people open their eyes in the middle of practice and talk, respond to the telephone, check and type email or text messages during the meditation or energy practice. This creates the same problem as when you stop once and restart again.

When joining in a group meditation practice, or with someone at home or a friend, sometimes one individual stops in the middle, moves around, talks, makes a phone call, makes noise, comes and leaves in the middle of the practice – all these interruptions will not only fail your own practice and interrupt others, but will also break the energy field generated in the group practice and disconnect with other higher dimensions.

On the other hand, a good practice is a complete practice, from the beginning to end without interruption, with the mind focused and empty, eyes closed, postured correctly in a still position or smooth movement, and one will never fall asleep. Such a complete practice will give you a total rejuvenation and transformation of life.

§10.12 Intermediate Break: Healing Music • Meditation

EHM10: Eternal life after many lives *(Yin, Fire, Wood)*

This music is composed with focus on the relatively yin energy of earth and fire elements to strengthen your stomach and heart energy. However if you feel you are weak, cold, have low energy, or unhappy, unconfident, or at a low mood emotionally (yin type of condition), then you can choose the following CD (yang type of the healing music) to practice.

EHM09: The Sea of Happiness *(Yang, Fire, Wood)*

[*Start to play Energy Healing Music #10*] Visualize the ancient longevity masters (such as Peng Zu, Lao Tzu, etc.) living multiple hundreds of years, and yourself meditating in the early morning and night (and sometime in the noon or afternoon) every day, and keeping a high goal – e.g. you want to live for your own longevity practice in order to accomplish your cultivation toward the highest goal of eternal life destination while you meditate deeper and deeper.

§10.13 Exercise Questions

1. What was the original purpose of meditation cultivation in the history of human civilization, and how did it spread in the human world and become health and longevity practice? Is meditation practiced only by monks or nuns in the temple? Can everyone practice meditation? How much do you know about the story of ancient longevity master Peng Zu and how he lived with his cultivation meditation lifestyle?

2. What are the core principle, form and methods of meditation, and what is your experience with such guided meditation practice?

3. What are the benefits of meditation practice and how has it helped you in your life?

4. Can you meditate with a quiet mind? Describe this component within your own experiences.

5. Do you have some difficulties in your meditation practice or in keeping your practice consistent? How can you improve your meditation quality and the body-mind-spirit strength you glean from your own practice?

6. How do you understand the fact that meditation cultivation improves health and heals diseases? Why do people today sometimes disbelieve or misunderstand the idea of spiritual power? How do you understand the higher energy, resonating with the higher spirit, and the integration of the body, mind and spirit?

7. How do you understand mind-body-spirit practice such as meditation in regard to improving and strengthening immune system?

8. How do you balance your spiritual practice with daily life and physical exercise, and achieve health mentally, emotionally, and physically?

9. What is your understanding about how and why health, beauty and longevity help to motivate your cultivation practice and do you see your own improvement in health and beauty?

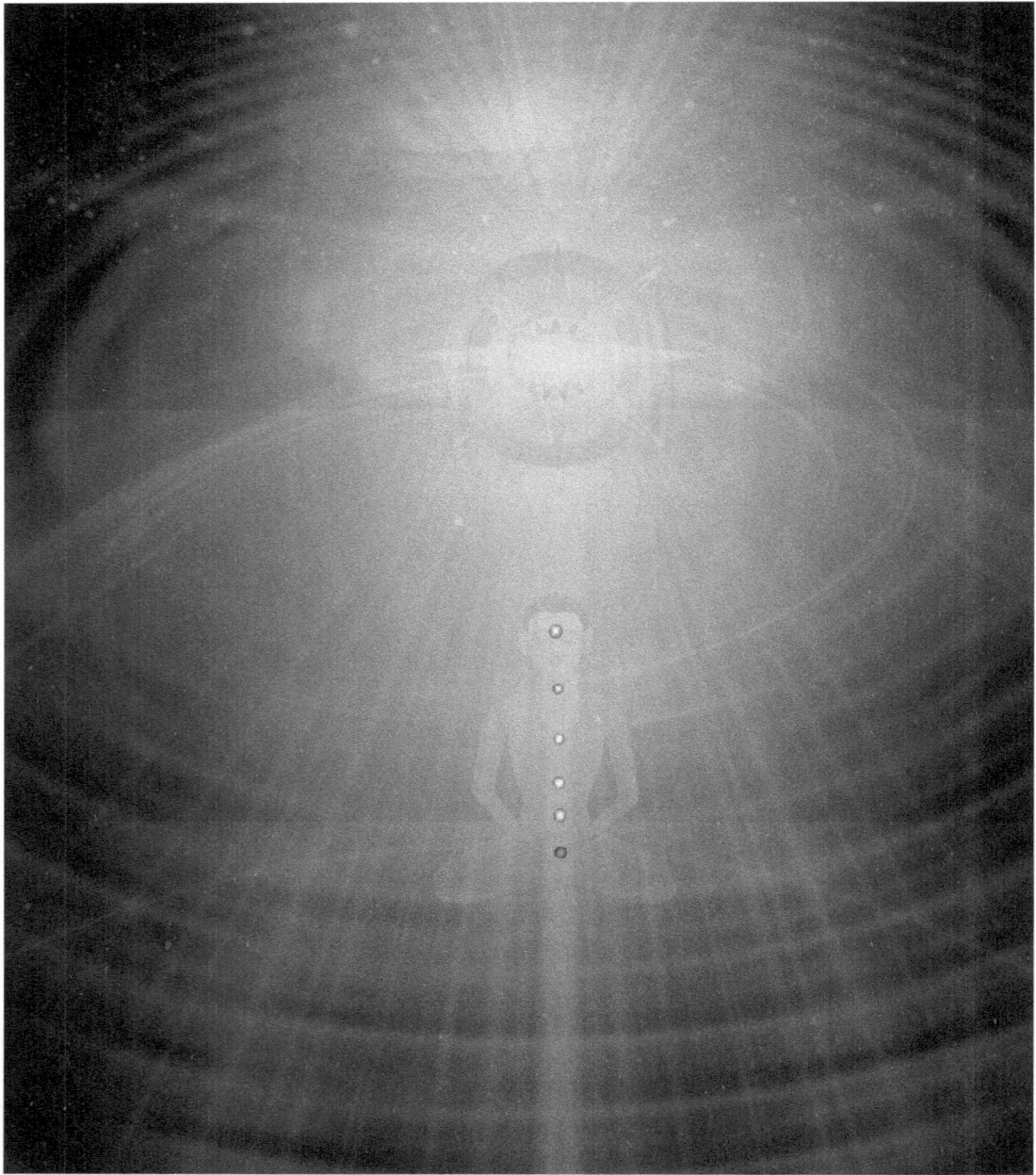

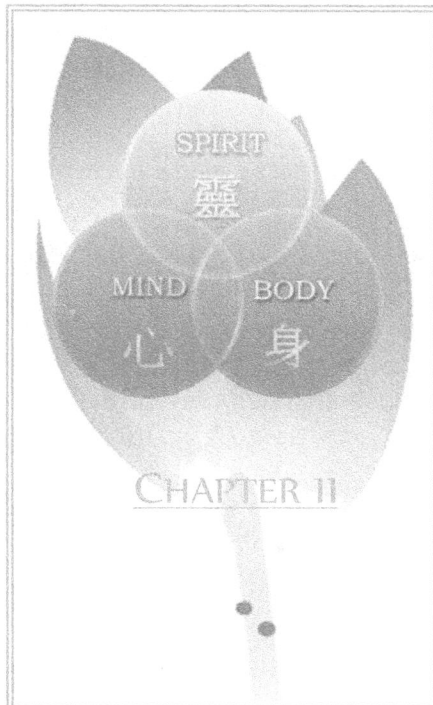

Energy Music Therapy – An Application of Mind-Body Medicine

§11.1 About The Name and Why Energy Music Therapy

Energy Music Sound Healing discussed in this chapter has several different names depending on the particular emphasized aspect of this musical healing modality. For example, it is sometimes called Non-Needle Acupuncture Music Therapy or simply Acupuncture Music Therapy, meaning the therapy is based on the principle of traditional Chinese medicine acupuncture, but uses music instead of needles or herbs. Therefore sometimes we just call it Chinese Medicine Music Therapy or TCM Music Therapy.

Other times, we wish to emphasize the music works from the point of view of energy medicine and therefore refer to it as Five Elements Energy Music Therapy or Five Elements Music Therapy, or even simply call it Energy Music Therapy.

Since we incorporated brainwave frequencies into this Five Elements music to help resonate the energy vibration and enhance the healing power, we sometimes refer to it as Brainwave Energy Music Therapy. Furthermore, since the energy music works on the acupuncture meridians, we, at time, also refer to it as Brainwave Meridian Music Therapy.

When we combine other techniques such as hypnosis, psychological healing conversation, eastern philosophical and human cultivation teaching with this treatment, we use the term, Brainwave Meridian Therapy (BMT) which will be addressed extensively in next chapter.

In this chapter, however, all these names simply refer to the same type of therapeutic music therapy and present it as an energy therapy modality or an application of the mind-body medicine. Please be aware, however, this music healing therapy is not the same type of music therapy that is referred to by the Western medicine society. Let's take a look.

As discussed in the previous chapters, any physical or mental disease, sickness or discomfort is a reflection of the conflict or disharmony of the energy vibrations in the body, mind and spirit, and the conflict is caused by energy blocks, imbalances, energy deficiency, or diminishing energy within or between the body, mind, and spirit or their yin and yang and five elements.

Therefore, to heal the cause and then cure the symptoms, we need to remove the blockage, balance and smoothen energy flow and increase the energy level of energy within the body, mind and spirit, such that the energy integrates all life components, resolves the conflicts and imbalances, harmonizes and unifies mind-body-spirit into one synchronized life unit, and thus the whole being is healed.

Question is: How do we achieve this goal? The key is energy. This means we need to produce good healing energy to cancel or correct the conflicted sick vibrations or disturbing messages, cleansing the excessive elements or tonifying the deficient elements of energy within the mind and body. Its application is called Energy Medicine.

As a note, when we say mind-body medicine, this is the general term that identifies us as healing science. The term energy medicine, then, is (and refers to) the practical solution, tool, practice and technique of mind-body medicine. Energy Medicine, however, has many different modalities.

Among these energy medicine modalities, probably energy music therapy is one of the most effective and comprehensive approaches.

Here I am going to introduce the Energy Music Therapy (EMT) developed in our clinic as an application of mind-body medicine. This therapeutic energy music is also used in the brainwave-meridian therapy (BMT) that will be introduced in next chapter. In this chapter, we mainly introduce this energy music as a standalone therapy and self-healing or self-improvement practice.

§11.2 Five Elements • Five Tones • Five Organs • Five Emotions

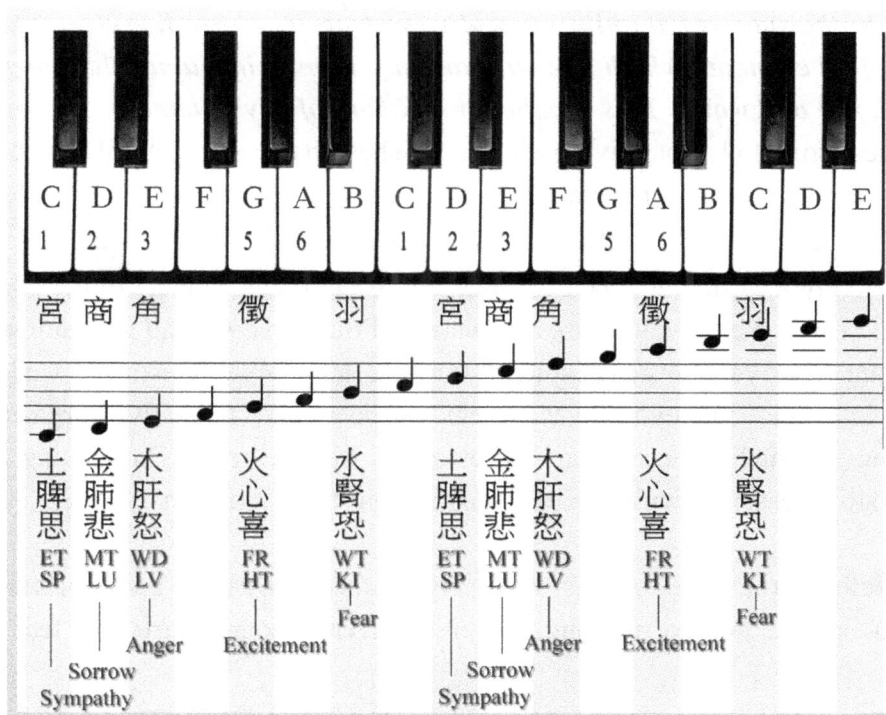

Fig. 11.2. Diagram showing five elements of musical notes on the keys of piano (C, D, E, G, A), syllables (1, 2, 3, 5, 6), ancient Chinese characters of the five music notes (宫，商，角，徵，羽), Chinese pinyin of the five notes (Gong, Shang, Jiao, Zhi, Yu), Chinese characters of the Five Elements, Five Organs, Five Emotions, and the English abbreviations of the Five Elements, Five Organs and Five Emotions: ET (earth) / SP (spleen) / Sympathy, MT (metal) / LU (Lung) / Sorrow, WD (wood) / LV (liver) / Anger, FR (fire) / HT (heart) / Joy (over excitement), and WT (water) / KI (Kidney) / Fear, respectively.

Energy healing music (EHM) is composed based on the principle of Yin-Yang and Five Elements that we have addressed in the previous chapters. Compared to other types of five-element music, this energy healing music we created has distinctive advanced features and healing benefits, after experience over 20 years in its composition, production, application and research of this Energy Music for mind-body healing. This healing music now is available in a set of musical CDs, which covers each of the elements and addresses all organs and emotions. The basic healing set includes 10 titles that are featured with yin and yang natures for each element: water (yin and yang), wood (yin and yang), fire (yin and yang), earth (yin and yang), and metal (yin and yang) covering the energy meridian systems of kidney (KI) and urine bladder (UB), liver (LV) and gallbladder (GB), spleen (SP) and stomach (ST), heart (HT) and small intestine (SI), lung (LU) and large intestine (LI), respectively. An additional healing series has also been made available with more newly developed pieces that address more health issues commonly seen today.

Based on the ancient cosmological conception of Tao (Dao), we look at all phenomena in the substantial universe as alive systems that have five elementary features of energy – five elements which are substantially named in human language as earth, metal, wood, fire and water. This is called the Theory of Five Elements. According to this theory, musical sound also has five basic tones. These basic elements of music tones were named in ancient Chinese pronunciation (musical tone, syllable, numbered tone) as Gong / 宫 (C, do, 1), Shang / 商 (D, re, 2), Jiao / 角 (E, mi, 3), Zhi / 徵 (F, so, 5), and Yu / 羽 (G, la, 6), respectively (see the table below). These musical tones connect to the corresponding five elements (earth, metal, wood, fire and water) of the universe, and resonate with the five yin organs and five yang organs (spleen/stomach, lung/large intestine, liver/gallbladder, heart/small intestine, kidney/urine bladder), respectively. The five organs store the corresponding spiritual essence: heart stores spirit, liver stores yin soul, lung stores yang soul, kidney stores essence, ambition, will, and spleen stores emotion.

Therefore, the five organs relate with the emotional and spiritual features: sympathy in spleen, sorrow in lung, anger in liver, joy in heart and fear in kidney, respectively.

§11.3 Five Elements Mutual Generating & Restricting Relations

The five elements (organs, tones, emotions) have mutual generating and mutual restricting relationships. The mutual generating cycle refers to the mechanism in which the elements generate one another cyclically and endlessly: Wood → Fire → Earth → Metal → Water → Wood. This mechanism reflects the power of the universe and its life force. Based on this mechanism, the five elements automatically and generically create, transform, promote, nurture, support and enhance one another as energy source and production in the order of the cycle.

5 Elements	5 Tones	5 Organs	5 Emotions
Earth	C, 1, Gong	Spleen, Stomach	Sympathy
Metal	D, 2, Shang	Lung, Large intestine	Sorrow
Wood	E, 3, Jiao	Liver, Gallbladder	Anger
Fire	F, 5, Zhi	Heart, Small intestine	Joy
Water	G, 6, Yu	Kidney, Urine bladder	Fear

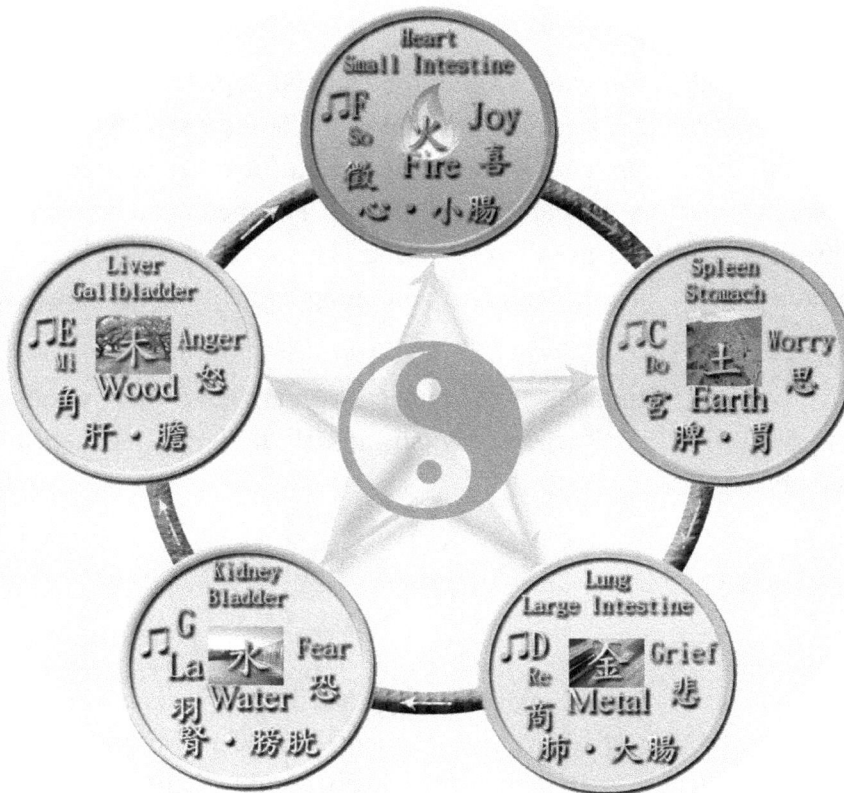

Fig. 11.3. Diagram that shows the generating and restricting relationships of the Five Elements of the universe and their corresponding yin and yang organs, musical tones, and emotions. The arrows on the circle in clockwise direction show their generating relationships (Wood → Fire → Earth → Metal → Water → Wood), while the arrows on the five star show their restricting relationships (Wood → Earth → Water → Fire → Metal → Wood).

Specifically, the wood element burns and makes fire, and fire produces ash, generates soil and forms the earth. The earth contains all kinds of minerals and forms metal. When the metal is heated and cooled down, then water droplets are formed over the metal as a result of condensation; this is the process by which metal generates water. The water grows the trees or plants that are wood. Similarly the five elements are associated with the five organs of human body; the five kinds of emotions, as well as the five tones of musical sound which themselves are also in the same mutual relationships.

The mutual restricting cycle of the five elements refers to the mechanism in which the elements restrict, inhibit and control one another continuously in the order of Wood → Earth → Water → Fire → Metal → Wood. This restricting mechanism provides the opposite force to balance the generating power and prevent the generating mechanism from overwhelming and over-functioning, so that it stabilizes the whole system in a balanced, stable and healthy state.

Speaking in detail, wood can break up the soil and deplete the nutrients of the earth, thus controlling earth. The earth contains, maintains and holds water, forms dams to prevent flooding, and thus the earth can control water. Water, on the other hand, can extinguish fire and control its spread, and the fire can melt the metal. The metal can be made into a tool to cut wood, controlling the wood from overgrowing. This restricting cycle repeats from one to another continuously, balancing with the generating cycle and preventing it from rising overwhelmingly.

The five organs, emotions and musical tones have the same relationships accordingly based on the mutual generating and mutual restricting mechanisms of the five elements as described above.

§11.4 Five Elements Music Composition and Energy Features

The composition of Five Elements Energy Music is a special musical composition skill that is based on the idea that the five elements (earth, metal, wood, fire and water) correspond to the five musical tones (Gong / C / 1, Shang / D / 2, Jiao / E / 3, Zhi / F / 5, Yu / G / 6), respectively, and when one of the tones is focused or entered as the major tone throughout the composition, the melody will naturally present its particular pattern and specialized feature in terms of musical energy, emotional expression, mood, vibration frequency and healing effects. For example, the water tone music composition uses water tone (羽 / Yu, G, La, 6) as its major tone, and the most musical sentences are written to end with the water tone, or are often composed with other tones surrounding the water tone as the center note. Music composed in this way generates the specific energy pattern of water element. We called it water element music, water tone music or simply water music.

A major tone is not only often used as the ending tone in the musical sentence, it is also often technically emphasized (and heard as well as felt or absorbed) as the stronger, longer, or vibrating tone of musical performance. Each element of the music carries its particular elemental energy features, healing energy, emotional, psychological and physiological effects – and healing benefits.

Considering the mutual generating and restricting relationships of the five elements, when we compose a specific element of the music, not only the major tone, we also pay attention to its associated element tones. For example, when we compose water element music, besides the water note (羽 / Yu, G, La, 6) as the central tone, ending tone or major tone in the musical sentence, prolonged, strengthened or emphasized tone, sometimes we also add more metal tones (金 / Shang, D, Re, 2) as water tone's generating or promoting tone to additionally support and enhance water tone energy. As the melody flow progresses, at a certain point – and this is an important distinction of our model – we incorporate some earth tones (宮 / Gong, C, Do, 1) as the restricting tone of the water element, to prevent the water energy from overwhelming and causing an imbalance of energy. Therefore the entire piece of element music – in this case the water energy music – sustains balance.

A piece of music is not just a rigid arrangement of a series of musical notes. Indeed musical melody expresses and evokes emotional feelings and spiritual energy through interactions between sound wave vibrations and neuron systems as well as entire biological body. The mechanism of music-human interaction remains unknown as a mystery in modern science. From the perspective of mind-body practice, however, we believe that music is a heavenly gifted powerful and joyful tool that transforms energy from spiritual and mental dimensions to living beings throughout the process of music creation, appreciation or application. A piece of energy healing music carries and transmits the vibration energy from the composer, producer and therapist, during all processes of composition, creation, production, performance, guided meditation, hypnosis induction, and clinical application, depending upon his/her cultivation, energy state, and mental and spiritual connection with the higher spiritual energy source.

Our set of energy healing music for the mind-body healing treatment was composed, produced and energized in the author's energetic meditation state and based on many years of personal cultivation and clinical experience in mind-body healing. The music contains messages from the compassionate universe and its great natures of love, truth, forgiveness, peace, and wisdom. The energy was featured with the balanced five elements of universe vibrations and an emphasis on one or two of these elements in each piece of the series. The musical waves resonate with your true nature, and help you get rid of the conflicts, confusion, and negativities in your mind and body while you listen and practice with it. This reestablishes the peaceful, energetic and balanced energy field within you, removes the energy blockages in your body, mind and spirit, opens all energy channels (meridians), and enhances energy circulation through all meridians in different dimensions. At the same time, it purifies your body, mind and spirit, inspires your soul and mind, heals and rejuvenates your whole being, and elevates the level of your life physically, mentally and spiritually.

§11.5 Earth Element Music and Its Healing Benefits

The earth music is composed with the earth tone (宮 / Gong, C, Do / 1) as a major tone that is used often as an ending note of the musical sentences, and is prolonged and emphasized in the instrumental performance. Sometimes the composition also gives proper attention to both the fire tone (徵 / Zhi, F, Fa, 5) as the earth element's energetically generating source and the wood element (木 / Jiao, E, Mi, 3) as earth element's restricting tone, in order to balance the energy of the earth element.

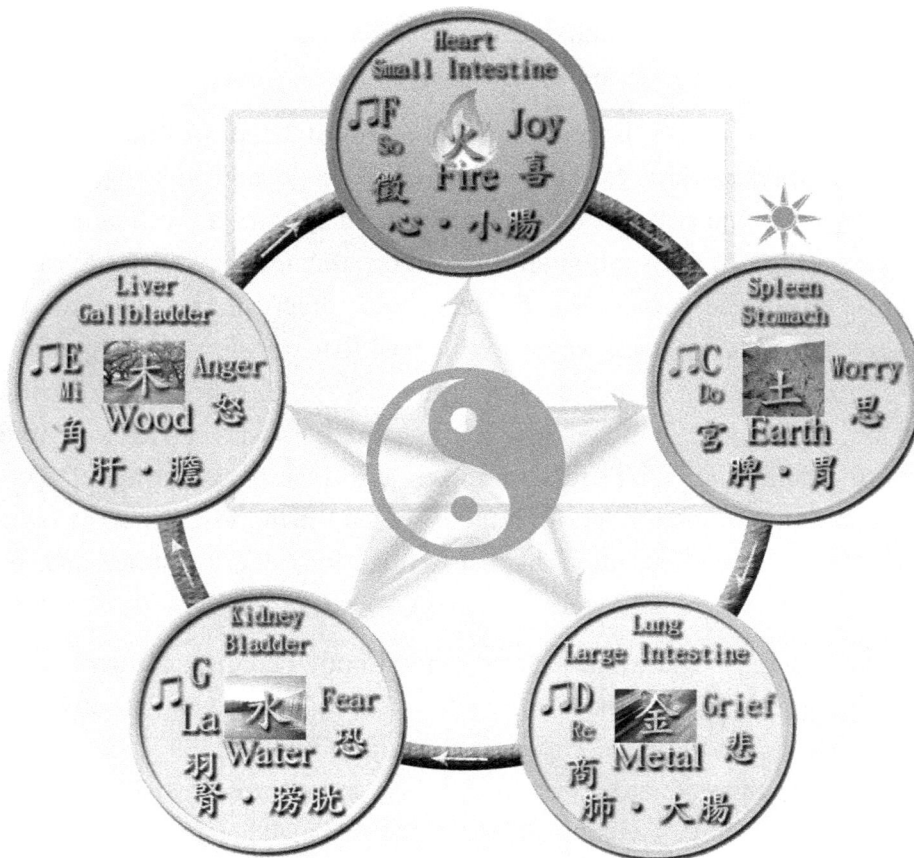

Promotion: Wood → Fire → Earth → Metal → Water → Wood

Restriction: Wood → Earth → Water → Fire → Metal → Wood

The sound waves of earth music enter the stomach and spleen meridians, support lung and large intestine meridians (metal element), cleanse the liver and gallbladder meridians (wood element), and balance the kidney and bladder meridians (water element). The tone color is featured as low, deep, slow, stable, strong, solemn, rich and broad as if the waves come from the remote sky, vibrating with the big land of earth. The vibration is resounding broadly as spring is coming to the land, and it is warm and compassionate as the motherland nurturing and nursing lives on the earth. All lives are rejuvenated with vital life force.

In the set of the Five Elements Energy Music, the earth music is very deeply and broadly vibrating with the entire space between earth and heaven; bringing the earth vibration energy to the stomach and spleen; establishing a vigorous and vast energy background to promote digestion and absorption of nutrition, nourish the blood and appetite; strengthening heart and lungs; supporting and balancing emotions; and eliminating negative emotions such as worry, sadness, fear, frustration, anxiety, and anger. This piece of energy music especially generates warmth, as well as heals and prevents you from getting cold.

§11.6 Metal Element Music and Its Healing Benefits

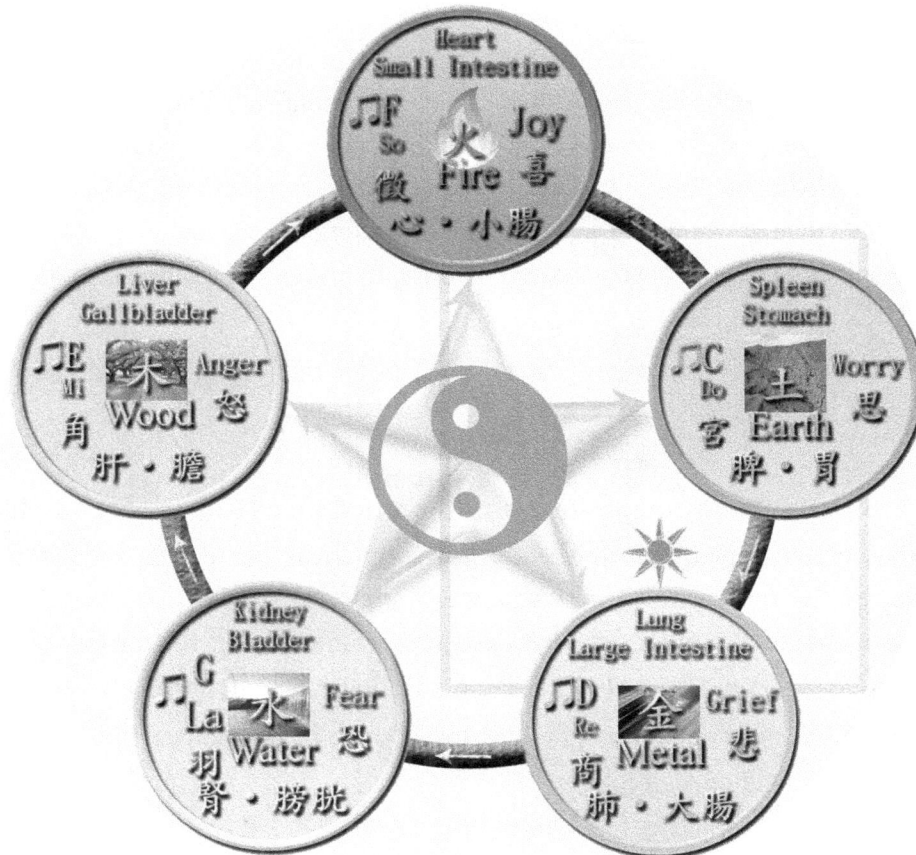

The metal element music is composed with the metal tone (商 / Shang, D, Re, 2) as a major tone that is used often at the end of the musical sentences, and is often prolonged and emphasized in the musical performance. As metal element's energy generating source, we sometimes give proper emphasis on the earth tone (宮 / Gong, C, Do, 1), and as restricting tone we also give attention to the tone of the fire element (徵 / Zhi, F, Sol, 5) to balance the metal energy in the energy music healing.

Promotion: Wood → Fire → Earth → Metal → Water → Wood

Restriction: Wood → Earth → Water → Fire → Metal → Wood

As a meridian energy therapy, the sound waves of metal music enter the lung and large intestine meridians, support kidney and bladder meridians, cleanse heart and small intestine meridians, and balance the liver and gallbladder meridians. It improves associated emotional aspects such as grief, sorrow or sadness; enhances the health of lung and large intestine; cleanses lung and large intestine; supports kidney and strengthen kidney essence; relieves depression, sorrow sadness, grief and fear by bringing a bright joyful emotion. The tone color of metal is: bright, fresh, crystalclear, crisp, transparent, high flying, far-reaching, broad spreading, euphemistically "up and down," and spiritually vibrating.

The metal music in the set of Five Elements Energy Music contains two pieces. These are the yin and yang metal music. The yin metal music is soft, clear, soothing and cooling, while the yang metal music is high and far reaching, broadening the lung capacity and energy, cleansing the heat and fire of liver, and enhancing the kidney energy. It is pleasing emotionally, bringing joy and bright feelings, releasing depression, grief, sorrow and sadness, restoring the energy of soul and mind, and rejuvenating the body.

§11.7 Wood Element Music and Its Healing Benefits

The wood music composition uses the wood tone (角音 / Jiao, E, Mi/3) as a major tone that often appears at the end of the musical sentences and is prolonged and emphasized in the musical performance. Using the water element as wood element energy's generating source, the composition sometimes gives proper emphasis to the water tone (羽 / Yu, G, La /6). And as restricting element, some attention is also paid to the note of the metal element (商 / Shang, D, Re/2) to balance the wood energy in the music's energy healing.

Promotion: Wood → Fire → Earth → Metal → Water → Wood
Restriction: Wood → Earth → Water → Fire → Metal → Wood

The wood sound music therapy functions by entering the liver and gallbladder meridians, supporting the heart and small intestine meridians, cleansing stomach and spleen meridians, and balancing the lung and large intestine meridians. This energy music improves liver associated emotions such as anger, overwhelming stress, anxiety, impatience, frustration, and overheated liver Qi mood. Its music waves enhance the health of both liver and gallbladder, cleanse the fire in liver and gallbladder, support the heart and harmonize the stomach and spleen.

Emotionally this wood element music eliminates liver anger, stress and frustrations, and brings peace and joy to the mind and body.

Wood music's tones are melodious, far-reaching, gentle, lyrical, positive, uplifting, warm and sunny like spring, flowing upwardly and downwardly, and are emotionally and spiritually vibrant.

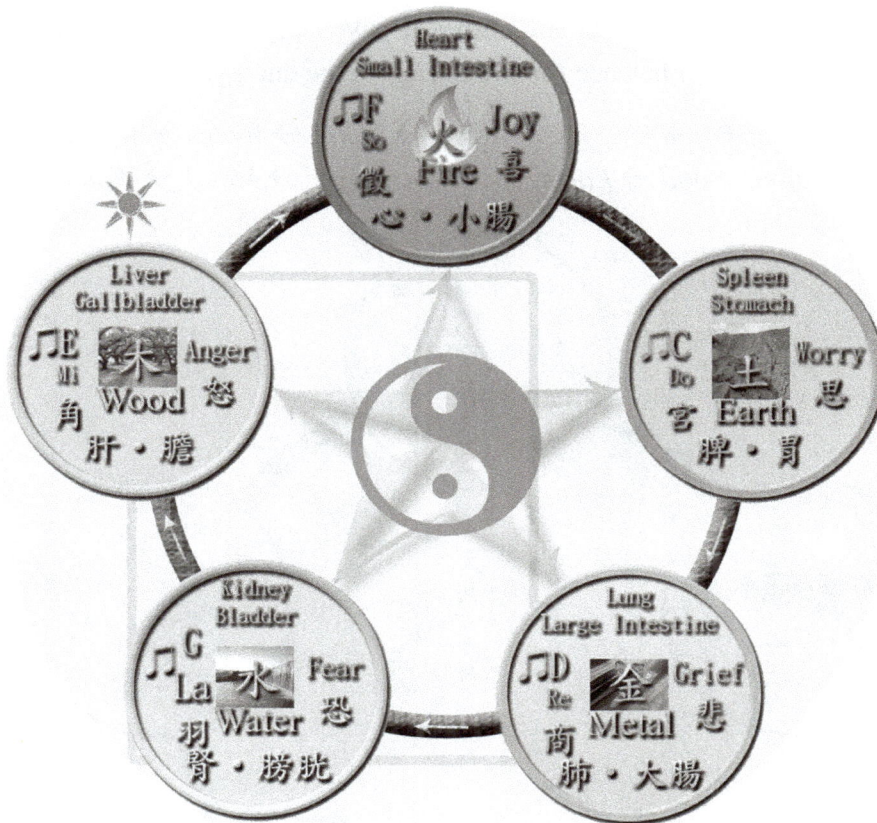

The wood music in the set of Five Elements Energy Music contains two types of compositions. These are yin wood music and yang wood music. The yin wood music is musically and emotionally soft, gentle, comforting, encouraging, nurturing, nursing, soothing and calming. Yang wood music is positive, uplifting, high and far reaching, broadening the liver Qi and blood flow, brightening the eyesight, stabilizing blood pressure and blood sugar, cleansing the heat and contamination of lung and large intestine, strengthening the heart energy, calming the spirit, pleasing the emotions, bringing a peaceful and soothing mood to the liver, releasing anger and stress, and balancing the body and mind and emotions.

§11.8 Fire Element Music And Its Healing Benefits

The fire element music uses the fire tone (徵音 / Zhi, F, So / 5) as a major tone, so that the fire tone often appears at the end of the musical sentences, and is prolonged and emphasized in the musical performance. As the fire element's energy promoting or generating source, the composition sometimes gives emphasis to the note of wood (角 / Jiao, E, Mi / 3), and as its restricting tone, sometimes it pays attention to the note of the water element (羽 / Yu, G, La / 6) to balance the fire energy in the energy healing.

*Promotion: **Wood** → **Fire** → Earth → Metal → Water → Wood*
*Restriction: Wood → Earth → **Water** → **Fire** → Metal → Wood*

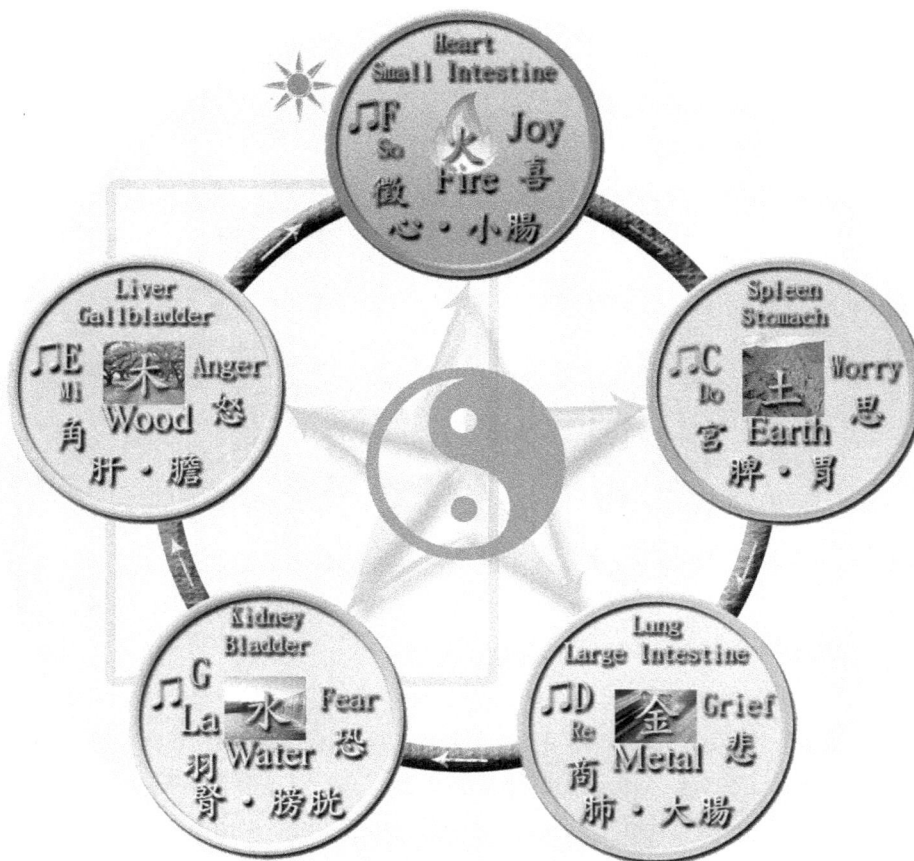

The fire music waves enter the heart and small intestine meridians, healing heart and small intestine as well as their associated energy system, supporting the spleen and stomach meridians, cooperating with the kidney and bladder meridians, and balancing the lung and large intestine meridians. The fire energy music improves the health of the heart and small intestine and related health issues of the entire energy system. These issues may include the: blood, tongue, throat, sweat, facial complexion, adrenals, thyroid, prostate, and pituitary. At the same time, according to the mutual relationships in the five elements, this music cleanses the lung and large intestine, harmonizes stomach and spleen, and increases appetite and digestion. Emotionally this fire music enhances heart-associated emotions such as love, happiness and joyfulness, as well as eliminates depression and sadness, and brings positive thought and mood to the mind and body. The fire music tone is colored with features of joy, love, warmth, kindness, crispness, brightness, melodiousness, positive energy, and confidence and is gradually and relatively fast paced and encouraging.

Within the set of Five Elements Energy Music, fire music contains yin and yang compositions. Both have positive and happy melodies and rhythms, but the yin fire music is relatively calming, and gradually deeper, softer and gentler in expressing the energy of love and happiness. The yang fire music is relatively stronger and straightforward to express its positive, uplifting, confident and happy energy. Listening to the fire music, you will become more open minded, positive, active, happy, worry-free, confident, passionate, loving, enthusiastic, and yang energy enhanced. You find your blood pressure stabilizes, kidneys strengthen, and spirit boosts.

§11.9 Water Element Music and Its Healing Benefits

The water music employs the water tone (羽音 / Yu, G, La / 6) as a major tone, and most of its musical sentences end with this musical note. The tone is prolonged and emphasized in the musical performance. As a water energy generating source, the composition sometimes also emphasizes the metal tone (商 / Shang, D, Re / 2). As a restricting tone sometimes it pays some attention to the tone of earth element (宮 / Gong, C, Do, / 1) to balance the water energy in the healing composition.

Promotion: Wood → Fire → Earth → Metal → Water → Wood
Restriction: Wood → Earth → Water → Fire → Metal → Wood

The water music sound enters the kidney and bladder meridians, heals these energy systems and related organs and emotions. It also supports the liver and gallbladder meridians, balances and works together with the heart and small intestine meridians, and cleanses the heat of the stomach and spleen meridians. The water energy music improves the health of the kidneys and bladder as well as the health of their associations in the energy meridians such as ears, bones, urine, head and pubic hair, brain, and marrow. Regarding its mutual relationships in the five elements, this water music also strengthens the liver and gallbladder, improves and harmonizes heart and small intestine functions, cleanses the heat of the stomach and spleen, and helps them digest food and absorb nutrients.

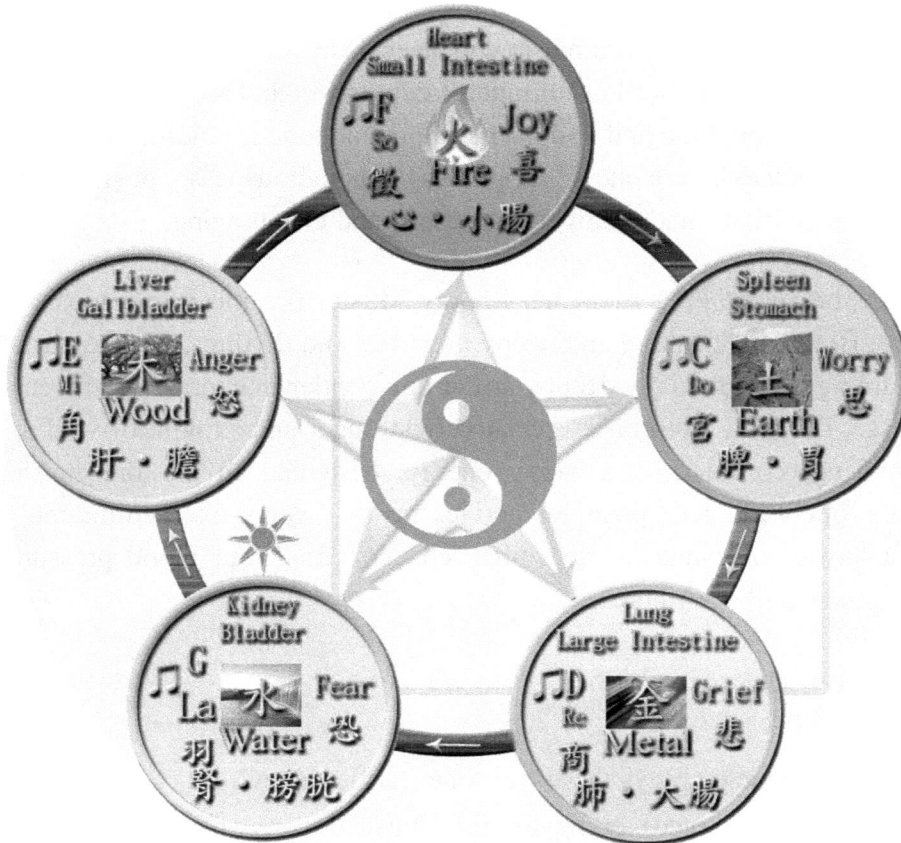

The sound waves of water music carry the water energy and express water energy natures of: elegant softness, fluidity, calmness, coolness, peacefulness, heavenliness, purification and purity, clearness and transparency, emotional and spiritual expressiveness, compassion and kindness, creativity, flexibility, and intelligence, wisdom, femininity, and adaptability to any situation. Listening to water tone music helps nourish the kidney essence, supplies kidney yin and yang energy, eliminates negative emotions such as fear, depression, low confidence, overwhelming stress, anxiety, frustrations or anger, and especially helps improve conditions such as tinnitus, insomnia and other symptoms caused by yang excessive, kidney essence deficiency.

The water music supplies the kidney essence, enhances kidney yin and yang, improves all kidney energy associated conditions including back pain, sciatica, hearing difficulty, hormone imbalance, female problems (irregular menstruation, dysmenorrhea, pre-menstrual symptoms, etc.) and male problems (impotence, premature ejaculation, etc.), menopausal syndrome, and other symptoms caused by kidney Qi deficiency.

§11.10 Music Selection upon Yin-Yang Five Elements Theory

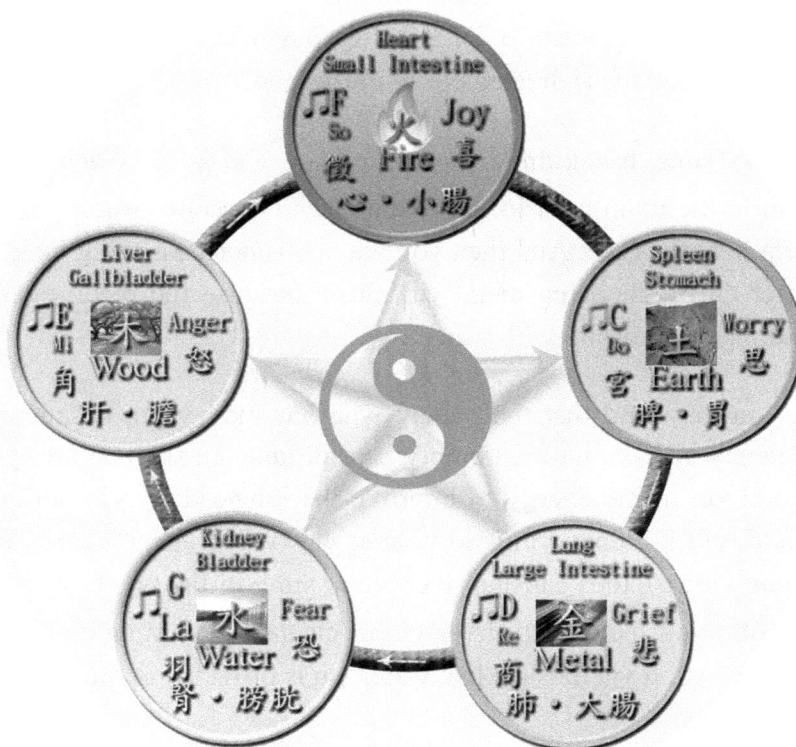

The Theory Of Five Elements teaches that the five elements form a dynamic system that has an internal mechanism of mutually generating relationships and mutually restricting relationships. In this five elements system, each element is not independent, but related with other elements: some of them promote the element, while some of them restrict it.

For example, the water element is promoted by the metal element and restricted by the earth element, while it generates and nurtures the wood element and inhibits the fire element. The other elements also follow the same principles as they associate with other elements in a mutually promoting and restricting relationship.

In addition and on the top of this Five Elements Theory, the ultimate underlying principle is the law of Yin-Yang as we discussed in the early chapter. It means that each element itself has yin and yang, the two opposite natures of the life force that are depending on each other in a balanced way for their supporting and restricting relations.

Therefore, when we use The Five Elements Music to treat disease or improve health, we have to simultaneously apply the principle of Yin-Yang and The Five Elements Theory in order to manage the selection and alternation of music titles so that they can effectively deal with an individual's specific condition. The initial diagnosis of the person's energy status is based on the eight principles of TCM as discussed in the previous chapter and is very important to help choose the right element of music title.

For example, if one has kidney yin deficiency (腎陰虛 *Shen Yin Xu*), then, tonifying kidney yin is the main goal in the treatment. Therefore, water yin music is the first selection to help heal the case. And then you may consider enhancing lung metal yin to support kidney water Qi by choosing metal yin music because the metal element has the generating or promoting relationship with water.

Sometimes you may find that the patient who has kidney yin deficiency may also have lung yin deficiency or have internal empty heat in lung. In such a case, you certainly need to provide metal yin music energy to improve the lung-kidney yin deficiency. Since water generates wood, when kidney yin is low, liver yin (wood element) may also become deficient (肝陰虛 *gan yin xu*), thus causing liver wood yang to fire up (肝陽上亢 *gan yang shang kang*). Therefore, you may tonify liver yin to cleanse liver yang and cool down the liver fire by giving some wood yin music while water yin is provided at the same time.

Sometimes, due to a liver yin blood deficiency, the heart is also lacking in blood according to wood generating fire, therefore causing heart yin deficiency. In such a case, you need to address the heart yin deficiency by giving fire yin music.

You may check to see if the patient has spleen heat that can damage kidney Qi according to the restricting relationship with water element. Otherwise, too much worry and emotional stress can also disturb the spleen function and cause the spleen to heat up. In such a case, you need to give some earth yin music to cool down the spleen heat (yang) and improve digestion function, thus strengthening kidney yin energy. In fact if the patient has low energy in the kidney yin for a long time, then he/she may also have kidney yang deficiency because of yin and yang dependency. In such a case, you may use both water yin as well as yang music alternately or simultaneously.

Considering other relationships of the water element with other elements, when kidney yin deficiency causes the high liver fire, it may also cause spleen/stomach upset, disordered Qi or cause Qi deficiency because the liver wood restricts the earth element (stomach and spleen). In such a case, you may have to provide earth music to improve spleen and stomach function. Furthermore, you may discover that the patient may also have heart fire rising up and heart yin deficiency because of the wood yang firing up the fire (element) of heart and the low yin energy of the water kidney unable to suppress the rising fire. As such, water cannot restrict the heart fire, causing heart yang energy to become overwhelming and the patient to become overly emotionally sensitive, as well as experience difficulty in sleeping (insomnia). As heart fire burns, and eventually the heart yang may also become deficient. This is also called disharmony between the heart and kidney or failure in communication between the heart and kidney (心腎不交 *xin shen bu jiao*). In such a case, you can provide fire yin element music and water yin element music to treat the patient for heart yin and kidney yin, respectively. This is the way to help heal the emotional over-sensitivity and insomnia.

When the health condition is improved and all the elements of energy are balanced to the original healthy level in their mutual generating and mutual restricting relationships, then you may use the Five Elements Energy Music in a rotating routine throughout all elements in order to maintain and strengthen a individual's overall energy and health condition, physically, mentally and spiritually. This is also a means of preventive healing/care to strengthen all organs, systems, and immunity as well as emotions in order to prevent future sickness or discomforts.

The above is just an example that gives you an idea about how to consider the elements based on the theory of Yin-Yang and Five Elements so that you can dynamically help with some complicated conditions in the healing process. Using Five Elements Energy Music is like using Chinese herbs, such that you need to consider the patient's condition, energy status and their dynamic changes during the healing process, making adjustments accordingly at each stage. The difference and also good thing with regard to energy music healing is that the healing music dynamically interacts with the patient's body, mind, spirit, (including emotions) all at once, so that the entire being is involved in the entire process, automatically transforming and transferring energies within and between multiple levels or multiple dimensions, creating feedback loops and making adjustments right away. Therefore, issues of balance can be achieved much more readily, easily and effectively.

Also important: The energy healing music introduced here was created with balanced elements with consideration of mutual promoting and restricting relationships surrounding each element, so listening to such healing music will automatically balance the entire being without much concern about specific increments and the effects of such increments that can result with the use of herbs.

§11.11 How to Listen The Five Elements Energy Music

We have discussed how a doctor or therapist uses The Five Elements Music as an art and practice to heal a patient or improve an individual's health of mind-body-spirit. While in this section, we will talk about how a person can best listen to the music to heal. This information will also help a doctor/practitioner to further understand the principle and application of this energy healing music composition. Please note that the energy healing music set that a doctor or therapist uses in our clinical setting to treat a patient is completely the same as the energy healing set that is provided for individuals in their self-healing practice. But the doctor's set is medically stronger and more effective, and requires the therapist to have diagnostic and other mind-body medicine training in order to generate and administer treatment. While for the purpose of individual use, the general music set is balanced, safe, and effective for common, everyday use. The principle with which the energy healing music is created is the same, however; therefore this chapter is suitable for both a mind-body medicine doctor and self-healing practitioner to read.

§11.11.1 Understand the Principle, Mechanism And Purpose

First of all, you need to understand that the healing music is a media which bridges, connects and merges you with the universe's energy source. Through the resonance or communication of your soul, emotions, heart, spirit, organs, nerves, hormones, and brain with the musical energy frequency, you reconnect your body and mind to the universe's nature, your original life force, and balanced Yin-Yang Five Elements energies that were originated from the universe. As such, you reopen your energy meridians and receive the universe's healing and compassionate energy. And as a result, you achieve healing benefits at all levels of body, mind and spirit.

By understanding this, during your music healing process, you can fully relax yourself, let go of human notions, attachments, narrowed mind, stubbornness, rigid logics, and analytical or skeptical attitude - all of which prevent you from resonating with your true spirit, the universe's nature.

In short, energy music healing is a process of helping you let go of all the conflicts, confusions, negativities, worries, angers or other mental blocks; open your energy channels (meridians) at the physical, mental and spiritual levels; and synchronize your entire being with the universe's nature. As a result, you are transformed, healed, energized, and enlightened at the higher energetic dimensions. To reach this goal, you do need to reset your mindset and completely get into and enjoy the world of spiritual healing and daily cultivation living produced by the energy healing music and guided by its teaching principle.

§11.11.2 Choose Right Music from the Energy Music Set

If you are a doctor then you diagnose your patient and choose the music as we addressed in the previous section.

If you are interested in self improvement/cultivation and wish to give yourself a music healing session, then you can choose a piece of energy music, from the musical set, based on your understanding of this book. We suggest that first you choose the element of the healing music directly related with your major concern about your health condition. For example, if liver yin deficiency and overwhelming liver yang, then choose wood yin music, while if kidney yin deficiency then choose water yin music. If spleen heat is high, then you choose earth yin music first, and so on. After a session or some sessions, you may further consider alternating other related elements, as we have discussed in the previous section.

Once you choose the specific music title based on your common understanding, you just go with that. In most cases you won't have any problems with that because the music is created in a relatively gentle, soft, and balanced pattern for general usage.

Your mind and body will tell you what you need. You should feel good if the healing music you choose is right. If you don't feel the selection is right while listening, however, you can change it. Just make sure, though, that you don't worry "too" much or get bogged down wondering about every possible nuance regarding the different musical selections as that may overwhelm and confuse you.

You should trust your selection or the doctor's selection without wondering or doubt, so you can relax and resonate with the music in a peaceful mood for the best result. You should understand that the key is in your mind. If your mind relaxes, stays calm and quiet, and you look into your own mind inwardly to cultivate yourself, then the music vibrations will resonate with you, and you will feel good. Otherwise if you focus on external things and concern yourself too much about the music selection, then you will feel stressful and nervous, and that will inhibit you from getting into the energy state produced by the healing music.

Please do not keep changing from one CD to another without having some experience and healing benefits. Try, instead, to stay with one element from the beginning to the end and absorb the energy while relaxing, meditating or being hypnotized or self-hypnotized. When you feel you have gotten enough from one title, then change to another. As you experience the healing music more, you will feel more confident in choosing the right music each time.

After awhile with the music healing practice, each person can have his/her own experience and identify more precise ways the healing music works on them personally. You can meditate, self-hypnotize, practice Taiji, Qigong, Yoga, gently move, walk, or even sleep with this energy music. But be aware, you should never drive with the music as you have been training your mind to operate in different spaces. Besides, if you should get drowsy, you definitely do not want to be behind the wheel for obvious reasons.

When listening to the music, focusing and quieting the mind is important. Talking on the phone, watching TV or doing other things while listening to this energy healing music will not be beneficial or effective. Therefore these are not recommended.

Your continued overall practice with this healing music will bring you further self-experience, information and personal benefits. Some of the following mentions, however, will be commonly experienced by many practitioners, yet are worth pointing out in order to step benefits up a bit sooner. For example, if you are feeling any pain, then use a relatively lower pitched music instead of high-pitched music because the latter will tighten the nerves, and you may feel that the pain gets worse. If you feel cold, then you should use rich, thick, deep, low pitched, warm music, while if you feel hot or are having internal heat, then you choose the music that is relatively thinner, lighter, cooler, calmer, slower, and higher pitched. The volume of the music is also an important factor when you listen to the music, depending upon your mood each time. Please be open-minded, and experience different volumes to receive best benefits.

§11.11.3 Getting Ready for The Session

Make sure you adjust your sound equipment appropriately at the right volume or have a remote control on hand for easy adjustment. Have a quiet environment in which to listen to the music, and no one or anything – e.g. telephone, TV, radio, pet, visitor – interrupts you during your music healing session. Have a comfortable temperature where you do not feel hot or cold, and can relax fully. Make sure not to have too much light so you can relax well, or sometimes you want to completely turn off the light in the room. Of course in case you want to have some sunlight or be outdoors, it is fine to meditate or relax with some comfortable sunlight with your music healing. In such a case, however, you still need to make sure you're not getting too hot or too much sunlight, or risking sunburn or UV damage to your skin. You may want to go to the bathroom once before starting the healing session, so you will not get up for bathroom in the middle of the session. Please wear relaxing and comfortable clothing or get into your bed with light covering, keeping warm, but not hot, and then get ready for your music healing session, giving yourself a very relaxing and joyful healing treat. Again the key is to fully relax your mind and body. It is the most important thing in getting yourself ready for the music healing.

§11.11.4 Practice Position - Sitting, Lying Down or Standing

Choose the best comfortable, relaxing and energizing position to practice energy music healing. Remember energy music healing is not just for relaxation or rest, but it is for healing, correcting, energizing and transforming the body, mind and spirit. Therefore, the position must be right as the part of mind-body-spirit health and cultivation practice. The position can be different, depending on the person and/or your time of day. The music healing position can be sitting, lying down, standing, or sometimes doing slow movement, exercise or walk. If you are tired, feel sleepy or have no energy to sit up, or for some elderly people or some individuals with a difficult condition, you may lie down to practice the music healing.

If you sit too much - worked all day in your office or you have been lying down too long, after a whole night sleep – and you feel you want to stand up, then you can use the standing posture. Most of the time, the sitting position is your best bet.

As we have previously discussed, the sitting position can be either the formal lotus meditation posture, which is the best or your everyday relaxed-sitting position, which is fine too.

If you lie down to listen the healing music, you should, then, make sure you feel comfortable on the bed (or couch etc.), with your whole body fully relaxed, overlapped palms on your belly area (about 2 inches below navel, called Dantian in Chinese or Qigong terminology or Qi Hai, in Acupuncture terminology).

If you use the standing position, you stand with feet at shoulders width apart, knees slightly bent, entire body relaxed, neck and shoulders relaxed, both arms stay down and hands overlapped on the Dantian point. Whether standing or lying down, your mental and physical relaxation state should be the same as the sitting position as described above.

Besides the still positions as described above, as an alternative, you may want to listen to the healing music while practicing a gentle movement, exercise, or take a walk outdoors or indoors. That said, however, please note: formally using music healing in the still position as in a sitting meditation or trained energy movement practice is going to be the most effective for daily practice.

When getting ready to start the healing practice with your chosen energy music, an induction (if a doctor doing the treatment for a patient) or self-induction (if you are doing self-healing practice with the music) will help you get into the deep dimensions of the healing energy vibration frequency. The induction is not quite the same as hypnosis induction, but here we borrow the term as one important procedure at the beginning of the energy music healing practice.

In this section we briefly introduce the induction technique in order to achieve the best healing benefits.

Induction is a verbal or silent wording script that the therapist or the subject uses (him/her self) as a guide into a relaxed, peaceful and positive conscious state for healing. In our music healing practice, we use a simple script for the induction. The following is an example of induction script for therapists to use with a client and can work for you as well if you are practicing self-healing.

This induction can be used at the beginning of the session. Start with it before playing the music, and after, just one or a few induction sentences. When the subject starts to get into the mood, start to play the music and continue the induction. During the induction try to visualize how the music waves vibrate and resonate all over the body and mind, and how it relaxes each part of the body and mind. With this visualization, the induction words can be easily remembered and every word of the verbal induction will carry the energy to influence the subject.

Please completely relax your body and mind, so you are ready to enjoy this wonderful and transformational healing session with this powerful energy healing music. [*Start to play the healing music.*] Now gently read the following:

You are part of the universe and now merge to its energy source through this energy healing vibration. Relax your mind and body. We are going to have a very long, peaceful and joyful healing journey.

Relax yourself from the top to the bottom, every part of you – relax your head, neck, back, and shoulders ... down to your arms and legs and feet ... until all parts of your body are relaxed.

Relax all organs, your heart, liver, lungs, stomach, and kidneys, and relax all your cells, nerves, muscles and joints. Breathe slowly and deeply, bring a peaceful smile to your face. Feel the energy that is like the fresh air and bright light flowing into your body and mind. Your soul is shining and flying in the beautiful golden space; you are out of this time-space dimension, and you can get into the multiple spiritual dimensions.

You have disappeared physically, but your spirit is clear, crystal, transparent, and totally free, flying everywhere in the vast cosmos. This is the original you.

Stay with your true pure nature – truthful, peaceful, loving, happy, compassionate, open minded, patient, resonating with the universe's characters and energy frequencies. This energy opens all your energy channels, removes all blockages, feel it circulating all over your body and mind, balancing you, healing you, energizing you, rejuvenating you, and unifying you. You get deeper and deeper, deeper and deeper...

You may add a few words somewhere in the induction to suggest that the subject take an inward look into the area of his/her body of concern, particularly if a specific health issue is of concern (emotional or physical). This will allow the individual to relax that area and communicate with it, so the music vibrations can resonate with it to heal.

It will also be helpful for the subject to feel relief from the worry. For example, if liver fire and anxiety or anger was the concern, then in the induction when suggesting that the client/patient relax all the parts of the body, you add: Especially relax your liver, smile at it, let the music waves flow into it, so your liver is relieved of blocked Qi and fire and lets go of anxiety and frustrations and replaces them with peace and happiness.

As your healing teaching goes deeper and gets connected with the patient spiritually, you may choose deep spiritual and emotional energy music and talk to the patient while both of you are listening the music and meditating:

You came from the vast universe, being part of it and protected by its great power, and being loved by its immeasurable compassion, and you never should worry about anything. We came to this land with nothing materially and will leave it one day without anything; why should we attach on all material things?

We have attached to all these heavy material things of this world and get too tired to even have a moment of feeling free and relaxed.

Now, wake up and no longer attach to them. Let go of all these heavy materialistic attachments and enjoy the freedom and peace of your mind.

You are connected to the entire universe, and to your true Self. Now and from now on, you just stay with this true you, cultivate yourself and travel your life journey forever...

If you are practicing self-healing with the energy music, the induction above can be naturally converted to a self-induction script by replacing the word you with I. You don't have to vocally speak out to perform your self-induction; actually you can just silently induct yourself in your mind.

When you use different musical titles selected from the five elements music set, the induction script can be slightly different because of different musical images. The above induction, however, gives you an idea about how to guide your client or yourself into the energetic vibration dimension that is produced by the healing music sound.

For each different healing music title and session, your induction or healing teaching talk can be performed differently based on its musical energy pattern, emotional mood and spiritual messages, and the patient's ability of understanding or acceptance. With the energy music, the session goes deeper and deeper very easily and naturally because its energy field reaches deeply into other mental and spiritual dimensions layer by layer, helping the patient understand and resonate deeper and deeper. Every patient comes in with different problems and different personalities, but they walk out of the clinic with the similar result: They feel good, healthy and clearheaded because they are assimilated and unified with the same universal characteristics and balanced energy state.

Don't get too complicated or too detailed or specific in the induction. The key is to help the subject relax and empty the mind and body, and after that, the music will take over. The induction should only take a few minutes and then the subject (you or your client) should get into an empty state and stay with it during the entire healing practice.

§11.11.6 Individual Experiences

As the beautiful melodious music healing vibrations are flowing into your cells and soul, you feel you are embraced by the infinite free space and time of the immeasurable compassionate cosmos and riding on the melodious rhythms and vibrations, floating and flying. You are blowing through the soothing and comfortable spring breeze and rain, passing all places that are filled out of the silky sunlight and white clouds, flying over one and another, over the Castle Peak of mountains, enjoying the colorful magnificence and heavenly spectacular wonders. You feel fully relaxed, worry-free, freely flying, floating, expanding, and fully enjoying the mysterious spaces and peaceful lighting of the world in deep transcendence, static emptiness and eternal infinity. Your body, mind and spirit are totally purified, energized and transformed to a new state.

As you go deep with the music or meditate with it time after time, you will have more and more amazing healing results, sensations, feelings and positive changes. The key is that you totally let go of your human thoughts and attachments, and explore your godly Self, so you will fully resonate with the musical vibration frequencies that carry the universe's spiritual nature and superpower of the energies.

Each individual may have different healing sensations, feelings, benefits and experiences with the music healing practice. Certain aspects of these wonderful experiences are unique to you – and the "you" at the moment. You may, for example, even experience some different nuances each time you listen to the same healing music. This is because your body, mind and spirit are transformed into a different level, in a different depth, of spiritual healing dimensions.

§11.11.7 Upgrade Healing Level and Spiritual Growth

While you practice healing with the energy music set, you are recommended to come back to read this book (or listen the audiobook) again and again, so every time you read (or listen), you will understand its concepts and tools better, resonate with the music deeper, and your healing benefits and spiritual growth will progress further. Reading this book repeatedly will also motivate you to have great interest and joy with the practice, grow with the practice, and be enlightened and transformed by the divine messages during the practice.

As you acquire more experience in healing longer with the energy, you will know this healing practice as an endless joyful journey. You should keep elevating your healing level and spiritual growth continuously, and eventually you will find that this does not just benefit you in healing or health, but also help you develop wisdom, intelligence, and open the mind to clearer and higher quality ideas, creativity, and spirituality. Since we mention growth of spirituality here, we may need to be clear on one thing in order to avoid confusing you: There is no concern if you have your own belief system or religion because this music healing is a natural method for you to increase the health of mind, body and spirit, but not a religious practice or belief system.

Music healing only helps you grow in a balanced way physically, mentally, emotionally and spiritually, but won't add anything to your belief system or interfere with your personal belief practice. There are no religious requirements, procedures, or object(s) of worship in this music healing practice. It is purely a health and healing system, and there is no need to worry about affecting your own religious belief and practice.

§11.12 Intermediate Break: Story • Healing Music • Meditation

A client's healing story on severe depression

BMT Saved My Life – My Severe Depression Healed

- Eva C

When I first came to Dr. Liu for treatment of my severe depression and anxiety, I had already completely stopped menstruating for 3 months. My energy was low, and my circulation was so bad that my hands and feet were always cold. My blood pressure was constantly as low as ~95/55. I felt hopeless in my life. I couldn't work and didn't know what to do. Many times I suddenly started crying uncontrollably.

According to Dr. Liu, all my symptoms were due to a combination of deficiencies in kidney yin, excessive liver fire, hormone imbalance, and mental blocks. My mom saw Dr. Liu's article in the newspaper, and made an appointment with him, for me. When I started seeing Dr. Liu, I began to feel better and better each time. I felt energy start flowing within my body; my hands, feet and whole body were growing warmer during the sessions. With each session, I could feel positive changes. I was happier and more peaceful. After the first month, my period resumed, but I still had some emotional frustration, which Dr. Liu indicated was a positive reaction, as emotional blockages were being released.

We continued sessions for another month, and now my depression and anxiety are completely gone. My period returned to normal, with no discomfort. My blood pressure is normal, and my circulation is much better; my hands and feet are no longer cold. I feel very peaceful, and am very appreciative for Dr. Liu's help. He brought light and hope into my life. Right after I finished my sessions, I got a new job.

Meditation with Energy Music

Based on conditions, such as those experienced by Eva – deficiencies in kidney yin, excessive liver fire, hormone imbalance, and mental blocks – choose a suitable piece of energy music from The Five Elements Series. Play it and meditate for one hour.

Before ending the meditation, with a clear conscious mind, visualize the five elements picture presented in this chapter. Then, consider other elements from the healing music that you might use to heal Eva's specific case, and make your choices based on the mutual promotion and mutual restriction relationships of The Five Elements.

1. What is Energy Healing Music?

2. What are The Five Elements, and how do they correspond to the five tones of music, five organs of the body and five emotions of human beings?

3. What are the relationships of the five elements and how do you understand them in the context of mutual generating and restricting relations in the five human organs, emotions and music tones? Use the picture of Yin-Yang and Five Elements to explain the relationship cycles.

4. What is the theory by which the Yin-Yang and Five Elements Energy Music is composed, and what are the energy features for each elemental music pattern?

5. Describe the earth, metal, wood, fire, and water element music and their healing benefits?

6. How should you dynamically use the Yin-Yang and Five Elements Music based on the Yin-Yang and Five-Element Theory? Use an example to explain how you would choose the appropriate element music for treatment/healing?

7. How do you listen to and practice with the Yin-Yang and Five Elements of Energy Music – in terms of getting ready, selecting title, position or posture, and induction at the beginning of the healing practice?

8. What is your personal experience with regard to energy healing music?

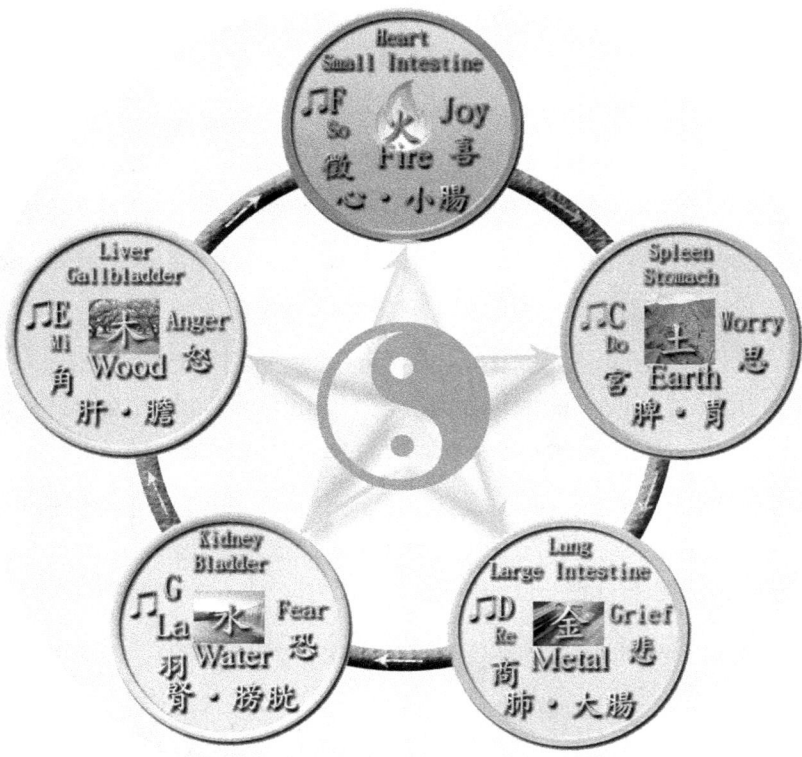

CHAPTER 12

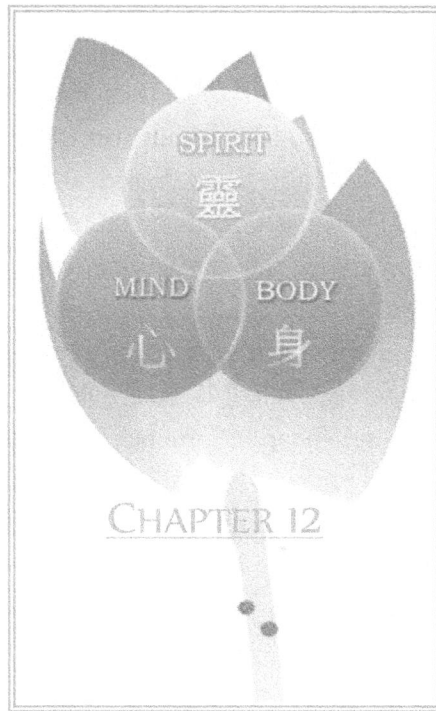

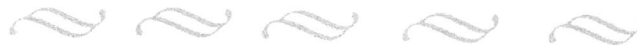

Brainwave-Meridian Therapy
– An Application of Mind-Body Medicine

As an application of the mind-body medicine, this chapter introduces the technique called Brainwave-Meridian Therapy (BMT). BMT is an integrative mind-body medicine developed and practiced in our clinic over years. The author of this book developed this practice based on the principles and techniques of traditional Chinese medicine, Qigong, meditation, psychological and spiritual healing, neuroscience, brainwave science, Yin-Yang and Five Elements of energy music sound therapy with brainwave incorporated, hypnosis, ancient mind-body-spirit cultivation, and principles and concepts of mind-body medicine addressed in this book. These are synthesized into one, simple practice with comprehensive energies, covering multiple levels to achieve the total health and wellness of the whole being, the body, mind and spirit.

339

BMT directly addresses the root causes of health problems without medication, herbs or needles. Root causes commonly found are (1) emotional and spiritual confusions, conflicts, disturbances, distractions, noise, overwhelming stress and hopelessness, and (2) physical and mental energy imbalance, blockages, deficiencies or weakness, with variations depending on individuals. Both categories of causes involve many factors in a person's lifetime and sometimes also past lives, depending on the individual. BMT consists of a series of procedures linking (1) diagnostics based on Traditional Chinese Medicine principles, and followed by (2) psychological consultation based on the ideologies and principles of mind-body-spirit medicine and energy medicine (some of which are addressed in this book), (3) Yin-Yang and Five Element energy music composition, production and brainwave incorporation, (4) treatment with the energy healing music in combination with (5) meditation and (6) hypnotherapy, and (7) HeartMath technique, (8) acupressure, (9) exercise, (10) teaching patient self-healing practice and daily improvement. BMT uses natural laws to effectively remove physical, mental and spiritual blockages, circulate energy along the meridians (energy channels), empower the vital life force, enhance physical, mental and spiritual energy levels, balance and rejuvenate the mind and body, and uplift the spirit, achieving whole being health.

BMT includes several components and procedures to integrate the healing into one system as a holistic treatment for the body, mind and spirit as well as all daily life related health practices.

I will address some major points to draw a picture about how BMT treatment is practiced and how it works. I will keep in mind that this may help some young students in this field learn mind-body healing consultation. So the following contents will share some clinical experience, to a certain extent, and will also discuss necessary healing principles involved with the implementation of BMT.

§12.2 Doctor's Passion, Compassion and Good Energy

A good mind-body health practitioner has great compassion, passion and a sincere heart with which to listen to and treat his/her patient. This is the most important and the first thing we need to address and practice seriously. This and only this can guarantee the success of the healing work.

From the practitioner's first word greeting the patient, in the very beginning of the session and initiating conversation about the person's health problems, the doctor should put heart into carefully listening to the patient as the individual tells his/her story. The practitioner needs to listen very carefully even more than the patient's closest friend does.

During the session, your heart is always with the patient – your eye contact, expression, wording, voice, smiles (natural and appropriate for each case), mood, thinking, questioning, answering, talking, every detail is all naturally flowing with the patient. You are relaxed, implying your patient can relax and feel comfortable. Your sincerity while listening to your patient makes him/her freely open their mind to share personal stories and true feelings with you.

On a personal note, as a mind-body-spirit cultivator, I do meditate everyday and get myself fully energized before my day starts. This is very helpful and extremely important for success in the healing work of my day. Therefore, during a session, I stay very calm, energetic and passionate, and enjoy hearing from my patient. Not just listening, but also keeping my mind and focus on the conversation, thinking about what are the causes for the problems, in regard to his/her growing history: family, parents, living and working environment, daily life, emotions, character, habits, relationships?

At some point, the doctor can naturally add a few words as guiding posts to lead the conversation towards the core causes of a health concern, preparing the patient to understand and self recognize the cause in the next step of the session. In fact, many patients are confused about their issue. So when telling you their story, they easily get very emotional, and sometimes get into a myriad of unrelated topics. On one hand, you calmly and patiently listen to their story, let them release their emotions, and collect enough information, never dogmatically force them to cut off or interrupt the patient's talk, so that you can truly understand the issue and the patient's concerns. On other hand, however, you also need to make sure the conversation is not going all the way out to unrelated topics or that the patient does not get uncontrollably emotional, either of which will confuse the patient even more, so the session will not head off in the right direction.

If you are a student practitioner in this field, this is something you need to put effort into practicing. As a mind-body doctor, you are not just listening to the patient's story, but also importantly you are naturally directing the conversation to focus on a clear and main line. Of course, you do this patiently, wisely and naturally without giving the patient an impression that you are trying to rigidly control the conversation or you are impatiently interrupting the patient's talk. During the conversation if you surely realize that the talk gets into an unrelated topic, then you can find a right entry point and naturally add a few words to lead it to the right direction. Therefore the conversation can help the patient reorganize his/her mind, thoughts and problems toward a clear understanding about why such incidents as those the person reports have occurred and how they are related to core causes. In fact, even this very initial conversation becomes part of the healing journey. The healing starts from the very first moment when the patient starts to tell you his/her story.

The first session is extremely important especially in the step of collecting information from the patient. Personally I do not suggest that you give a very long list of questions in the "patient form" for your patient to fill out. This is because too many questions in the form will make your patient stressful and nervous before the session. A simple form with some major questions is good enough. Different from modern medicine in the hospital, you should take a long enough time to talk to your patient in a comfortable and relaxed mood in order to have an inspiring conversation on various and useful details regarding your patient's: health concerns/condition(s), history, lifestyle, habits, relationships, family, education, work, and so forth. All these factors are related with his/her issues of mental and physical health. The doctor should be friendly and warmly approach the conversation with the patient regardless of his/her manner, attention, respectfulness, age, sex, race, nationality and cultural and religious backgrounds, as well as other personal aspects. Talk with your heart involved, so you will truly connect to your patient's mind and soul and better understand his/her case.

Getting to know about the patient's health issues and related information is the first step and an important procedure in BMT therapy. Due to the complication of many chronic conditions, the initial session sometimes takes longer than a regular session. In our clinic, the first session usually takes three hours including initial conversation and treatment. Regular follow-up sessions, however, are two hours long. So we do not believe in cutting these short either. It is absolutely worth taking a longer time for each session.

The session always includes two parts: one is a close conversation or teaching, discussion, which includes patient feedback with Q&A. This revolves around the emotional, mental, psychological and spiritual issues. The second part of a session is a full practice of BMT treatment with therapeutic energy music combined with hypnosis, meditation, biofeedback / HeartMath technique. Based on our many years of experience, this is the best way to heal most chronic mind and body conditions.

Many patients have suffered from mental and physical discomforts over years. In the first session, they often have a lot of things to tell you. They are sometimes confused themselves, so they may keep giving you overwhelming information or random talk regarding many issues in their lives. Sometimes they keep complaining about someone, others or everyone, or about a multitude of things or everything. Sometimes, the more they talk, the more they become emotional, over expressive, unable to make a clear point or they experience more difficulty articulating themselves.

They may think negatively and in strange ways. Listening to and understanding them may not be easy. Your patience, compassion, clarity and calming mind will help you have a smooth session in order to get to the point; finding the cause of the health problem, especially in the very first session. As a doctor of the mind, body and spirit, you understand your patients and calmly listen to them. At the same time, you understand deeper about the issue and the causes. Thus you do not just listen and echo along with your patient, but also, you use the right words to naturally lead your patient in the major direction of the core cause, solution and healing strategy. This way your patient's talk will get to the point, and your diagnosis or comments on the issue will be easier to summarize. You don't want to interrupt your patient's talk, and on other hand, you also want the talk to be focused in the right direction. You ask suggestive questions to lead the talk in a good flow, inspiring your patient to open their mind and understand the cause of his/her problem. Your queries tell the patient that you are very interested in their talk, so that you can understand how the details may relate to the cause of their problem.

§12.5 Diagnosis & Explanation to Patient

BMT uses the diagnostic methods described previously to evaluate a patient's energy status and in combination with psychological and spiritual conversations. This is an important procedure in BMT. It is using the principles and concepts of traditional Chinese medicine, but simplified in procedure and implementation. Please note that diagnosis as we mention it here is not to diagnose disease, but in fact it is to evaluate the energy status of the patient.

We go through the TCM four diagnoses, for example, including asking, looking, tongue diagnosis, and reading pulse. If you are not familiar with the technique of pulse reading, it can be temporarily left out, so by asking, looking, tongue diagnosis and psychological conversation, you still can know the basic problem and cause at energy level.

We believe that life energy is at multiple levels including physical, emotional and spiritual levels and reflected in many aspects. In traditional Chinese medicine, the four methods of diagnosis are typical and well used to determine the patient's energy. In our mind-body medicine practice, we simplify the procedures to meet our needs.

Usually we combine all these methods in the initial conversation process. The tongue diagnosis and pulse reading can be combined and followed by the initial conversation.

During the initial conversation, we naturally pay attention to the patient's body tone, fitness, gait, skin, facial expression, eye contact, emotional expression, and mannerisms, talking, voice, its volume and clarity, the way of speaking and use of words, and body language to know his/her energy state, mental and physical conditions. Compared to regular Chinese medicine doctor's practice, we are not only interested in the patient's energy state but also most importantly relate it with and put more focus on the patient's mental, emotional, psychological and spiritual state, mood, feelings and expressions, trying to get contact with the patient's true spirit. On other hand, different from regular psychologists or mental health practitioners, we involve the patient's energy state, energy frequency and healing energy vibration in the entire process of diagnosis, conversation and treatment.

When you are amidst your session, you can simply combine these concerns into the initial conversation.

We use the principles and concepts of TCM as energy medicine, observing the patient's energy state and mental, emotional and spiritual state as vibration frequencies within the body, mind and spirit. Through the energy vibration state, we can actually feel and understand the whole person in multiple dimensions. This "profile" helps us determine the energy pattern and mental blockages and how to deliver the right treatment.

Consider the following patient's case – let's refer to her as Kate, the case mentioned at the end of Chapter 3, – as an example. After the diagnosis by asking, looking, tongue checks and conversation, we got clear ideas about her problem(s). From the energy medicine principle, Kate apparently had a yang type of illness. In other words, she was lacking in yin Qi, and had excessive yang Qi, appearing as heat or fire. This excessive heat, however, was not the essence heat or fire (not a real one), but was empty heat or empty fire. It was the internal fire in the liver and spleen due to a deficiency of kidney yin. This condition had already gotten to the interior level and had worsened. In addition, she exhibited anger, stress, anxiety, depression, fatigue, and insomnia.

Physiologically she had digestive difficulty, constipation, dry skin and swollen feet. All these are related, in terms of the excessive fire in the liver, heat in spleen, and lack of yin in the kidneys, as well as her stressful life, anxiety, anger and irritated emotions and temperament. These factors are all causes of her physical and mental issues and they are also the results of each other. Usually the kidney yin deficiency is the original or initial cause, which results in other problems sequentially. In her case, however, it seemed her hyper emotions such as anxiety, stress and anger also became core causes that affected her physical condition, resulting in even more imbalance in the energy of yin and yang in the liver and spleen, as well as further deficiency of kidney yin. This created a negative feedback loop – the body and mind affecting each other.

Mental causes are often deeply involved. These may include childhood experiences, parents or family, growing and living environment and conditions, working and family relationships, social and cultural backgrounds and sometimes also related political and social stressors and pressure. As a mind-body health practitioner, you will find major, minor, or even subtle causes for health problems in regard to the patient's psychological, emotional and spiritual issues. For Kate's case, in fact her mental blockages were started from her very abusive childhood and followed by many stressful disturbances and difficulties in her life including relationships, jobs and inborn conditions.

Explaining your diagnosis result to your patient is very important. It will help your patient better understand his/her case, and help the healing directly and deeply resonate with your patient. When you explain how you see the case, what was the cause for the problem, the individual will usually be very interested in listening to you, feel connected with you, and can understand how you are approaching the treatment.

When you say something that touches his/her heart, matches his/her situation, triggers him/her to recall anything in his/her life, then the patient starts to resonate with your healing vibration and receive the healing energy. Different from conventional hospital treatment, holistic medicine such as mind-body healing, as we discuss it now, must touch the patient's soul by spending time communicating with the patient. After diagnosis, you certainly should kindly explain how you view his/her condition and causes. And then you describe your treatment principle and approaches (see in the next section), encourage the patient to keep positive thoughts and hopes, not to worry, and believe that their issue is curable or improvable as long as both patient and doctor work together. This is very important.

§12.6 Make a Treatment Plan & Explain It to the Patient

Based on the diagnosis and initial conversation as described above, we make a plan to treat the patient. The treatment plan focuses on the core cause first – and among all causes at multiple levels. In most cases, the health problem was caused by various factors at multiple levels and aspects, including energetic, psychological, emotional, spiritual, lifestyle, social, family, relationship, environmental, educational, genetic factors, etc. Therefore the treatment must reach multiple levels in order to heal from the root.

In mind-body medicine practice, we treat all these causes at multiple levels to pursue the total healing of mind, body and spirit. In the beginning, however, we start to treat the patient with the most effective and immediate and feel-good approach first, so it will give the patient a positive healing right away and help him/her gain confidence about his/her health and the treatment.

Most patients have experienced their health issue(s) for a long time without improvement through other types of treatments. Thus, they often do not have confidence that they can heal or they now doubt the results of any treatment. Therefore, taking the most effective way to treat the major cause and making the patient feel good first is the most important step at the beginning. BMT has such power because it can quickly empty a patient's mind by its very effective energy music sound vibrations, and then the energy quickly quiets the mind, opens energy channels, and stops the discomforts physically and mentally.

In fact, most patients who come to our mind-body medicine clinic have been in their "conditions" for a long time and are in need of quick effective, positive, encouraging, peaceful, caring, nursing and balanced healing energy. Their physical and mental discomforts are due to the blocks, disturbance and lack of energy within the body and mind. Therefore, immediately dealing with their energy is the key to quick relief of their discomfort and moving forward toward a deep healing. Note: the energy therapy must address and heal all causes (as aforementioned), at multiple levels. We have found BMT is an effective energy therapy for such cases.

Again using Kate's case as an example, we had a deep conversation about the causes of her illness, especially her childhood experiences that caused an entire lifetime of anger, depression, and being unfairly treated. These emotional negativities deeply rooted in her mind. Her emotional memories triggered physical and mental problems and tremendous painful experiences, which have continued to weaken her physically, psychologically, and spiritually. Specifically speaking, her emotional stress (anger, depression, etc.) caused her liver fire and kidney yin deficiency, which further induced insomnia, skin problem and swollen feet.

She fully agreed with our evaluation and was touched by the understanding and by finally rooting out the core cause of her issues.

She looked forward to using energy medicine principles to help her heal. She understood and was very happy for the treatment principle and plan that would focus on recreating totally pure, peaceful, effective and harmonious energy vibrations that would cancel out all the negative memories, messages, confusions, noises and disturbances of anger, anxiety, depression, and hopelessness, she had carried within and unleashed into her outside world. Then, we reestablish a peaceful mental environment and physical condition.

For her treatment plan, we used the BMT technique, especially the water element music waves combined with hypnosis, meditation and HeartMath technique to cleanse all the heat, fire, noise, confusions, anger and depression in all related organs and emotional organs, and deliver the soothing and cooling water energy into the kidney meridians and emotional brain, so she could feel calm, and peaceful, and have good sleep, rest and relaxation day and night, and whenever she needed. After we explained these treatment approaches, she was very happy and ready for her healing journey.

§12.7 Progress in BMT Treatment & Discussions

The BMT treatment starts at the second half of the initial session. As such, the first session therefore leaves the patient ideally already feeling better. Otherwise, if we are not seeing an obvious improvement, we will at least guide the patient to a much clearer perspective on their condition, the cause, and ultimate treatment goal, so emotionally they can feel lighter, positive and hopeful. We look for (and generally get, but not always) improvement with each subsequent session.

As the healing progresses in each session, the sick Qi is eliminated layer by layer. There are sometimes ups and downs in the healing result, that is not a linear slope simply rising upward all the time. But every up and down is all part of the natural cleansing and healing process.

The blocks and sick energy inside the patient's mind and body have many layers. We can see the "darkness" leaving from the patient during the BMT treatment. Once one layer of the sick Qi is eliminated, the patient feels better. And soon another layer comes out. The patient feels heavy and discomforted again. Emotional feelings and the patient's physical condition can fluctuate from up to down, then up again, throughout the healing cycle. Yet the cycle is not precisely repeated each time, but progresses layer by layer, with ups and downs, as the patient moves deeper and deeper towards complete healing.

After each treatment, a small discussion with the patient is very helpful and inspiring. The healing music activates the patient's soul and mind, brings forth many thoughts from the bottom of his/her heart. Sometimes patients automatically recognize their problems on their own and quickly make corrections in their mind, their emotions and daily life to heal themselves. As a doctor, seeing our patients grow and heal this way is the happiest blessed moment.

§12.8 Long Term Healing Benefit & Daily Practice

The discussion with a patient after each treatment is extended to stabilize healing results toward a long-term benefit. BMT energy is very powerful and effective, so the patient can get healed and feel good, but even so, this does not mean the healing result can last forever. The healing vibration created the strong healing energy environment that melded the whole person (body, mind and spirit), and washed away all sick messages within the patient's body and mind. This is good in regard to the primary success of the healing. But if the patient is not completely enlightened spiritually and not clear-headed about their own life, personality, character, mindset, and emotional management, then, the old thoughts, habits, addictions, attachments, and lifestyle remain unchanged, so as a result the problem will be back again.

For such reason, after a treatment or at the beginning of the next session, we have an open discussion and sharing of mind-body-spirit healing concepts with the patient. We look back on the entire process of this life and the healing treatment; discuss why their problem occurred, and how it is better now, and then how to prevent the problem from coming again in the future. The center point in the discussion is that one has to keep one's true Self aligned with the great natures of the universe by corresponding mindsets, personality, and daily lifestyle. We teach the patient meditation, self-hypnosis, exercise, healthy lifestyle, and encourage them to practice daily, for long-term healing and health benefits.

§12.9 Intermediate Break: Story • Healing Music • Meditation

The following healing story came from a natural herbalist and herb garden businesswoman who had multiple health issues such as severe arthritis, chronic pain syndrome, depression, insomnia, and stress. She responded to the BMT healing so well she no longer needed to take prescription medications.

BMT Has Really Helped Me Immensely

- Christina B.

I hadn't had a good night's sleep for 4 1/2 years. I was sure that part of it was emotional. It began after my sister died very quickly (within a month) in the hospital. The pain in my hip started the day we took her to the hospital; I could hardly get back into the house. Since then, I've been diagnosed with severe arthritis in my left hip, and have been taking pain pills. Being an herbalist, I teach about health issues, and advise not taking drugs; however, I was sneaking prescription meds on my own because the pain was so bad.

After my first treatment with Dr. Liu, I actually slept for nine hours! This therapy worked much better than the pain pills ever did! Nothing else has worked so quickly for me. I had tried a lot of different therapies and seen about 47 different practitioners. Although Dr. Liu scheduled me for the next week, I came back, instead, the very next day! It was doing so much for me, and I was anxious to recover 100%. After the first treatment, the pain was down about 30%, and after the eighth or so, it was down by 95%. It's just amazing, what a difference this made in my life! I was just at a medical supplement conference where there were many medical doctors, PhDs, medical researchers, and a few herbalists. I was very, very busy, and I didn't really rest all weekend. I was extremely tired yesterday, but this morning I'm feeling great! I know that before my sessions with Dr. Liu, if I had managed to get through three days like that, I would have felt like staying in bed for 3-4 days afterwards. This therapy has helped me immensely.

My friend and I have a small herb company; we grow plants to sell, so we do some manual labor. I had back problems before for trying to lift heavy things (I broke my back in 1983), and to be able to do as much as I am now and not have any pain afterwards is really amazing! I am telling everyone: "You got to try this! It works!! It really has worked for me!!!" To have something that works this well, and all you have do is lie down and listen to music... Hmmm... you can't beat that! "No pain, no Gain" - well, that's baloney! This therapy involves no pain, and I feel so much better.

Cultivate Yourself In Meditation

Whether you are a healthcare practitioner or an individual who wants to be healthy, cultivating to have higher quality of mind, body and spirit and good energy, is extremely important. Only when you have good energy in mind and spirit can your healing work well and can you cultivate yourself to a higher level. Before reading any further, let's meditate and cultivate more, charge your mind and spirit with great energy, so you will be motivated through this learning. Choose a piece of the energy music, which you like the most from the series you have and have a deep meditation with it for one hour. Empty your mind, sit upright in a still but relaxed position, go deeper and deeper while letting go of all human thoughts, attachments, desires, wondering, calculating, but fully connected with the vast universe and resonated with its great characteristics …

§12.10 Exercise Questions

1. What is Brainwave-Meridian Therapy?

2. How important are the doctor's passion, compassion and good energy in the mind-body healing practice?

3. How and what will you prepare for your patient for his entry into your clinic?

4. What do you do in your patient's initial session in regard to diagnosis and conversation to get to know your patient's condition, its cause and to help create a plan for treatment?

5. How do you finally diagnose your patient and explain your diagnosis result to him or her?

6. How do you make a treatment plan and explain it to your patient?

7. What do you do when the healing result has ups and downs and why is it like that? How do you stabilize the healing result by using the multiple levels of healing mentally, physically and spiritually?

8. How do you make sure the healing result is long-lasting by teaching your patient self-healing and preventive health?

SPIRIT
靈

MIND BODY
心   身

CHAPTER 13

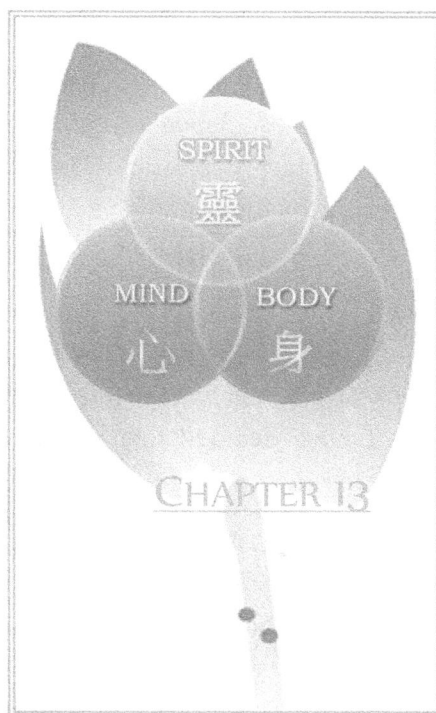

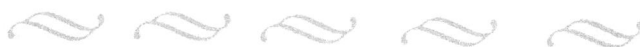

Preventive Health with Mind-Body Practice

The most well known ancient Chinese physician Bianque/real name Qin Yueren (407 BC – 310 BC) lived during the Spring and Autumn Period in the area of Bohai, presently Renqiu county, Hebei Province, China. He was the founder of the fundamental basis of traditional Chinese medicine (TCM), created the four diagnostic methods and established the entire practice system that has been practiced for many thousands of years right into present time.

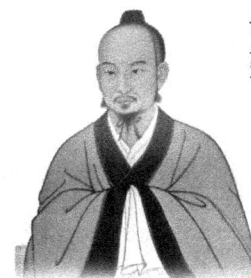

He was born in a family that was not wealthy, so he developed many diligent characteristics such as honesty, kindheartedness, passion and sincere enthusiasm. He was hard working and loved to learn new things. When he was a teenager, he worked in a small motel, kind of like a village inn. Because he was a smart and kindhearted boy and worked so diligently, everyone liked him very much. At the motel, he cleaned everyday to warmly welcome new guests, and he took good care of old customers. There was an old man who was a long-term guest living in the motel. His name is Chang Sangjun. He liked Bianque very much because of his good characteristics. Chang Sangjun knew this young man had so much good cultivated Virtue. Both the elderly man and Bianque were alike in that they were greatly respectful to others. Therefore they became very close friends and were able to exchange much on a personal level.

One day, Chang Shanjun secretly told Bianque, "I hold some secret herbs and herbal medicine books with me. They are my secret treasures in my life. Now I am old, maybe one day I have to leave this world. I look at you, such a decent, sincere, perfect, diligent young man, beyond your years really, so I have decided to pass all my secret treasures, these medicines and books, to you. Please keep them secret and make good use of them."

Bianque immediately knelt down and thanked Chang Sangjun as his teacher. Chang Sangjun gave him an herbal bag and explained to him: "You divide this medicine into 30 parts, and swallow one of them with dew each day, then just wait and see. Something will happen after 30 days." And at the same time Chang Sangjun passed to Bianque all the secret medicine books that he had held for many years in this life. Bianque carefully took the books, was so touched and could not help bursting into tears. When he opened his tearing eyes and wanted to kneel down to say thanks again, but Chang Sangjun had suddenly disappeared completely, and he never appeared to him again. Bianque followed Chang Sangjun's instruction; everyday he'd collect dew, and take the medication carefully. Nearly 30 days past, but nothing happened. Everything was as normal as usual.

As soon as he took the last medicine on the 30th day, unexpectedly and all of sudden, he could clearly see into the next room – right through the wall. He looked again more carefully and when he did, he could not only see through the wall, but he could see people in the room and more amazingly see "into" their bodies – organs and all – as if they were transparent. Bianque's heart was secretly glad, but he tried not to reveal his excitement. He knew his teacher Chang Sangjun was not an ordinary person. "He must be a divine being, what he gave him, was this super normal power to see through things," Bianque finally understood.

Since then Bianque very assiduously read the medicine books that his teacher Chang Sangjun left. Not long later, Bianque was able to diagnose and treat diseases for the people around him. With his skilled medical knowledge and extraordinary eyes, he eventually became an amazing doctor, and it was he who literally opened up the historical page of Chinese medicine.

Bianque traveled all over his country and other countries in ancient China to treat people who were suffering from many kinds of diseases. He treated people with his kind heart and great technique. His healing results were good and respected by all people. His patients included women and men, children and the elderly, poor people and wealthy people, ordinary people and even the emperor.

One day, The King of Wei Kingdom (Wei Wenwang) asked him a question: "I heard that you and your two brothers are all expert in medicine, so who is the best?" Bianque replied: "My oldest brother is the best doctor, and the second brother is the next, and I, myself, am the worst one." The King was very confused and did not understand why he said that because everyone knew Bianque was a good doctor the most famous. But they did not know that much about his other brothers. "Tell me what do you mean by that?" The King asked further.

Bianque explained: "My oldest brother has treated people before they became sick. When the person did not feel sick yet, he was able to eradicate all those root causes that may cause the person's diseases. Those people never got sick at all, therefore never knew they were cured by him. It's why my oldest brother has never been famous. Actually not that many people know him and appreciated him at all.

My second brother cured his patients at a very early stage. The patients just felt a little bit sick, had a few symptoms, and he gave them a little bit of herbal medicine, and they got healed. It's why those village people think my second brother can only cure minor ailments or simple diseases, but not big ones. They did not appreciate him much because his patients never really suffered from serious disease. Therefore he did not get famous either.

I myself always deal with those very serious conditions when the patient is in great pain, and their family worries so much. In such cases, people saw me taking actions such as needling their body, blood-letting, applying medicine on the affected area of the body, or sometimes even performing a major surgery. When patients' conditions improved or healed, they so appreciated me. In fact, they told people all around. It's why I got much more famous than my brothers. My first brother heals the root causes at highest level before people have a disease. My second brother cures the initial condition of the disease by treating the causes that started affecting the person. This is at the second highest level. While I only cure people when the disease has already fully come forth at surface level and become serious. I am at the lowest level." At these explanations, the King of Wei Wenwang smiled and understood.

The Yellow Emperor's Classic taught, "The medicine saint treats disease before it becomes disease, but does not wait until the disease has already become disease to treat." It was in the same period, the Spring and Autumn Period, over 2500 years ago.

Nearly 1000 years later, in the Tang dynasty, another famous Chinese doctor, Sun Sumiao, further classified the treatment into three levels as "The highest level of doctors treat the causes of disease before becoming disease, and the intermediate level of doctors heal the initial stage of disease, and the lowest level of doctors treat the disease itself."

The really good doctor and his practice should heal the causes of disease and not wait until people really get ill. This means to treat people, the person, the whole being, mind, body and soul, not just treat the disease itself.

People get very sick then receive medication, sometimes wind up in hospitals, and sometimes receive surgeries. This has been their M.O. for acquiring healthcare treatment, but they have suffered a lot in spite of the advancements of medical techniques.

Today, the drug-based direct treatments for diseases have become the mainstream medicine which is monetarily costly, but is also physically, mentally and spiritually costly as well – often resulting in a road of more pain, suffering, worries, fear and sometimes death.

We need to learn from those ancient ideas and practices and pursue the best, least invasive, low cost and preventive medicine. It is the goal of our mind-body-spirit medicine and healthology. Today's medicine seems to have forgotten about and actually reversed those initial three levels of healing practice. We would all benefit most by placing them back in their original hierarchy. That is: **The preventive medicine that heals the causes of illness within the whole being "before" they are able to cause health problems should be the main, highest-level practice. The practice that treats the condition as early as possible if the disease starts should again be placed as one's second choice. And treating the disease itself once it has manifested as serious at a hospital should be seen as one's worst and bottom-level option.**

§13.2 Heal the Causes Before Getting Sick

The mind-body medicine or healthology is the highest level and first choice healthcare practice as mentioned in the story above, and it eliminates the root causes of all kinds of diseases, including life-threatening diseases such as cancers, by treating and cultivating the whole being before the individual becomes sick. It practices positive thinking, peaceful mind, optimistic spirit, universal characteristics, and vibration energies as preventive healing and health.

We do not recommend the idea that people wait until sick and use invasive treatment. We try not to focus on disease because we believe the diseases can be prevented through daily healthy living and mind-body-spirit practice.

Helping people live a healthy meaningful, energetic, positive, beautiful and long life are our focus and ideal goal. We do not think the optimist's way is to live along a path that ignores preventive healthcare practice in his or her daily life, and as a result, just sit back and get sick, and then pursue curing one's sicknesses by using drugs and surgery-based medical procedures.

As optimists we believe that our mission is preventive healthcare, rather than defensive.

So far, however, we have not addressed that many specific diseases, and have discussed the preventive health practice and healing in general. In this chapter and the following chapter, though, we will discuss the prevention of some common modern diseases from the perspective of mind-body medicine and healthology.

We will use those worst diseases such as cancers as examples to discuss preventive practice in mind-body medicine and healthology. Although we talk about cancer, per se, the ideas, concepts, knowledge and practice can also be applied to the prevention and healing of other diseases that are usually related with lifestyle, stress, environment, and mental distractions in our modern times. These modern common diseases include: Cancers, Fibromyalgia (FMS), Multiple Sclerosis (MS), Tension Myositis Syndrome (TMS), major organ failures (heart, kidney, liver, lung, etc.), Cardiovascular Diseases, Chronic Respiratory Disease, Diabetes, Autoimmune Disease Symptoms, Depression, Anxiety Bipolar Disorder, Autism, Asthma, Back Pain, Eating Disorders, Stroke, Headache, Migraine, Stomachache, Common Cold, Flu, and other Epidemics, etc.

§13.3 Even Cancer Can Be Prevented

Many modern diseases are difficult to heal. As an example, cancer is one of the worst killers of life, but it is preventable. We discuss preventive health by using cancer as example, but in fact, prevention for other diseases follows a similar idea. First of all, instead of worry or fear about life-threatening diseases such as cancer, we should have courage to face it, identify and absorb good knowledge about it and put efforts toward preventing it.

Not only cancer, in fact any kind of disease, can be dealt with preventively. This practice is the idealist way, we know this, yet we highly encourage everyone to do it.

We absolutely do not suggest people wait until cancer is discovered and then rely on medical treatment. Every time when a cancer patient walks in our office for alternative care of their conditions such as mental fear and physical pain, we feel so sad and pained for the patients because they are really suffering physically and mentally. Once one has cancer, no matter how much medical technique has advanced, the treatment is always harmful to the patient's entire life system. After the cancer treatments such as chemotherapy and radiation therapy in the hospital, their life often becomes very difficult. Also, actually there is no 100% guaranteed cure for any kind of cancer. In most cases, cancer treatment is just to help the individual survive, manage the condition to a minimal level or extend a limited length of lifetime.

As holistic health practitioner, we want a much better, effective and comfortable solution for this difficult disease rather than the harmful and/or low success rate treatments of chemotherapy and radiation therapy. To find the best solution and prevent all of us from getting such terrible diseases as cancer, we need to know what causes such diseases and whether there is a way to prevent them?

Although modern medical science has no clear evidence to indicate what are the real causes of any kinds of cancer, the integration of the knowledge we gained from researchers and the practice and experience in the profound holistic mind-body-spirit medicine through its long history actually gives us great light for solution in terms of natural curing and prevention of these difficult diseases.

From the understanding of mind-body medicine and spiritual healing science and modern researches, we can address some important issues about why people get cancer and how to improve the condition (if it has already happened) or prevent it through daily mind-body-spirit health practice, healthy lifestyle, and natural healing approaches.

Some of the understandings addressed in this chapter are based on (1) the latest scientific researches, while some of them are based on (2) the principles and natural law that we have practiced, and as well as (3) the clinical experiences and facts that we obtained in the practice of mind-body-spirit medicine, or (4) the combinations of all these.

With this knowledge, experience, and approach within our preventive practice of mind-body-spirit medicine and healthology, even cancer can be prevented. Firmly believing in this will make a big difference, and only this belief makes all kinds of diseases including cancers preventable.

§13.4 Core Cause: Microenvironment Disorder of Mind-Body

The original life processes at all levels – e.g. physically, biologically, cellularly, molecularly, genetically, emotionally, mentally and spiritually – and is precisely designed and preprogrammed by the creator, the super divine power of the universe. These life processes are supposed to be in their preset order and balanced status in order to stay in the best healthy condition. Specifically speaking, for human beings, the energies of Yin-Yang and The Five Elements of the organs and all associated energy systems and mental/emotional states stay in their balanced mutual generating and mutual restricting relationships. At the same time, the mind, body and soul are harmonized and synchronized with the original spiritual natures of the universe. With such an ultimately balanced harmonious energy environment and spiritual energy environment, the living being remains at the best balanced state of life force, and all biological and genetic structures, functions, developments, metabolisms, behaviors and activities of living cells in the physical body are under the precise controls of genetic code, Deoxyribonucleic Acid (DNA) as the most important central unit of the cell, and at the same time the body, mind and spirit smoothly cooperate with and communicate to each other as one unified being crossing all dimensions.

DNA stores genetic instruction information that guides the cell as it produces proteins and makes an exact copy of the cell itself. This process must be very precisely conducted. Such complicated genetic process is very sensitive to any kinds of energy vibrations, and involves many microenvironmental factors within the cell and intracellular interactions, and cooperation between or within genetic and biochemical molecules, as known by many researches [65-66]. The microenvironment's natures does not only involve cellular and molecular factors such as biological, biochemical, and genetic factors, as well as foods, nutrition, blood pressure, blood circulation, hormones, immunity, and oxygen supply, but also involves emotional, mental, spiritual, family, relationship, social, cultural, educational, vibrational and energetic factors. All these factors are energy vibrations that are not only deeply involved with the cellular, molecular and particles' spaces, but also associated with and influenced by the entire body, mind and soul of the person, transmitting the vibrational energies into the microenvironment of the cellular spaces.

All life components are one. All parts of the body are one. Each part, each cell, each molecule (including DNA molecule) and each particle of the body is associated with others. The body is the physical container of emotional, mental and spiritual energy, and these components are associated with each other.

If we say a human being has emotion, mind and spirit, then we should also say that a living cell has emotion, mind, and spirit, and a molecule inside the cell has emotion, mind, and spirit too. DNA is one of the molecules inside the cell. So this means that DNA also has its emotional (mental) and spiritual state in its dimensional nature. Extensively speaking, even smaller or fundamental particles have their emotion, mind and spirit at their levels of dimensional environments. All these are a part of the entire living being. They are vibrated, resonated with, controlled and influenced by their own and others' minds, spirits, emotions. They are further determined, controlled and influenced by their growing histories, behaviors, vibrations, energies and environments at all dimensions and all levels – finally affecting the microenvironments of fundamental living units, the cells within which the DNA exists, and guiding, operating and involving not only the entire biological process as understood commonly by conventional science, but also emotional, mental and spiritual states and activities of cellular, molecular or even deeper levels of contents in the biological body.

In this way, we look at a DNA molecule as not just a chemical compound, but also an energy, emotion and spirit carrier inside the body. Such a genetic molecule is sensitive to environmental factors which are not just the factors of biochemical environment, but also factors of mental, emotional and spiritual environment. This no longer just sounds like a hypothesis without proven evidence, but in fact, it has been strongly suggested by many researches. It seems true that stress and emotional trauma can trigger cancer, very possibly through microenvironmental distractions.

The genetic research group of Prof. Tian Xu at Yale University, Medical School, published their research on *Nature*, and mentioned stress-cancer correlation and stress-sensitive JNK[15] cell interaction involved the process of cancer growth and invasion: "we show that clones of cells bearing different mutations can cooperate to promote tumor growth and invasion in Drosophila. We found that the Ras^{V12} and scrib mutations can also cause tumors when they affect different adjacent epithelial cells. We show that this interaction between Ras^{V12} and scrib clones involves JNK signaling propagation and JNK-induced upregulation of JAK/STAT[16]-activating cytokines, a compensatory growth mechanism for tissue homeostasis. The development of Ras^{V12} tumors can also be triggered by tissue damage, a stress condition that activates JNK signaling. Given the conservation of the pathways examined here, similar cooperative mechanisms could have a role in the development of human cancers." [67]. Many researches indicate that altered DNA methylation caused by microenvironment alternation is very likely one of the causes of

---

[15] **c-Jun N-terminal kinases** (JNK), kinase that binds and phosphorylates c-Jun on Ser-63 and Ser-73 within its transcriptional activation domain. It belongs to the mitogen-activated protein kinase family, and is responsive to stress stimuli, such as cytokines, ultraviolet irradiation, heat shock, and osmotic shock. They also play a role in T cell differentiation and the cellular apoptosis pathway.

[16] **JAK-STAT system:** a major signaling pathway to the second messenger system. It comsists of 3 components: (1) a receptor (2) Janus kinase (JAK) and (3) Signal Transducer and Activator of Transcription (STAT). This signaling pathway transmits information from chemical signals outside the cell through the cell membrane into gene promoters on the DNA in the cell nucleus, which causes DNA transcription and activity in the cell. Many JAK-STAT pathways are expressed in white blood cells, and are therefore involved in regulation of the immune system.

cancer development [68-70] (further discussion about these researches will be in the following sections).

Isn't it possible that the DNA methylation process is influenced by emotional stress? Isn't it possible that the DNA molecule has an emotional sensor that is sensitive to emotional struggling and can be affected or altered when the person has undergone emotional trauma?

From the perspective of mind-body-spirit science and practice, we think it is very possible. Think of this, we know human beings have emotion (and mind, soul/spirit as well), but does this emotion exist in any particular part of the body? No, obviously not because we know emotion belongs to the entire person, the entire being. So why don't we have a reason to say this emotion is pervading all over the body from outside to inside layer by layer, from organs to tissues, cells, and molecules, of course including the most important genetic unit, DNA?

But we do have such reason to say so. This is the real meaning of what we say when we say "Body and Mind are One." They – mind and body - are actually ONE THING overlapped, connected and in no way operate separately. Otherwise, it does not make sense to think: "There is a vividly living human being with emotion and feeling but his/her biological body is a rigid, hard, cold, emotion-less, metal-like body existing there separately or independently from the emotion (mind, soul and spirit)."

Now our question is: What makes modern people affected so deeply to the level of DNA so that finally a cancer develops?

Obviously and of course, not only emotional stress, but also other factors or their combinations can cause cancer or other modern diseases. We have to look at the issues such as lifestyle, living environment, mindset or thinking pattern, and social activities, in order to find out the complete answer. Today, it is not questionable that human beings are surrounded by many overwhelming disharmonies and distractions in the mind, body, spirit, and an entire environment and energy field that are harmful to our life systems. We have broken the balance of original life force, and finally poisoned the microenvironments of the cells and altered the key process of the DNA metabolism and genetic signaling, resulting in its alternation, mutation and function disorder. Not only cancer, in fact all diseases or discomforts can also be caused by sick vibrations such as disharmonies and imbalances of life force. But cancer is the most harmful impact that these disharmonies and imbalances cause. This impact ultimately affects the key part of the life system, the genetic code, but this is just the final result, as it must involve a series of processes in the body, mind, emotion and spirit intra-dimensionally and inter-dimensionally.

We believe that cancer involves all aspects of mind-body-spirit in modern lifestyle and environments. Cancer is the fatal disorder of the most crucial life process, the genetic signaling, that is caused by complicated microenvironment abnormalities involving multiple levels of mind, body and spirit. We will further explore this area in the following sections.

Regarding cancer development associated with the cellular and molecular microenvironments, many researchers have provided experimental evidences that support this hypothesis. The book titled *Genome and Tumor Microenvironment*, by Andrei Thoms-Tikhonenko, from the University of Pennsylvania Children's Hospital of Philadelphia included a lot of researches and analytical data in this area. These researches are very valuable and helpful for us in understanding the genetic process of cancer development.

It is very likely that cancer is caused by the body's microenvironmental toxins that can be induced by many factors in combination, including chronic inflammations, infection, chemical poison, daily stress, and emotional trauma. In short, cancer does not happen in one day. It is a long process that is going on within the body through all life components and processes which include body, mind, emotions, spirit, living environment, family, social and relationships, foods, drugs, overused and/or misused medications. This points to a path for prevention, meaning that we can prevent the occurrence of cancer development by carefully managing our daily life at physical, mental and spiritual levels, so that we will not allow such risky microenvironment factors to develop within our body.

§13.5 DNA Methylation Process & Microenvironment Toxins

One of the important genetic processes is DNA Methylation, the group methyl (CH_3) becoming attached to the specific section of the DNA molecule. This DNA Methylation is the key regulator of gene transcription. Evidence suggests that altered DNA methylation or DNA hypermethylation seems to be a *carcinogen* that leads to development and progression of human gastrointestinal malignancies. It was found that global hypermethylation (overall genome-wide reduction in DNA methylation) and regional hypermethylation in the CpG islands of specific gene promoters are associated with cancer development and progression. Question is: What makes the DNA methylation abnormal?

Although modern medical researches remain without absolute evidence on what causes cancer, the findings still provide us significant suggestions regarding what may be involved in the cancer development and progression, especially about the causes of altered DNA Methylation. In the following sections, we will address some possible cancer causes suggested by modern medical research, then we provide some solutions, discussions and suggestions from perspective of mind-body science in order to prevent the risks and stay away from this bad disease.

Researches indicate that aging itself may be the possible cause of developing altered DNA Methylation [68-70].

This finding is not surprising because it is a common understanding that aging is the phenomena that causes all functions of the body to become weak and senescent. As aging progresses, the cellular and molecular environments in the body become unstable, and immunity becomes weak, as a result probably the microenvironments of the DNA molecules become easy to be altered by the changes, challenges, stresses, disturbances, and damages biologically, genetically, energetically, emotionally and spiritually. This is the natural life phenomenon during the aging process. As well, some hidden potential factors in the microenvironment may not appear during younger age but can become active and potentially dangerous or harmful to your health as you get older.

Solution for Aging

Although aging is a natural process of life, from the history of human mind-body-spirit cultivation science, we know that a good mind-body-spirit cultivator can stay healthy and younger as a whole being throughout the entire life regardless of age. This is one of mind-body medicine's main considerations and goals.

The reason why mind-body-spirit practice can allow you to slow down the aging process and stay at younger age physically, mentally and spiritually is that the practice can repair, stabilize, rejuvenate, rebalance and strengthen the original life mechanism at all levels of the spirit, mind and body.

Your body is like a vehicle. If you just keep running all the time without maintenance and repair, if you do not provide good care to it, eventually it will have problems. Modern people are so busy all the time to take care of all material life issues, attached on so many things, but just do not give enough care to their own life; as long as this vehicle can run, they just keep running or even keep damaging it until more and more hidden damages and problems accumulated, and finally the entire system crashed.

We often see people who have worked so hard and earned a wealthy life materially. But they themselves are not really happy because not they have not to allotted enough care to their health and have lived an imbalanced lifestyle. This often gives rise to other detrimental issues that can then lead to further problems including: lack of communication with family members, relationship problems, lack of time to energize the soul, mind and body, joylessness, and sometimes even to severe sickness, and sadly, sometimes even to untimely death.

Life is both beautiful and fragile. If you just keep running it into the ground or letting it get prematurely old, then your life system and functions will automatically diminish, weaken and sicken. This is not questionable natural law. But you have the way to repair it, rejuvenate it, stop the aging process, and lock into a younger state. You have the way to make your whole being stay and feel youthful or perhaps even better.

How, then, is it possible to slow down or stop the aging process and prevent the risks of getting diseases due to aging?

In fact, the original life mechanism has a self-repair system to repair senescence and cleanse the contaminations, toxins or poisons, conflicts, noises, confusions, interferences, or negativities in the body and mind that affect the cellular, molecular and genetic microenvironments and cause diseases including cancer. This means the mind-body-spirit practice can constantly repair, refresh, renew, rebalance and rejuvenate the body, mind and spirit to remain in their original state from surface to the deep inside, including the microenvironments of cellular, molecular and genetic spaces such as DNA's existing dimensions, and as a result make your whole being stay healthy, young and beautiful.

Specifically speaking, with practice, your body and mind stay in the balanced state within Yin-Yang and The Five Elements – your energy channels within the body and mind remain at the opened state, so that the energy systems of your life can function healthily, smoothly and efficiently without the influence of aging. Through cultivation practice based on the universal law and energy principle, your mind, emotions and soul connect to the higher divine spirit and energy source, so your higher Self can play the leading role in your entire spirit-mind-body system from high to low levels, and guide your whole being – for the long-term – into a healthy living state, recognizing and filtering out the noise and distracting information from the contaminated environments and material world.

To achieve such an ideal goal, of course, you need to commit yourself to the practice, focus on your mind, and put daily effort toward cultivating your mind, body and spirit by seriously following the universal law and energy principle. Achieving a good health for your body, mind and spirit is a lifetime goal, daily task and fantastic and joyful journey, ever benefiting yourself, your family and society. It is worthy of your attention and the best thing you can do for yourself (and those around you) and will empower you throughout your entire life. The aging process progresses every day. If you do not practice daily health for your mind, body and spirit, then the effects of aging will be accumulated every day, and your risk and possibility of contracting sickness or disease, and succumbing to the progression of aging will rapidly increase. In reality, however, we often see everyday people relying on the drugs and surgery of modern medicine to maintain health instead of keeping a daily health practice, mind-body-spirit cultivation, meditation, Qigong, Taiji, music healing, and healthy diets, or other natural health practices.

Some people only see a doctor when they are sick or their doctor has diagnosed them with a disease. Sometimes people find safety in having health insurance, as if it is equal to having health, and they feel safe from getting sick. This, of course, is unreasonable because health insurance is only there to protect you when you have a severe disease and need medical treatment. Then the insurance will help you pay or partially pay for the medical treatment. But having insurance does not mean you will not get sick. When you are sick, no matter how good your insurance benefit is, you are still the one who has to suffer and struggle. Your best bet is not to get sick in the first place and to maintain your best health by implementing your own health practice daily. That is really insuring your health. That is the real insurance for your health. Some people very much rely on annual or periodic hospital checkups and think their health is fine if the hospital has not found any notable disease. This is also unreasonable because the hospital can find your health problem only when your disease has worsened enough to be detected. At the early stage or when hidden causes are in the growing state of disease, especially many types of cancers, the modern medicine cannot detect them.

The hospital only discovers the tumor when it is already a tumor, but cannot tell you the causes of the tumor before it appears as a tumor.

Preventive health and longevity practice are different. These make your body and mind healthy and strong, so that your own system can eliminate the causes or factors that may cause the disease. This is the ideal path toward healthy living. The key is to keep a strong message in your mind about daily health and longevity cultivation, and let go of human attachments and stressful lifestyle, and put effort into your cultivation practice every day. This is extremely important for everyone, especially today. Otherwise living a healthy and long life may be just a dream, but may never come true. **Do not let your desire-driven, busy day take your health and longevity away from you.**

If modern medical scientists tell you that aging is the risk factor for getting cancer or other diseases, we as mind-body preventive medicine practitioners want to tell you that keeping mind-body-spirit daily practice is the golden key for opening the longevity door, slowing down aging process, limiting and cleaning up the accumulating daily effects of aging and allowing you to stay young, and stay away from the risks of getting any disease, including cancer. It is doable, and it is absolute truth that the readers of this book should keep in mind and put effort toward, throughout your entire life and from now on as soon as you read this line at this moment.

Previous studies showed that stress, and psychological or emotional trauma, such as depression, anxiety, and so on can cause a long-term altered DNA Methylation, increasing cancer risk [68]. Researchers found that the oxytocin receptor gene methylation increased within the first ten minutes of the stressful testing condition, suggesting that the cells formed less oxytocin receptors compared to the relaxed situation. One and half hours after the test, the gene methylation dropped below the original level before the test, indicating that the gene receptor production was overwhelmingly stimulated, and its genetic activity became abnormal.

The oxytocin receptor gene (docking site for the neurotransmitter oxytocin) is known as the trust hormone or anti-stress hormone. This experiment suggests that under a stressful condition, the gene significantly altered, and its anti-stress functional expression could become permanently abnormal or dysfunctional. This means stress can cause loss of normal stress despondency. The stress in any form can transmit its violent vibrations into all levels including the molecular time-space dimension of DNA microenvironments, altering the DNA metabolism and genetic process such as DNA methylation. More extensive researches suggest that stress increases the risk of physical or mental illness. These findings strongly indicate that epigenetic processes are involved in the development of various chronic diseases such as cancer or depression. "Epigenetic changes may well be an important link between stress and chronic diseases" says Prof. Meinlschmidt, Head of the Research Department of Psychobiology, Psychosomatics and Psychotherapy at the LWL University Hospital, Bochum, Germany.

It is not hard to understand that stress and emotional trauma overwhelmingly challenge the mind, transmit disturbing vibration and messages into the body, and affect the nervous system, hormone system, immune system, cardiovascular system, digestion system, liver, kidney and other organs, and finally affect the microenvironment of DNA genetic molecules, enhance its abnormal methylation, and as a result possibly develop cancer. Over many years, increasing research data supports the viewpoint that stress is the most likely cause of cancer, especially mental stress or trauma, which depresses the entire being; the mind and spirit first, and then certainly, the body.

We have so many real examples in the clinic over the years, telling their sad stories of getting cancer because of emotional trauma. Years ago, Jane was our patient because of some chronic problems she experienced often, such as stomachaches and back pain. We successfully healed these problems with energy healing and mind-body medicine. She rejuvenated and could happily go back to her work and life as a middle aged, beautiful and energetic business lady.

We taught her preventive health practice such as meditation, introduced the advanced spiritual practice, and encouraged her to keep daily practice, however, after she finished her treatment she completely went back her busy lifestyle and did not seriously continue her health practices, as she herself told us. Some years later, she came to our clinic again with a totally different image, that of a very sick cancer patient, at late stage. She told us that she had encountered a business lawsuit with another business. Although she won the case finally, the very stressful and energy consuming experience over two years made her very sick, and she developed thyroid cancer. We could help her release pain and build up her strength to make chemotherapy and radiation treatment easier, but we are so sorry it was too late to save her life, although we had seen encouraging results from other cases when this disease is still at an early stage. It is difficult to heal any disease when it is at a very late stage, especially for a disease like cancer.

As a negative lesson, the case mentioned above can remind us to keep practicing cultivation in daily life, not attach on the material life issues, let go of human ego and personal interests, and take them easy, so we will not be stressed mentally and physically. As a result, Karma can be eliminated, trouble can be avoided, and health can be maintained.

Solution For General Stress

No question, stress reduction is absolutely important for modern people who want to live healthy and stay away from bad diseases such as cancer, depression, and heart failures, etc. Establishing a stress-free daily lifestyle and working condition is an ideal solution. As mind-body medicine doctors, we highly recommend everyone seriously learn a daily self-healing regimen for the whole being – the body, mind and spirit, and actually put forth efforts every day toward this practice. Like you eat breakfast, lunch and dinner every day for nutritional food, you also need energy cultivating practices such as meditation, energy music healing, Qigong, cultivation, exercise, and relaxation to charge energy for your mind, body, wisdom, inspiration, and efficiency. It is the only way to have a preventive stress-free health and live with a younger mind, body, spirit, and stay beautiful looking.

You must schedule the time to do it without any interference. You have to keep it as the first priority task in your mind and in your daily calendar. No excuses, no skipping on any day, for any reason. This way you will develop the good habits of daily energy healing and health practice, and as a result, the benefits will be the most blessed thing belonging to you.

Sometimes stress can also come from your job, career, business, financial pressure and daily life activities. Some jobs are very stressful and energy consuming due to the job's features such as tight schedules, long days, hard work, the demands of highly professional skills, multitasking, a fast pace working environment, and all this can be very energy consuming and stressful.

Modern life is very busy and stressful, thus increasing everyone's risk of sickness. You should be smart enough to not wait for a disease to develop and require healing, but instead prevent this from happening to yourself. Stress can be released, reduced and avoided, or you can do even better and have a stress-free life if you want. The solution is to practice cultivation of your mind, body and spirit and transform your energy, mind and body to a higher level.

As we have discussed in the previous chapters, an overloaded stressful life happens because (1) so many attachments on the material life drive people to become too busy and into working hard, but without (2) clear self-awareness of spiritual goals within this life (loss of Self), (3) without the understanding that cultivation of mind-body-spirit is the first priority task in this life, (4) without putting actual daily effort to practice cultivation, and (5) and without having a cultivator lifestyle and therefore running into a negative cycle of

Attachments → Loss of Self → Unawareness of Cultivation →
No Actual Effort Toward Cultivation → Low Energy →
Low Efficiency → More Meaningless Tasks →
More Busyness → More Loss of Self → More Attachments

Solution For Emotional Stress and Trauma

Emotional stress and trauma such as depression and anxiety come from many sources especially from relationships and family issues. This is a big problem today because people are living in a superficial material world and the minds of couples (or perhaps one of them) are outward-focused, but not inwardly cultivated. Conflicts arising between partners are not easily harmonized in a peaceful, loving, compassionate, patient and forgiving mood.

Sometimes arguments get worse, especially when couples start pointing a finger at each other instead of looking at one's own Self inwardly. Jobs, careers, or financial pressures – all these together – can make things even worse, causing communication and relationship problems as well as emotional problems, consuming mental energy and affecting health. In this section, therefore we discuss interpersonal relationships (especially that of a loving couple) from perspective of mind-body medicine.

The way to stay in harmony and resolve – or better yet avoid – relationship problems is for each partner to cultivate his/her own Self and improve their "own" mind nature, character, compassion, forgiveness, patience, and vibration energy. In this regard, serious spiritual cultivation and meditation practice will facilitate progress in spiritual growth and energy strengthening. These two elements combined are the best and most practical way to harmonize the situation, rather than arguing and blaming each other for problems.

Once the energy field is harmonized, the conversation, relationship, and understanding will improve. For the couple with similar characteristics and spirituality, the interpersonal situation may be better, but even they will still experience and have to deal with similar problems as described above if both do not cultivate well and evolve themselves to a higher-level energy and spirituality.

Of course the worst circumstance that causes major emotional stress in relationships is totally opposite characteristics that harbor within a couple. We often have one of them come to us (in most cases the wife) for emotional stress relief and energy improvement.

Consider one (of the couple) a spiritual person with many positive characteristics such as broad heart, bright personality, communicative, open mindedness, positive energy, high activity, optimistic, spiritual, compassionate, passionate, caring both for others and society, warm, loving, sharing, giving, forgiving, artistic, multi-talented, open to change and new things, flexible, having broad interests, and entertaining.

The other individual in the couple, however, is a materialistic person who has a narrowed mind, low energy, is uncommunicative, negative, passive, selfish, careless, cold, rigid in thought and logic, analytical and calculating, skeptical, stubborn, and refuses to change.

We often see such couples just like what we have described above. Of course, for the purpose of illustration, we have made these individuals extreme examples. In reality, however, one person may not have all of the positive or negative characteristics as described above.

Obviously the individuals in this couple have very different vibrations. One has the personality and characteristics we would associate more closely to the natures of the universe and has higher energy E_H with higher frequency f_H, while the other one is far away from the natures of the universe and has much lower energy E_L with lower frequency f_L.

The different frequencies of their energy vibrations cannot resonate with each other, but can certainly cause many big conflicts and troubles, and consume a lot of energy. The consumed energy ΔE_C is depending upon the difference of their frequencies.

$$\Delta E_C \propto (f_H - f_L)^n$$

Where $n \geq 1$ is the power of the difference $(f_H - f_L)$ that is determined upon how worse the situation between the couple. It can be further expressed as

$$\Delta E_C = C (f_H - f_L)^n$$

Where **C** is a constant, expressing each couple's situation. If they have absolute tolerance, understanding and caring toward each other or one completely forgives the other one, or through long years of efforts and caring for each other, build up a good loving relationship, then C = 0 or C → 0, meaning the consumed energy between them is nearly zero even though their frequencies are very different. Otherwise if they work out the problem by changing themselves to get closer in character, thought, value system, interest, and lifestyle, then their frequency difference (f_H - f_L) will become smaller or nearly zero, thus the consumed energy ΔE_C will become smaller or nearly zero.

If two of them do nothing to improve themselves and the situation remains unchanged, they will consume a lot of energy in their life. Usually the first person (who has higher energy frequency) gets very stressful, has so much energy driven down by the other person (who has lower energy frequency), the energy level drops down more and more, and finally the individual gets very exhausted, depressed, angry, frustrated, and even finally gets very sick.

$$E_H \rightarrow E_L$$

It's why we often see such a couple has a lot of pain and struggles over years. Eventually one or both got sick. This kind of emotional stress must be resolved to prevent further harmful impact to the mental and physical health including some serious diseases.

The solution for this kind of case is to work on the person (the one with positive characteristics) first, helping her (or him) to improve overall energy, clarity of mind, release anger, anxiety and frustration, and broaden the scope of view, and understanding the natures of both partners as we taught in this book, so she/he can see the entire situation as a third party, but not as one inside the relationship.

This takes a lot of work to transform the person out of the dark hole of their emotional trauma, and let her/him feel good energy, get into a good mood, have more compassion and broader mind to view things and objectively understand what original natures human beings are supposed to have. They also need to grasp their (and their partner's) good and bad characteristics and why things turned out as they have. After all this and with clear understanding, he/she will see the solution and hope from outside of their own world, from the broader spaces – of higher mind and spirit.

The key is that you detach with the low energy field and low energy person in the mental and spiritual dimensions. Originally human beings get engaged in a relationship with the intention of becoming happy, but because of low spirit, low energy, ignorance, lack of knowing the truth, and shortness of wisdom and sharing of wisdom, and less good Virtue and luck, less higher quality of being, and less shining attractive spirit, mind and body, the accumulated result is not happiness, but the opposite: troubles, problems and pain. This is not someone's intentional fault, but it is because we human beings really need to learn this lesson, wake up and know the truth, then cultivate and elevate the level of our own life as whole being of mind-body-spirit, and improve the quality of our own Self as a living spirit.

Insofar as our hypothetical couple is concerned, the one with relatively higher energy and better character, need no longer attach on the other person emotionally with human sentiment, but can have compassion (much higher than human love) in mind and objectively look at and treat the other person with compassion and understanding. At this level, there is no more anger, complaining and depression because of the other person. This is because the individual has started his/her own improvement cultivation and as his/her energy is getting better and better opportunities for positive changes manifest.

The mind-body medicine with energy healing practice is very powerful and effective for this kind of case because we work on the body, mind, emotion and soul by changing the energy at all levels and at the same time. In fact, this is our process of teaching and enlightening the first person in the couple and helping her/him to return to her/his true Self.

Coming to this point, the person often realizes that this was a lesson they somehow missed at a very early age. Once their energy changes to a higher and more positive level, the person's mind, worldview and emotional mood are also changed. As a result, the treatment helps rejuvenate the person in many aspects, including overall energy, self-recognition, understanding of another person; less confusion, anger, emotional blocks, grievance, complaining, as well as fewer feelings of being treated unfairly. So she/he can see the solution and have hope for the future, with positive goals and opportunities. After the first person is improved, we will try to help the other person if he/she is willing to get help and wants to change.

If it is possible, eventually we get the couple together in the same session and have them receive energy healing, meditate to communicate silently at a spiritual level, and connect their souls and emotions. We teach both of them meditation and ask them to practice it at home as well, meditating deeply together every day towards the same higher goal of cultivation in this life, so all conflicts at the human level will be gone. This is very beneficial for the couple. As a result both of them become happy, open minded, bright, energetic, communicative, more understanding, healthy, youthful, and attractive to each other. We have had many such couples as successful healing cases in our clinic.

If the couple has different characteristics and spiritual energy like the couple we just described above, of course, they absolutely need this practice to work out their issues. However, even if the couple has the same spiritual belief and similar personal characteristics, they still need to practice meditation cultivation together. Otherwise, eventually they will get tired, bored, stressed and conflicting at the human level because the human-human connection is at lower energy level, and sometimes is very self-centered, ego and desire-driven, and therefore very energy consuming.

Different from the human-human connection, however, spiritual cultivation helps the two connect to the same higher spirit and merge into one spiritual source, have the same good energy vibration, spiritual and mental characteristics, same ultimate goal in this life, same lifestyle, daily living schedule, shared compatible interests, ideas, mentality and feelings. Therefore as a result, they resonate with each other and love, care about, share with, communicate with, understand, help, cooperate with, tolerate, accept, forgive, and get along with and feel close to each other.

This is the secret to why many couples have problems and how to resolve them from the root. In fact, the vibration energy is the medium, like the air we breathe, that exists between people and determines how they feel and how they relate. The energy is like water flowing from a higher place E_H to a lower place E_L. Here the "high energy" we mention is based on the nature of the universe as we taught in the early chapters. It, of course, does not refer to a person who has a hyperactive character as people at nowadays may use the term.

If there is no sharing of good and higher energy coming from both sides of the couple, then the higher energy person does not feel good when being with the lower energy person because his/her flowing energy feels like it is being hijacked and then dropped to a lower level.

$$E_H \rightarrow E_L$$

The lower energy person, in contrast, can feel good because being around the higher energy benefits the lower energy person, but he/she may feel some emotional pressure as a result or loses self-confidence around the higher energy person. You probably often see such a couple: one loves the other one, but the "other one" does not care or may even want to run away from the relationship. Sometimes even though the first person tries so hard to please the second person, the second person still cannot be happy. Why is that?

In most cases, it is because the second person has higher and good quality energy, but the first person does not. Therefore the first person looks up to the second person and looks forward to staying with the second person. This is a natural phenomenon: lower energy being wants, yearns, envies, and longs the higher energy being. Attractive force (F_A) of a person is totally depending upon the person's energy nature and quality according to the criterion of the universal law and energy principle.

$$F_A \propto E$$

$$E_H \rightarrow F_{A.H}$$

$$E_L \rightarrow F_{A.L}$$

A person with higher energy (E_H) has higher attractive force ($F_{A.H}$), while a person with lower energy (E_L) has lower attractive force ($F_{A.L}$). This energetic attraction force includes the factors on the surface dimension such as appearance, physical conditions, fitness, health, beauty, expressions, language, voice, and dress, and all possible forms of visible energy vibrations, and also includes the factors in the invisible dimensions such as mental and spiritual energies or vibrations, personality, value system, characteristics, talents, spirit, caring heart, compassion, passion, spirituality, interests, talents, creativities, and all other vibrations or energies in this life and past lives (fate connection in past lives is also an energy form that can be carried on to this life), all possible forms of invisible energy vibrations.

The key for a couple to improve such a relationship and enjoy a healthy and happy life companion is not about how much human desire-driven activities you can amass, but it is really about how each of you cultivates your own Self, elevates your own energy to a higher level at all aspects and dimensions, and improves the quality of your own body, mind and spirit. This increases your ability to give your lover and yourself a good energy environment, inspiring frequencies, deep and bright moods, and true happiness. Only when both of you cultivate together and connect to the higher spirit in such an energy generating state, will your relationship be stress-free, energetic, meaningful, joyful and healthy mentally, physically and spiritually.

Consider this:

Because of some superficial attractions, desires, family and social factors, without clear reason really, two individuals land into in a relationship. At the beginning of this relationship, things may go well, because 1) The basic attraction between man and woman is so powerful and no matter what, that much is part of the relationship, 2) Both individuals naturally show the best parts of themselves, 3) Relatively higher Self, imagination, and spiritual mind get involved.

After a while, however, if both keep behaving only at the level of this physical realm, the energy drops low, boredom settles into superficial daily routines, and the couple's problems become superficial. Lower energy results in lower attractive force. Therefore both are no longer as attractive to each other as when they started the relationship.

If each person has no inner connection with his/her own Self, if each has no time to energize his/her own Self, if there is no mutual connection and understanding at a deeper spiritual level between the two, and if each is not sometimes in his/her own space for self-healing and energizing as well as in a shared mutual space, at times, for healing, cleansing, inspiring, energizing, and cultivating, then the two beings will have no way of having an exciting, interesting, happy, and loving relationship. Again cultivation of Self is the key.

Sometimes when two people stay apart and each one has some time alone with mutual agreement to do so, you probably feel better. And when you come back together, both of you become more attractive to each other. It is because both individuals are charged with higher Self energy. Then after being together for a while again, the two interact at human level and consume a lot of energy, so that the energy runs low yet again. Therefore, temporarily being apart and back again is a temporary solution, but not really an absolute solution. Sometimes going on a trip and getting some contact with nature or getting out of your own world – e.g. both individuals go to a dance club or on vacation away from home – seems these things can get a relationship better for a while. It is because both individuals pay attention to something outside of their relationship for a while, so they temporarily detach from the band of the two, and release some of the tension that has built up between them. But when they return from the outing or the trip, the same old, problematic issues return. Therefore, this activity is also only a temporary solution. So the question is: What is really the best solution?

The best solution is that two people practice spiritual energy cultivation – sometimes on their own, and sometimes together. Sometimes you may read and cultivate by yourself. Other times, you may read, meditate, practice energy movement, and share cultivation (and other) activities together to inspire each other. Note: Whether you are together or on your own private time, the cultivation practice cannot be just superficial, but must actually be done with effort and personal responsibility as well as your own joyful interest as an important part of your life. Only in this way will the energy be improved, and will you have good energy to share.

The energy I am speaking about is (as we have cited throughout this text) beyond this physical world and not visible, but it actually contains real substantial vibrations extends its influence into the entire space you are living in and beyond. These vibrations are available to any of you consciously and unconsciously at every moment. Everyone has his/her vibration energy behind his/her physical being and that has an impact to your surroundings – good energy gives people good feelings and positive influence, while bad energy gives people bad feelings and negative influence. A good spiritual cultivator brings good energy to surrounding environments, which is attractive to people and benefits others.

If two individuals carry higher, good and similar level of energy, then you will both feel great and the energy will be multiplied and rise to an even higher level.

If both of you have low energy, then many more problems will irritate the two of you. If one has higher, good, positive energy, and the other one has lower, bad, negative energy, then each of you will have problems, but in the different ways, as described above.

Now that you know this secret, I highly suggest that partners in intimate relationship understand each other and make an arrangement and commitment to peaceful meditation and spiritual energy cultivation practice in your daily life. You will develop a deeper, more meaningful and more joyful relationship, with less emotional stress and you will gather the benefits of good health and spiritual growth. This energy mechanism of which we speak can also be applied to the relationships within or between families, friends, groups, and communities.

3. Folate, Dietary Fat, DNA Methylation & Cancer Risk

Beyond stress, some researchers suggest that epidemiological factors like unhealthy dietary patterns such as folate deficiency or excessive folate intake, dietary fat, fried foods, over eating and high pH foods dietary habits may increase cancer risk.

Researches show that folate intake might strongly influence DNA methylation patterns. The findings indicate that polymorphisms of genes involved in folate metabolism are causally related to the development of cancer [71]. The currently available data from animal, human, and *in vitro* studies suggests that colorectal cancer may be involved in folate deficiency and higher dietary intake or blood levels of folate seems to reduce the risk of ulcerative colitis-associated colorectal cancer or its precursor, adenoma [72-77].

But not all types of cancers are necessarily involved in folate deficiency or maybe the opposite. According to the report published in March 10, 2009 in the Journal of the National Cancer Institute, a 10-year study found that men who took folic acid supplements faced more than twice the risk of prostate cancer as those who didn't take the supplements [78]. The incidence of prostate cancer in the study, however, was slightly lower in men who simply got adequate amounts of folate in their diet. It seems that effects of either excessive folate or folate deficiency on DNA methylation are highly complex, depending on cell type, target organ, and stage of transformation, and yet are gene and site specific.

So what do these researches tell us? What should we do to prevent cancer in terms of folate diet? In fact, we are all confused and don't know what to do. Should we take more or less folate in diet or supplement? It seems either more or less can cause problems, so theoretically we may want to say it is good to take right amount of folate nutrient. But the question is: What is the right amount of supplement to take in, and how much folate enriched foods to eat in your diet? This will be an extremely difficult question to answer for anyone, at least at this stage with the limited knowledge or complex yet confusing data obtained from modern medicine research.

Solution For Folate Intake And Dietary Fat

In mind-body medicine, however, we could have a better solution regarding how much nutritional folate supplement or dietary foods to take. Remember, artificially supplying the right amount of any kind of nutrient is difficult because we do not know how much the body needs. Additionally we don't know how much it can absorb and how the absorbed nutrient is metabolized in the body, organs, tissues, and blood. Nor do we know how such nutrients work in different areas of body or how they work for each different type or condition, age, sex, nationality, and whether other living conditions or working scenarios play into the picture.

Folate isn't the only problem. Other nutrients have the same problems when we try to exactly quantify them for the need of our body. Modern medicine tries to quantify the right amount of nutrients in attempting to achieve nutritional health, but it is very hard to do. Therefore many attempts often fail or only come up with a partial answer – and not the perfect solutions, for each individual.

We are not against what nutrition professionals practice in helping people have a balanced nutritional health, especially in terms of holistic nutrition knowledge, concepts, ideas and practice. These are still very helpful for us to manage daily dietary health.

We also encourage our patients to balance dietary nutritional foods from the understanding of energy medicine as we are going to cover in a different chapter. In regard to quantitative nutrition practice, however, the problem is that we cannot really exactly calculate and weigh all kinds of foods or nutrients everyday upon the needs of each individual with various changeable personal data. The complexity, uncertainty, variability, inconvenience and individual specificity make the quantification of nutritional practice impractical, stressful, difficult and sometimes incorrect and unsuccessful.

We know that the human body is an amazing life system that has its own power to live in its most healthy condition if we follow the natural law to strengthen the life mechanism and keep it functioning well. What to eat, how much to eat, how much to absorb, how it metabolizes, and where to go to meet the need of each part of the body and each organ of the body, and so on, all these are automatically and dynamically adjusted by the life mechanism, as long as the precondition is met: the whole system of the mind-body-spirit is healthy and functioning correctly.

Therefore the key is to keep the life mechanism functioning well and strong all the time. This goal can be achieved by mind-body medicine, energy medicine and mind-body-spirit cultivation practice. In these practices, we use different concepts to work with the body and mind. For example, we use energy principles to balance energy and circulate energy and blood, produce hormones and deliver them to the right regions of the body, so that our body will stay in the healthy condition. As a result, you will naturally and automatically eat well, sleep well, cleanse toxins efficiently, and have immunity strong enough to prevent diseases.

If the mind is healthy and has good energy, then it does everything and knows everything correctly, including having a healthy diet lifestyle. When the mind, however, is lost, confused, stressed, depressed, anxious, angry, frustrated, blocked, or in any negative mood emotionally, you will see people often eat without intention, eat and drink unconsciously no matter what or how much, without care about health, or they will eat and drink completely upon desire and emotion. Sometimes they may overeat, but other times forget to eat and drink, or never eat on time. Some people keep busy all the time, all day, and never even feel thirsty and want to drink water. Some people keep attaching on certain foods and keep eating the same food all the time, causing imbalances in nutrition. At times, people can eat and/or drink at expensive restaurants for hours making body overloaded, but then the same individual will eat unhealthy fast foods – that will both imbalance the body and eventually cause health problems. Many people nowadays are busy and eat at outside restaurants and fast foods places all the time, but hardly have time to cook at home and eat family dinner together, eating imbalanced additive-stuffed foods outside while missing out on an opportunity to establish a good tradition for family communication.

In contrast, as a mind-body health cultivator, you will pay attention to your diets, and eat natural foods with balanced varieties, different fresh vegetables and a reasonable amount of proteins.

However, you do not need to be too nervous about how many nutrients to take in every meal or try too hard to quantify it. This is because your mind and body as a mind-body-spirit cultivator always stay clear, peaceful, calm, tranquil, with no attachment and no addiction. Your body stays in a balanced and energetic state, so you will naturally have a healthy lifestyle and dietary custom, stay in the best state at all levels, biologically, nutritionally, energetically and emotionally.

As a good health practitioner and cultivator, your mind and body know what you need and how much you need to eat. You will not attach on certain foods such as heavy oily foods, too much meat, or overeat in every meal. Your mind and body will talk to each other and know what and how much to eat and absorb upon your needs.

A cultivated body also has a wide range of flexibility, resiliency, adaptability, and strong tolerance to some changes in foods, living environments and stress. As you reach such a state of Being One with the Universe, you are assimilated and synchronized with the natural law, so the system of your body and mind will function smoothly and healthily as the original mechanism is meant to work. Refer to separate chapter about dietary foods for preventive healthcare and combine these with mind-body meditation practice and exercise, to help you achieve the best health of body and mind.

4. Chronic Inflammation and Cancer Risk

Cancer development is the process of genetic lesion accumulation in cells. Researches suggest that chronic inflammation may lead to the altered microenvironmental factors such as DNA methylation and cause cancer development. Some researches and clinical observations indicate that many chronic inflammations could result in cancer sequelas or promote cancer development. Some common relationships between inflammation and cancer types are, for example, bronchitis and lung cancer, reflux esophagitis and esophageal cancer, intestinal inflammation and colorectal cancer, chronic pancreatitis and pancreatic cancer, cystitis and bladder cancer, UV-caused skin inflammation and melanoma (skin cancer), and so on. In addition, many cancers seem to be associated with chronic infection, such as, carcinoma and hepatitis B or C (virus), cholangiocarcinoma and cholangitis (liver fluke), gallbladder cancer and cholecystitis or cholelithiasis (bacteria), gastric cancer and gastritis or stomach ulcers (helicobacter pylori), skin cancer and chronic osteomyelitis (bacterial), cervical cancer and chronic vervicitis (HPV, papilloma virus), and so on.

It seems many types of cancer occur in the same site where infection, chronic irritation and inflammation occurred. These sites are highly associated with viruses, bacteria, or other causes of inflammation or infection. Some metabolic diseases such as obesity, non-alcoholic fatty liver and other newly discovered liver cancer risk factors, may also lead to cancer.

Recent studies indicate that if the inflammation or infection continues without being controlled or becomes a chronic problem, the immune response will become deleterious, and the inflammatory microenvironment becomes carcinogenic. Inflammation can cause the expression of genotoxins such as reactive oxygen species (ROS), reactive nitrogen species (RNS), and lipid hydroperoxides. These genotoxins are known to bombard and damage the cell's membranes, proteins, and DNA functions including gene repair mechanisms such as non-homologous end joining (NHEJ), homologous recombination (HR), base excision repair (BER), and (mismatch repair) MMR collaborate. These gene repair mechanisms are important genetic processes to maintain the fidelity of the original DNA sequence. When these mechanisms, however, are damaged or altered, it can cause gene misrepair, create DNA mutations and promote genome instability and inability, and, as a result, develop cancer.

Solution For Chronic Infection and Inflammation

Antibiotics: Urgent Use Only – Not Best Choice

For some acute or severe infections and inflammations, modern medicine can give quick relief by prescription medications such as antibiotics. There are different types of antibiotics widely used in modern medicine for both inpatients and outpatients with a doctor's prescription. Depending on the types of antibiotics, some of them, such as penicillin, kill bacteria by either interfering with the formation of the bacterium's cell wall or its cell contents, while some of them like bacteriostatics (bacteriostatic antibiotics) stop the bacteria from multiplying. Either type of these antibiotics can effectively stop the infections or inflammations, but sometimes they do have bad side effects that can be harmful to your body for either a short or long term, depending upon the dose and term of its usage or upon individual patient's condition.

These side effects of antibiotics include: stomach upset, diarrhea and severe watery diarrhea, abdominal cramps, vomiting, vaginal itching or discharges, growth of white patches on the tongue, allergic reactions such as hives, swelling of tongue, lips or face. The popular antibiotics oral fluoroquinolones, Cipro (ciprofloxacin), Levaquin (levofloxafin) and Avelox (moxifloxacin), increase your risk of developing a retinal detachment by five times compared with nonusers [79]. FDA placed a warning label on fluoroquinolones because these antibiotics are toxic to tendon fibers and may decrease blood supply in tendons, and cause tendon ruptures [79]. The estimated data show that over 142,000 emergency patients visit hospitals each year because of antibiotic-associated side effects and most of them are allergic reactions related [80]. The leading author of this study, Daniel Budnitz, M.D., at the Centers for Disease Control and Prevention (CDC) wrote: "This number is an important reminder for physicians and patients that antibiotics can have serious side effects and should only be taken when necessary." In fact some patients can lose life due to the antibiotics side effects. Especially antibiotic-associated diarrhea (AAD) can lead to pseudomembranous colitis, clostridium difficile colitis, which is a severe colon infection [81]. This colon infection is often seen in those patients who took the antibiotics during hospitalization.

Sometimes a problem with the antibiotic doesn't occur for 2-10 weeks after released from hospital. One of my dear patients and friends lost her life because of the clostridium difficile colitis caused by antibiotics. The hospital did not give the patient any instruction or warning on this risk after she was treated with antibiotics for 2 weeks and then released. Four weeks later after her release from the hospital, she got severe acute diarrhea. Regular antibiotics cannot cure this colon infection because it originally caused the infection. Vancomycin is the correct and most effective antibiotic used to treat this kind of colon infection, but sometimes if a hospital is delayed or as a result of faulty misdiagnosis or procedure, waiting test result or misused antibiotic, they can miss the best time to save the life. There are many concerns and problems with the side effects of antibiotics, including those life-threatening side effects.

Question is, do we always need antibiotics to deal with infection and inflammation? Should we rely on those prescription medications to relieve infection and inflammation? Answer is no, not always, at least sometimes it is not the first and best choice – only when it is an acute and severe case that our body's immune system alone cannot fight off. In fact, when our body is infected by bacteria or before the bacteria multiply and cause symptoms, our body's immune system will automatically send out a special type of white blood cells to attack the harmful bacteria and destroy them. In most cases if our body is healthy and strong enough, even if the symptoms occur, our immune system can still fight off the infection. Occasionally, however, when it is too much and our body cannot fight it off, then we need some help with antibiotics.

Often we see that many people visit their doctor whenever they get some health issue. Even when getting a little common cold, they immediately see their family doctor and get antibiotics to take. Frequent use of antibiotics for quick relief of common health problems can accumulate the antibiotics side effects and cause problems later. In fact, when you have a common cold, as an example, you may simply take off from work, have a complete rest and relaxation, practice meditation, music healing, natural diet, drink hot ginger soup and get a deep sleep, let your body deal with the infection and get healed naturally. Actually this is the way to exercise your body and make its immune system stronger, and as a result, your body will become even healthier. As long as you are not going to an extreme to challenge the immune system to the extent of its limitations, this natural way is the best healing choice.

There is an important concern worldwide that antibiotics are being overused. Antibiotic overuse is one of the major contributing factors to the growing number of bacterial infections that become resistant to antibacterial medications. In addition to many side effects as we discussed above, the antibiotic resistance continues to be a serious public health threat worldwide.

Not all infections (and associated inflammations) are caused by bacteria, actually many types of infections are caused by virus. Most upper respiratory tract infections including common cold and sore throat are generally caused by viruses – antibiotics do not work against these viruses. A virus is a piece of DNA or RNA, and it can enter into a living cell, host cell, attach itself to the cell, and make the host cell reproduce more viral DNA. Antibiotics can do nothing about such virus. Each type of virus has a different nature, and they sometimes affect different parts of the body. Therefore, the modern medicine has developed different types of medication called antivirals to deal with specific viral infections as well as associated inflammation. In fact these medications have limitations in their effectiveness and also have side effects. The ideal way is to preventively avoid virus infection.

Viruses are usually transmitted in a numerous ways: 1) through contact with an infected person, 2) foods and drinks through swallowing, or sharing foods, drinks, cup, bowl, or other dining table tools that are virus contaminated, 3) air through breath, inhalation, 4) through body fluid such as kiss, unsafe sex, 5) through touching virus-contaminated objects, tools, etc., 6) poor hygiene, eating and drinking habits. Depending age, body condition, infected part of the body, viral infections can have various symptoms in common such as fever, coughing, running nose, headache, muscle aches, chills, diarrhea, vomiting or nausea, rash, weakness, and fatigue. In severe cases the following symptoms may be seen: dehydration, limb paralysis, seizures, back pain, neck stiffness, personality changes, confusion, loss of sensation, impaired bladder and bowel functions, progressive sleepiness that can lead to a coma or death.

Natural Healing For Inflammation and Infection

The natural protection of our body from virus infection is the innate or natural immunity. Many virus-caused diseases can be improved or healed naturally by our body's immune system if it is healthy and strong. Daily meditation, energy healing, natural health practice and spiritual cultivation for the body and mind are the most important and effective solution for viral infection and inflammation. Natural diets and herbs are also the ways to help heal chronic inflammation. Unlike drugs, these natural approaches do not have negative side effects and addiction, so they are the best choices instead of taking medication unless absolutely necessary.

The process of inflammation is an important biological and immunological reaction that the body responds to injury and infection. From the point of view of energy medicine, inflammation is the symptom of excessive heat or fire generated within the body while it is fighting with viruses or bacteria during infection. The excessive fire appears as yang hyperactivity and yin deficiency. It means that there are disturbances, irritations, disharmonies, fights, conflicts or challenges inside the body that generate fire, heat, or cause damage within the cellular or molecular microenvironments in the body. It's why the writing character of inflammation in Chinese (炎) is structured as two characters of fire (火) overlapped in the upper and lower part. Fire or heat is yang and water is yin. Therefore inflammation is excessive yang and yin deficiency. The energy imbalance between yin and yang, cool and heat, water and fire, is the real issue going on during the inflammation. Inflammation is the outcome or expression of the excessive heat, fire or hyperactive yang energy, therefore, balancing energy, increasing yin (cooling, water energy) and reducing yang (fire, heat, called cleansing heat and tonifying yin) is the way to calm down the inflammation and infection, harmonize the microenvironments of the body, and heal the problem.

Deep meditation or a combination with energy music healing is an effective way to heal infection and inflammation. You can choose Water Yin Music for kidney (kidney, bladder, ears, bone, joints) system infections, Metal Yin Music for lung/pulmonary or respiratory system (lung, large intestines, skin, nose, hair) infections, Wood Yin Music for liver system (liver, gallbladder, eye) infections, and Earth Yin Music for spleen system (spleen, stomach, muscles, nerves, abdomen, overall energy and health) infections, Fire Yin Music for heart system health (heart, small intestine, cardiac vascular system, central nervous system, sleep and overall health). The Water Yin Music is also for all kinds of infections and inflammations in general because the water element of kidney yin energy is governing over all systems as yin energy system.

Meditating with this healing music is every effective to heal infection and inflammation because it does two things at the same time: (1) it calms down the body and mind to build up yin energy that cools down the fire, and at the same time (2) it strengthens the immune system that fights off the viruses or bacteria. Especially for chronic infection and inflammation, long and deep meditation with the energy vibration makes a big difference. Even if it doesn't completely get rid of the infection or inflammation, it will help your body heal much easier and faster. It is also a good opportunity to exercise your immune system and make it stronger. Most importantly this practice can deeply cleanse your microenvironments in the cellular, molecular and genetic dimensions, and detoxify the factors at the microenvironmental levels that may cause any worse diseases such as cancer. This is very important preventive practice for any diseases including cancer.

Since infection or inflammation causes excessive heat or fire inside the body, you can take some cooling and detoxifying herbs or dietary foods such as vegetables, fruits and teas which cleanse heat and fire to help heal infection and inflammation. For example, green beans, green tea, oats, berries, loofah, and bitter melon, salmon, etc. can calm down fire, cleanse heat, detoxify and sooth the body. These all have effective anti-infection and anti-inflammation benefits. For the infection or inflammation which is caused by cold Qi (for example, a common cold causing fever, sore throat or infection in other areas), some hot or warm diets can help eliminate the cold Qi to heal. Drink hot ginger soup with brown sugar added, meditate with the healing music, and have a good restful sleep, then the cold Qi will be eliminated and your health is recovered. As the Chinese saying, "Cold is the initial source of all kinds of diseases," indicates, cold can weaken your entire system and cause other sicknesses. Avoiding getting a cold can prevent other diseases.

5. Pollution of Environment and Foods

Environmental pollution and contaminated foods are big concerns as causes of modern diseases including cancers. Due to industrial environmental pollution, water, air and foods are widely contaminated and poisoned with life-threatening dangerous chemicals such as (1) arsenic, chromium, nickel, other heavy metals and their compounds and asbestos, (2) polycyclic hydrocarbons such as coal tar, bitumen, paraffin wax, creosote oil, products that contains 3,4 – benzopyrene, (3) dyes such as azo dyes, B aniline, benzidine, (4) and nitrosamines. All these chemicals are carcinogenic.

The higher inorganic arsenic level of drinking water and foods especially rice is of concern as a cancer risk. This is based on a research that raised the issue recently as reported by AFP, July 23, 2013 [82]. Other arsenic poison sources can be pesticides, herbs, semiconductor products and related manufacturing industries which directly involve workers.

It seems currently there is no effective and practical way to lower the level of arsenic retained in the rice, which we rely on in daily diet. An alternative for rice can be flour or other grains such as millet, sorghum, maize, soybean, green bean and other beans, potato, and sweet potato. I would like to suggest that using these varieties in a balanced way makes the most sense.

Pollution of environments and foods is a social problem that is mainly caused by the overwhelming industrial production and imbalanced development between economy and humanity, moral improvement, political advance, social and political system reform, crossing the globe. The loss of mind and soul must be paid off with the serious pain of many lives. From the perspective of mind-body-spirit science we are quite concerned about this issue and highly suggest that humankind from all levels seriously cultivate mind, body and spirit, while performing all other activities, including economic, political, scientific, entertainment, and daily living.

As a follow-up to our discussion on genetic and life-style contributions to various cancers, we will now address some of common cancers and their prevention from the perspective of mind-body medicine and healthology.

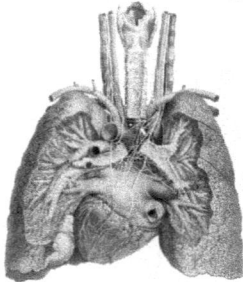

Lung Cancer: Smoking or a smoking environment is the most direct cause and highest risk behavior toward contracting lung cancer. We highly recommend you absolutely do not smoke and stay away from smoking environments. If someone smokes in your family or you live or work closely with someone who is a smoker, you also have high risk of getting lung cancer.

Another risky cause is environmental pollution. Depending on where you live, the quality of air differs. In general, the less population, the more nature surrounded, the farther away from industrial districts and central area of a big busy city, the better quality of air and healthier environment you have, so that you have a lower possibility and risk of getting cancer especially lung cancer. But you really need to check on an area you may be thinking of moving to, as some pretty high profile, pristine areas have been falling victim to industrial waste dumping (current and from years ago) and other forms of industrial pollution, affecting both water and air. You can run a fairly quick and accurate check using online sources such as http://www.airnow.gov/ that offers information about Air Quality Index (AQI) in the United States. If you live or travel to other countries, check the AQI over there. In the US, big cities, coasts and some cities in the northeast fall into the moderate region of AQI (50-100) that is acceptable but may be moderate for air pollution sensitive people, while most other places have good AQI (<50). I would like to warn readers that some other countries can have very bad air quality that goes beyond AQI > 200 or > 300 that is classified as very unhealthy or hazardous air pollution area, respectively.

Air purifiers and indoor plants may be used to improve your air quality. This is especially necessary in an isolated room without good air circulation. For a newly painted room or a house, no matter if it is new or old, you certainly should move in after the smells from the painting materials have completely disappeared as those painting materials are very toxic and harmful to your body, especially for your pulmonary or entire respiratory system.

Many chemicals used in construction, including lawn chemicals, are quite hazardous to air quality. Besides avoiding environments plagued by air pollution, you can practice 5 minutes of natural deep breathing each day, listen to your Metal Element Energy Music and meditate daily, as well as eat one or two stewed pears every other day or practice other preventive natural diet healing for the lungs (see separate chapter). This will help you keep your lungs very healthy and strong, preventing lung cancer, asthma and other pulmonary diseases.

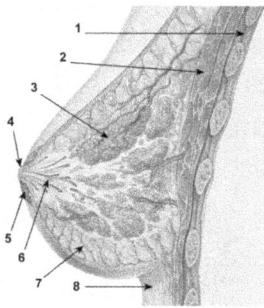

Breast Cancer: Women can prevent breast cancer and stay away from it if you do the following things: Stay in a stress-free life, especially no mental stress and emotional trauma. Reading this book, practice mind-body-spirit cultivation every day, such as meditation, Qigong movement exercise, energy music healing, and have no worries and attachments on work, human life issues, and emotional issues. Stay positive, happy, bright, stable, and peaceful emotionally, attitudinally and in your lifestyle. Don't overload yourself with works or overwhelm yourself with family and social activities or tasks. Balance your time between work and relaxation. Take some time to learn and practice arts. Get involved in relaxing cultural activities, but don't make your schedule to busy. Plan to have daily energy practice, exercise and health improvement. Live with an organized schedule each day and get enough sleep, never staying up late, especially not later than 11 p.m. or staying up long hours at the night working on your computer or for other activities. The best way to do this is to go to bed early and wake up early for health improvement practice or exercise every morning.

Eat healthy, such as vegetables and fruits as major dishes and less or no fatty and high calorie foods, and do not smoke and/or drink alcohols. Make sure you have a regular menstrual cycle (for women before menopause age) and balanced hormonal function, otherwise see a doctor for advice. We do not recommend hormone therapy, or it is not the first choice. Traditional oriental medicine has a natural way, using herbs to balance your hormone system. Many cases with irregular menstrual period are caused by mental stress or negative emotions, so you need to practice relaxation and mind-body cultivation by following this book's instruction, in particular: meditation, music healing, more contact with nature and more relaxing activities such as enjoying the arts (but not busily scheduled). No teenage marriage or delayed childbearing. You can perform breast self-check monthly under instruction of your gynecology doctor. Annual breast examination in the hospital is recommended. But, again, daily preventive practice of mind-body-spirit is the best effective way to stay aware from breast disease.

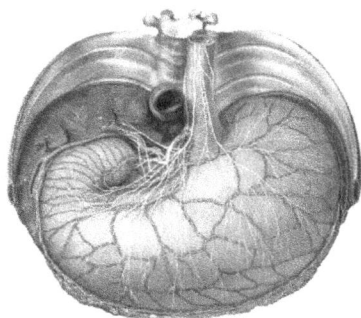

Gastric Cancer: Gastric cancer is the fourth most common cancer in the world. To stay away from it, beside all general issues on cancer prevention already described, please especially try to 1) Avoid preserved or salted foods, hot pepper – e.g. red pepper, processed meats, smoked foods, barbecue animal foods, animal internal organs that may have any disease, oily fried foods that seem to cause gastric mucosal changes, strophic gastritis, and resulting in gastric cancer. 2) Try not to eat until you are "too full" or overeat. Instead eat until you feel around 80% full and never overload your stomach. 3) Try to eat on time by following the body's natural clock, 7-9 a.m. for breakfast, 12-1 p.m. for lunch and 5-6 p.m. for dinner, and never eat at late night or right before your bed time. 4) Try to eat well-cooked foods, especially meats. Vegetables and fruits must be well washed. Make sure there are no chemicals, bacteria or dirt on them, especially if you make salad without cooking it. A recommended way to wash vegetables or fruits: mix water, vinegar and salt (3 cups : 1cup : 2 teaspoons), and soak the vegetables or fruits for 3~5 minutes, then rinse with water to remove bacteria such as E. coli and salmonella. You might also wash the vegetables once with boiling water or for best and safest results, boil the vegetables for a moment before making the salad. 5) If possible, try to eat home-made foods instead of eating out, or at least limit how often you eat away from home, so you can have control of your healthy lifestyle. 6) In every meal, have a minute of meditation with a grateful mind before starting to eat, and eat with a peaceful and relaxed mind, so your body will absorb the food well. 7) Remember to drink hot or warm water or room temperature water after meals and during the day, and it is better to drink less or no soft drinks. You need to drink water (in ounces) = Your Weight (in pound) x 1/2 ounces. 8) Taking a relaxing walk after meal will help digestion, and never do stressful work or tense activities, or slip into an emotional mood or have an argument after eating. 9) 10~15 minutes after a meal, take one minute to practice a small meditation: close your eyes, relax yourself, and put your right hand on your lower stomach area, lightly (very lightly never press hard) massage your stomach by moving your hand clockwise 36 times and then counterclockwise 36 times while slowly and naturally breathing. 10) Eat healthy foods associated with dietary healing, as we will discuss in a separate chapter. 11) At least once a week, in your daily meditation, listen to the Earth Element Music while you practice meditation.

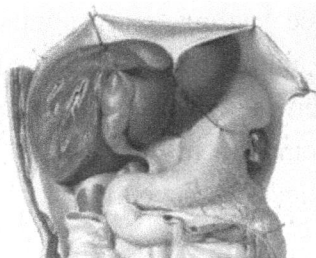

Liver Cancer: Liver cancer is the sixth most common cancer in the world. The liver is an emotionally sensitive organ. As such, you should keep your emotions peaceful, positive, happy and calm all the time, stay stress free, no anger, no bad temper, and practice your daily mind-body cultivation and meditation, and at least listen to the Wood Element Music twice a week, so your liver will be in good condition of health. Go to bed not later than 11 p.m. because (cyclically) it is a good time for your liver to rest and restore energy in order to function well. Heavy alcohol drinking or long-term drinking can cause liver disease especially liver cancer, so you should limit your consumption of alcohol. If you have such an addiction and cannot stop by yourself, visit your mind-body medicine doctor or other mental health practitioners such as hypnotherapist to help you quit. There is some evidence that contracting hepatitis B virus, or eating cereals and beans that have aflatoxin contamination may put you at high risk for liver cancer. For one who already has a liver health condition, you will especially need to give extra care to your liver. For people who often stay up late night – face looks dark, low circulation, low or high blood pressure, fatigue easily – you need to take care of you liver as well and can start by going to bed early (no later than 11 p.m.). Daily meditation and gentle movement exercises with wood element healing music will help you improve these conditions.

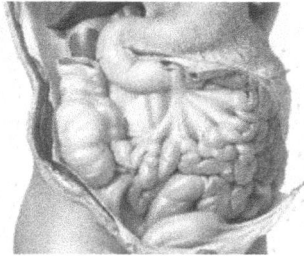

Large Intestine Cancer / Colorectal Cancer: Large intestine cancer is the third most common cancer in the world. Red meat, heavy drinking of alcohols, deeply fried foods, holding back stool for lengthy time periods, and constipation are likely to lead to colorectal cancer. In addition to referring to the stomach cancer prevention, we also suggest that you 1) Eat enough vegetables including fiber vegetables and fruits like celery, Chinese leek (Allium tuberosum), okra, bananas, apples, prunes, and the like. Eat two cooked green apples (remove the central part and seeds, boil in water and cook the apple until soft, then remove the skin and continue to cook until it becomes very soft or like apple jam) each day. 2) Eat more liquid foods such as soups including rice soup or porridges. 3) Drink enough water every day. 4) Drink honey water. 5) Sleep early and long enough hours, 6) Exercise and take a walk every day. 7) Self massage everyday: with overlapped hands, massage lower abdomen area clockwise 36 times and counterclockwise 36 times in the morning after waking up and at night before sleep, especially if constipated. 8) Defecate about twice a day, but not less, otherwise eat more fiber vegetables and fruits, especially apples, raw or cooked. 9) Practice meditation and energy movement every day, and listen to the Metal Element Music and Earth Element Music at least twice a week. Or do both daily.

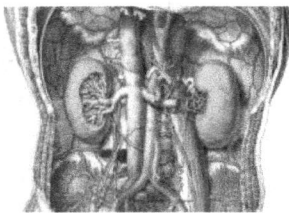

Kidney Cancer: Kidney cancer is the fifth most common cancer in the world. Body over-weight with fatness, contaminated arsenic levels in the drinking water and smoking are some of the well-known factors that lead to kidney cancer. Other possible causes are chronic kidney infection, kidney failure, or other kidney diseases. Protecting your kidneys throughout your life is very important. Besides all the general concerns with the cancer prevention issues we mentioned above, you should give good care to the following issues: 1) Good sleep after 11 p.m. and have a time-scheduled, organized lifestyle. 2) Try not to hold off when needing to urinate. 3) Drink enough water. 4) Make sure not to get constipated. 5) Often swallow saliva, especially during meditation. 6) Keep your feet warm. Every night before going to bed, soak your feet with warm water for 20 minutes and then massage the central area of your feet (Yong Quan acupoint) with your two thumbs 36 times. Sleep with your feet warm, not against air conditioning or cold wind, and don't walk barefoot on cold floor. 7). Good diets for kidney care include such foods as black sesame, black fungus, black beans and so forth. For kidney yin deficiency, tonify kidney yin with sea cucumber, cordyceps, wolfberry, turtle, or white fungus; while for kidney yang weakness, tonify kidney yang with lamb, deer antler, psoralen, cistanche, cinnamon. But visit your Chinese doctor before you decide to take these dietary supplements. 8) Don't over-work physically; that hurts Qi, do not work too hard mentally that hurts blood, and do not overdo having sex that hurts your essence of kidney. 9) Be careful not to over take medications, either Western medicine or Chinese herbs which can overload your kidney for detoxification. 10) Practice meditation and energy movement every day and listen to the Water Element Music and metal element music at least twice a week.

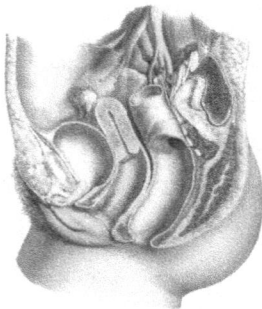

Cervical Cancer: Cervical cancer is the second most common female cancer in the world. In modern medicine study, we know that cervical cancer can be caused by sexually transmitted Human Papillom Virus (HPV) infection. Therefore first of all, to prevent cervical cancer, safe sex is the most important and effective approach to take. In addition, there are many reasons that can cause this cancer, such as staying up late, disordered (unorganized) living schedules and lifestyle, stress, overloaded work, emotional trauma (depression, anxiety, fear, etc.) and relationship difficulty. These may cause endocrine disorders/imbalanced hormone conditions. Other causes can be starting sexual life at early age (teenage), and unhealthy sexual life and sexual relationship. Other female diseases also can cause cervical cancer (also refer to Breast Cancer prevention in the forthcoming pages). Daily meditation cultivation, energy movement exercise, and energy music healing are recommended for any woman to maintain the health of female organs and prevent cancers, especially cervical cancer and breast cancer. Water Element Energy Music and Wood Element Music are effective for women to maintain hormone balance, health of female organs, and manage emotions with ease and peace.

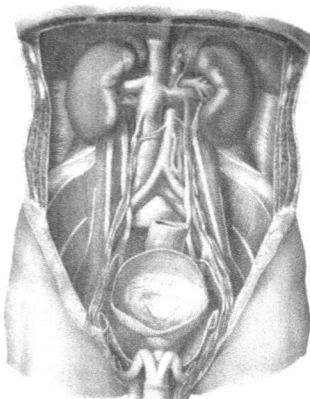

Bladder Cancer: Bladder cancer is the 10th most common cancer in the world. Studies show that arsenic contamination in drinking water is one of the causes of bladder cancer. Holding urine and delaying urination for extra long can increase the risk of bladder cancer. Other likely possible causes for bladder cancer include smoking (smoking is believed to be related with ~50% of bladder cancer cases in the USA.), aging (low rate of cancer development under 40 years of age, but much higher rate after 65 years old), bladder defect (people who were born with a bladder defect have high risk of bladder cancer), bladder infection and chronic inflammation (e.g., a parasitic infection can cause bladder chronic inflammation and result in squamous cell carcinoma risk), women receiving radiation therapy for cervical cancer (show high risk of bladder cancer), and exposures to arsenic or the chemicals that are used in the manufacturing of rubber, dyes, textiles, plastics, paints and leather. The bladder belongs to the same set of meridians as the kidney, but it is a yang organ, so kidney yang deficiency can cause bladder problems (refer to earlier section on kidney cancer prevention). Meditation, energy movement exercise and water element music healing keep your bladder healthy and strong as well as promote kidney health for longevity.

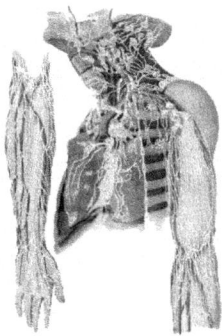

Lymphatic and Hematopoietic Cancer: Lymphatic and hematopoietic cancer includes lymphoma, leukemia and multiple myeloma. These cancers and liver cancer tie for the sixth most common cancer in the world. Although the cause for these types of cancers remains unclear, some researchers reported that some chronic infections and inflammations as chronic gastritis might be the partial trigger of malignant lymphoma. The malignant lymphoma wakens or even damages the immune function of lymphocytes.. Your immune system is an overall organ covering the entire body as an extremely important system physiologically. Modern sciences are not so clear about how lymphatic and hematopoietic cancers are developed, but it is very clear that all factors associated with stress, environments, and emotions are involved in these cancers. We highly suggest that modern people stay vigilant about their daily meditation cultivation, natural healing, healthy diet as well as simplifying their lifestyle and having a relaxed living schedule, so you can maintain a healthy mind, body and spirit, and stay away from the risk of getting all these cancers. Using energy music healing meditation cultivation and alternating each title to balance your energy when needed will help you maintain a strong and healthy immune system and reduce your risks.

Pancreatic Cancer: Pancreatic cancer is the 13th most common cancer in the world. Individuals with obesity or diabetes may be at higher risk of this cancer. Imbalances of metabolism, hormones, nutrition, and emotions are all involved in this cancer development. The key to prevent this cancer is to eat healthy with more vegetables and fruit, but less fatty and oily foods, and to maintain a regimen of daily energy movement exercises, walks, energy music healing, emotional stability practices, peaceful relationships, healthy environment,

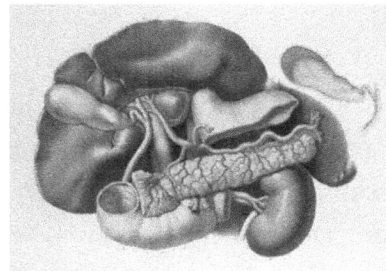

organized living schedule, simple and relaxing lifestyle, and mind-body cultivation and meditation.

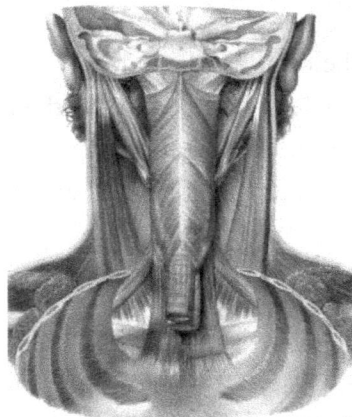

Esophageal Cancer: Esophageal cancer is the 8th most common cancer in the world. The main reason for esophageal cancer is the eating of hot food, such as the excessive consumption of hot drinks such as teas and the like. Other causes are smoking, obesity, and eating processed meats. These are most likely the direct cause of esophagus cancer. A healthy, aware diet (see previous discussions), living smoke free, and daily cultivation practice can lower your risks and again strengthen your body's healing mechanism.

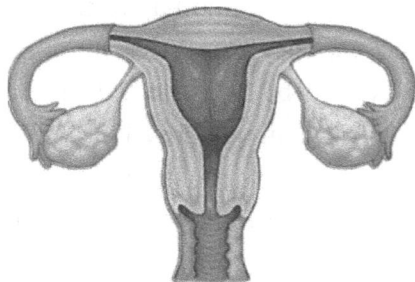

Ovarian Cancer: This is the 7th most common cancer affecting women throughout the world. Many causes have been identified, such as with breast cancer and cervical cancer. Please refer to previous sections on breast cancer and cervical cancer preventions. The key to prevent this cancer is, again, emotional and hormonal balance. The mind-body cultivation meditation, exercise, energy healing and preventive health practice will help you stay away from the risk of getting this cancer.

§13.7 The Effort You Put in Equals the Happiness You Get Out

Cancer is a life-threatening disease and no one wants to get it. So who determines it? The answer is that each individual can participate in warding off this terrible disease. It is under our control if we put effort into its prevention. The environments we create, the foods we prepare and eat, the stress we experience in daily life, the work we do, the thoughts, emotions and desires, attachments that we have, are all up to us.

To prevent cancer or heal cancer, or other diseases, one has to seriously cultivate the mind, body and spirit, so that the super powerful energy we accrue can refresh the contaminated or altered microenvironments of genetic molecules and restore the balance and harmony back for the original life mechanism. The difficulty in this effort is that as human beings we have become used to attaching to so many things in this physical realm (level) which keep the mind away from true Self and lose connection with the soul/spirit. As such, modern human beings are exposed to the very high risk of getting serious diseases including cancer, depression, and heart failure. The causes include but are not limited to: human attachments, ignorance, not knowing the truth and meaning of this life, misleading information and an incorrect understanding about the health of the whole being, relying on the drugs or surgery of modern medicine, not looking at our own Self inwardly, excessively pursuing and focusing on the superficial world and material interests, the overwhelming use of left brain and the entirety of its associated education systems from elementary school through graduate schools, and the very stressful lifestyle and working environment as well as complicated and difficult relationships we live with and among. All these elements increase one's risk of cancer or other severe physical diseases and psychological disorders.

We human beings tend to pursue all kinds of success in many aspects of this life such as education, degrees, careers, money, relationships, family, research, science, politics, power, fame, business, and so on, but sometimes we do not care about our own health, or don't have enough time and knowledge to have a healthy life mentally, physically and spiritually. We often see that people are busy all of the time, for all kinds of things and reasons, and just do not have the time to improve their health and cultivate their own life. It is important for you to witness (in the pages of this book and now in actual daily life) the impact of these kinds of human decisions and attitudes that keep people on the superficial level of living.

You can, however, follow another path. You can, for instance, take effort to make corrections in your journey and live a simpler, natural and healthy and peacefully joyful life. This is the path upon which everyone's true spirit stands out and clearly understands the true meaning of this life and what is the most important thing to do in this lifetime. From here, we will all take good care of the health of our mind, body and soul, and have a much better life.

From today onward, if you think it is important to have a healthy mind, body and soul, then start to practice meditation, energy music healing, and cultivate your body, mind and spirit. The amount of effort you put into this aspect of your life will equal the happiness you will glean.

My Stroke Recovery With Dr. Liu's Needle-Free Acupuncture

- Bob Z.

I had a stroke over a year ago which caused the right side of my body to become paralyzed. I felt pain when I tried to lift my right arm, not to mention writing or driving. Walking also consumed a lot of my energy. My memory began fading, sometimes I stuttered, and I had difficulty calculating. My doctors recommended surgery. However, after viewing my X-rays, they couldn't identify any problem with my muscle tissue. They offered only tests and medication. I went to two other practitioners who were physical therapists, but they could not significantly improve my condition.

Then, through a friend of my wife who had wonderful healing experiences, I found Dr. Liu. So I began my stroke recovery journey with Dr. Jason Liu and his Brainwave-Meridian (needle-free acupuncture) Therapy.

After my first session, the swelling in my swollen right arm was reduced by about 70%, so I could move my arm and fingers much more easily. I could close my fist, which was something I could not do before. After four sessions, I stopped all my medication (4 kinds for high blood pressure and 1 for blood sugar). Without medication, my blood pressure this morning, for example, was 118/76 (before it was over 160 without medications), and my blood sugar was 108 (it was over 140 without medication before). They are now normal and stable after Dr. Liu's therapy. All these changes occurred in less than two months with Dr. Liu's therapy.

Meditation to Cleanse Darkness

The goal of MBM and MBH is to heal all causes of sicknesses before they become sicknesses. The Karma darkness within and surrounding a living being is the real cause of diseases. The darkness of Karma masks the true Self of the individual and prevents him/her from connecting to the universe's nature and its energy source, causing energy blocks and deficiency or imbalance. Because it is in other dimensions, conventional medicine cannot reach it and eliminate it completely. The practice of mind-body-spirit cultivation such as meditation works with other spiritual dimensions and can purify the mind and spirit in other dimensions.

Now I invite you, my dear reader, to join me and have a deep meditation as last session to conclude this book.

Choose either of the following energy music titles *as your preference* and sit in a cross-legged position or whichever you are able to comfortably maintain, to meditate.

EHM07: Let Go and Stay High *(Yang, Earth, Fire)*

EHM08: Assimilate with Earth & Heaven *(Yin, Earth, Fire)*

We have traveled a long way throughout this book to search the truth of the universe and our Self, answering many important questions about mind, body and spirit, such as: why do we human beings get sick, how to heal the whole being of mind-body-spirit, where did we come from, what is our original nature and energy state, how do we return to the original Self to heal problems, maintain health and prevent future sickness, why do we need whole being medicine especially today, and why do we all need mind-body-spirit cultivation practice and how can we go about it? No more confusion and wondering; now we are clear about all these. From now on we need to put our effort into daily practice in order to achieve the goal: true health of our whole being and a good quality of life by focusing on a journey of mind-body-spirit cultivation (self-improvement and exploration) toward the bright future and eternal life.

We connect to the powerful universe and with great compassion and righteous thoughts to clean up all messages and sick information inside us and which are surrounding our living and working environment as well as the human world.

Cultivate, strengthen, and live healthy.

§13.9 Exercise Questions

1. Please describe the three levels of healing as defined in the ancient time, and what is the situation of today's modern healthcare if considering these three levels of healing?

2. How do you understand the concept: *heal the disease before it becomes a disease?* Why is preventive medicine important today?

3. How do genetic researches find out about the cause of cancer? How do you understand the microenvironment disharmony causes altered DNA and increases in the risk of getting cancer?

4. How do you slow down aging and prevent altered DNA methylation and cancer risk?

5. How do you deal with stress and prevent altered DNA methylation and cancer risk?

6. How do you avoid folate and dietary fat that may alter DNA methylation and increase cancer risk?

7. How do you heal inflammation and infection to prevent altered DNA methylation and cancer risk?

8. How do you prevent common cancers in your daily life?

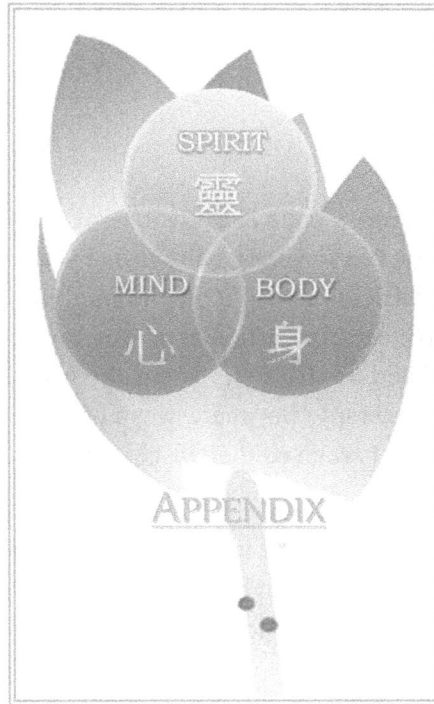

Healing Stories – Case Testimonials

Some of the healing stories have been shared in each chapter above. With some more healing stories, we list them all together in this chapter for your convenience and easy searching and discussion.

As an application of mind-body medicine and healthology, BMT has helped many people reduce suffering from chronic health problems mentally and physically. After the patients regained health through natural healing, they were happy to share their stories in hope of helping others understand how the mind-body medicine could work for more people to achieve mind-body health. All testimonials described in this chapter are contributed from the actual patients who had a great healing success with BMT. These healing stories are not for telling how great the doctor is personally, but for helping readers understand how the mind-body medicine and healthology works, and help you maintain an open mind to explore the profoundness and benefits of this field.

Note: to protect our patients' privacy, all names in the testimonials are nicknames.

An Admiring Of Healing Art – BMT Energy Therapy Healed Me

- Jeffery S.

I have been surfing since I was a child and it is one of the most important activities in my life. Unfortunately, my left hip started feeling very painful five years ago, and it bothered me quite a lot, and it gradually made surfing difficult. I went to the hospital to check what went wrong. After a series of tests, the doctors gave no clear explanation about the cause, but suggested that I undergo a hip replacement surgery. I refused and wanted to try some alternative therapies. I tried acupuncture, chiropractic, shiatsu, and massage therapy, but there was not that much improvement. Because I was under such a severe pain, finally I received the left-hip replacement surgery by paying $23,000 for the two-night stay in the hospital.

After three weeks, just when I got rid of my walking stick, the pain had transferred from my left hip to my right hip and even my lower back! This made me feel very disappointed about the surgery, not only because of so much money spent without results, but also because the degree of the pain worsened after the surgery.

As this condition became worse every day, the physical pains became emotional pain as I realized that I would have to give up my favorite hobby in my life. I went to some other doctors, physical therapists and alternative medicine practitioners, but they couldn't help me until I came across an ad placed in both the Yellow Pages and the Vision Magazine about Dr. Jason Liu and his needle-free/drug-free Brainwave-Meridian Therapy.

During my first visit, Dr. Liu's diagnosis clearly pointed out that the major cause of the pains was associated with some long-time energy blockages, which had existed even before the replacement surgery. He explained that the surgery hadn't removed the blockages, so that was what caused the pain in my right hip and lower back.

Dr. Liu's meridian energy therapy is very effective. I could feel the energy flow through my back, hips, and legs and noticed the pain reduction right away at the first session. I scheduled appointments with him every day for two weeks and felt better and better each time. After the first two weeks, I could surf again! In order to get healed completely, I visited him 3 times a week, and then reduced to 2 times a week, then once a week. The results are stable. Recently I had a vacation for two weeks and went surfing in Hawaii. I surf almost every day and never feel any pain. My daily life also has become much easier because this pain is completely gone.

Through my healing experience with Dr. Liu, I now understand more about his energy medicine. It seems that he is working beyond the physical realm to heal the cause – energy blockages. It may be hard to understand, but I do know the energy blocks existed and that they couldn't be removed by surgery. Now they are gone, so I am completely healed. Thanks for Dr. Liu's healing art.

BMT Ended My 8-Year Illnesses – Fibromyalgia

-Rose R.

"Rosario, you are really looking different now." All my friends have been telling me this for the last week, especially my husband, who was out of town for one week and called me: "Honey, you sound happier now." Yes, I do look happier and feel a lot happier, for the first time in years. I am sure the positive changes occurred because of Dr. Jason Liu.

I had been seeing different doctors and hospital staff for the past 8 years. I started with high blood pressure, developed fibromyalgia the same year, and the list continued: high cholesterol, amnesia, diabetics, tension, insomnia, depression, abnormal liver function, weight gain, 24-hour pain, swollen feet, fear, worry, anger… I had 18 things on my list before I went to see Dr. Liu. I had 13-14 pills taken every day. I knew these drugs had many side effects and made me sicker, but without them I was unable to control my high blood pressure and couldn't sleep. Doctors told me walking would be good for my diabetes, but I could only walk 10 to15 minutes due to lack of energy. I couldn't have normal family life with my husband, we wanted to do things together, but I was always telling him, "No, I am tired, I have pain in my body." He worried about our family and me a lot. I couldn't even drive from Chula Vista to San Diego, because of the pain in my neck that prevented me from seeing straight; I had to ask people help all the time… This was torture every moment, and I was constantly in a bad mood and I would fight with everyone around me.

Thank God for helping me find Dr. Liu who took away my pain and all my pills! I would like to emphasize that Dr. Liu's healing does not involve needles or medicines, only his composed brainwave-meridian music, which is customized for each individual. All I needed to do was to lie down and enjoy his beautiful music. I could feel dramatic changes after the 3rd session. After 6 weeks, I stopped taking all medications except vitamins. I was able to walk 40 minutes every day last week; my blood pressure is 117-78 after walking, which is normal! I can now sleep 8-9 hours, but before I could only sleep 1-2 hours. I feel more energy during the daytime; I lost 8 pounds during the past 2 weeks, without the burning stomach caused by the medicine I was taking. My swollen feet became normal, and I can drive by myself now, without having to bother others.

The most important thing to me is that I am able to calm down and handle things and to talk to people without fear or worry about my kids. My husband is very happy to see these changes in me; we now can go out and enjoy activities together. Everything has changed, and so dramatically that I can hardly believe it; it seems like a dream!

I am telling everyone what Dr. Liu has done for me, how great this therapy is, and how lucky we are in San Diego. I owe it all to Dr. Liu, who took away the pain I endured for eight years and all my medication without needles or surgery. He did it just with his music. Thank God for Dr. Liu's knowledge and compassion.

BMT Really Reunified Me

- Kate W.

Last fall, I was going through some very difficult physical problems: my hands and feet were very swollen, bleeding, and oozing; I could barely walk and it was very distressing. It seemed like a cross between an allergic reaction and a toxic reaction, so I started detoxification treatments. I used Oxygen Light and other therapies, which helped, but couldn't eliminate the problem. When my urine pH level reached 4.2-4.5, coupled with my back pain, I realized it was Kidney related, so I drank cranberry juice. There was something extreme going on with my body, and it got to the point where I finally realized that what I was doing was not addressing it sufficiently.

Throughout my life, the medical industry has made me ill, literally. I was born ill, and their medicines made me more ill; they were injecting me with cortisone when I was 6 years old! I've probably had kidney channel damage ever since I was young. I have studied many therapies; I have tried, almost everything. I have been interested in and done lots of research about healing with sound, color, lights and vibration frequency. I was looking at the Light Connection Magazine when I came to Dr. Liu's advertisement for Acupuncture-Music Therapy, using sound. This really fascinated me, so I went to his website. What intrigued me most is that Dr. Liu's therapy is primarily based upon sound/vibration energy healing, utilizing no needles or medicine.

I called Dr. Liu and made an appointment, and the results were amazing! All I had to do was lie on a magnetic bed (under a nice comfy blanket), put on headphones, and listen. Dr. Liu's voice would guide me in the beginning, and then I would go on a musical journey. Dr. Liu encouraged me to allow the music to carry me away into the inner dimensions of my soul, and while it did, he hooked me to a 2nd computer with brainwave and HeartMath technologies that measured my brainwaves, heartbeat and brain-heart synchronicity.

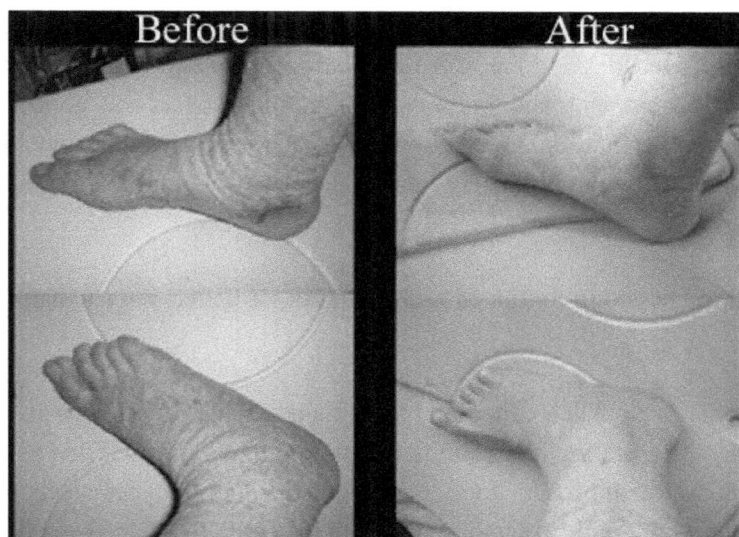

My dramatic improvement started within 24 hours. I went twice a week for 4 weeks. What surprised me most was that I went in for physical problems, yet Dr. Liu's diagnosis pointed out that my physical problems were really the result of emotional problems. I was going through some relationship problems, which caused my kidney and liver energy channels to block. As he skillfully tweaked the music he composed for me, my progress was both subtle and dynamic, and deeply unifying beyond my wildest imagination! Session-by-session, I watched, felt, and realized that I was integrating into a "New Me", literally.

My feet are now terrific. You can see the difference before and after in these slides. My hands are great, my skin is great, and even my income has doubled. Before my treatments, I felt very disconnected from spirit, very splintered. Now I feel unified, complete and very connected to Spirit, which has a great impact on physical well-being.

Those of us in San Diego are truly fortunate, as Dr. Liu is the only person offering this therapy in the United States! Although this type of music therapy dates back thousands of years, Dr. Liu goes way beyond what has been written in the Yellow Emperor's book of "Chinese Internal Medicine. Dr. Liu is a very gifted man; his enthusiasm is contagious; his varied degrees are extra-ordinary, which all add up to an exceptional person with a truly distinctive and profound therapy!

My 9-Year Pain Gone!

Alice suffered from chronic pain in her lower back, legs and feet for the past 9 years. She could only sleep for 2 hours each night. Her conditions have complicated factors, including elephant legs (elephantiasis), depression, anxiety, anger, insomnia, and severe pain. Her daughter, who is a nurse, took her to all kinds of the doctors she knew, including pain management specialists, psychologists, neurologists, acupuncturists, but she was told they couldn't do anything to help her.

When Alice came into the clinic, she was in a wheelchair. Her posture was bent over, and she was very tense. Her legs and feet were swollen so badly that she could not take off socks. After 30 minutes of BMT treatment, she found that the pain in her feet was gone. Her screams of joy and the scene of the mother and daughter embracing each other were so touching. Alice could stand straight and walked to the bathroom by herself. Vera told us that she found us through one of her co-workers, whose mother had been healed by BMT.

A few more sessions continued and she felt a lot better, but she had to go back to her home in Texas.

Six months later, Alice called and said thanks while telling that she had continued to heal after the sessions. The healing had automatically progressed by itself and as a result of her ongoing efforts. Her pain was completely gone, depression healed, and her sleep was very good, weight balanced, and she was totally transformed to another person. "My 9-year Pain gone!" Alice told everyone. Her families and friends saw how dramatically she had changed her condition and could not believe she could be so happy.

My Fibroid Healed - Saved Me from the Surgery

- Iris C.

My name is Irene. I came to the U.S. from Russia a few years ago. I was diagnosed as fibroid and advised by my doctors to get an immediate hysterectomy, a surgery that removes the uterus. The condition caused heavy bleeding (8 days each period) for 2 years. I even had to have emergency care due to losing too much blood that resulted in anemia and low blood pressure (85/50). I became very weak, physically and mentally. I thought I would die in this way as the condition was getting worse and worse. However, I didn't feel ready to go through the surgery, as that's a lot of money, for the operation and the after-care cost, and I was also afraid of the side effects of removing this main female organ. I heard many complain that a hysterectomy could cause female hormone imbalance, speeding up aging process and other related problems. I also read some information from online medical advisors that said that many physicians and women's health advocates argue that 75 to 80 percent of hysterectomy surgeries are not necessary because alternative ways could help. For all these reasons I had kept looking for a natural healing way to help.

Luckily, I found Dr. Jason Liu, from a magazine. When I met with Dr. Liu, I was emotionally depressed, looked pale, and not sure how he could help me in stopping the bleeding. But an amazing thing happened. The bleeding volume reduced right after the 1st session. It was unbelievable! I continued another 20 sessions and by then my period returned to normal - 3-4 days with regular amount. The fibroid is healed so I don't need the surgery anymore!

My life is changed because of Dr. Liu's healing work. I have become not only physically healthy, but also very positive and happy mentally and emotionally. I feel a strong confidence to recommend Dr. Liu's natural healing to anyone who is in needs.

My Stroke Recovery with Dr. Liu's Needle-Free Acupuncture

- Bob Z.

I had a stroke over a year ago which caused the right side of my body to become paralyzed. I felt pain when I tried to lift my right arm, not to mention writing or driving. Walking also consumed a lot of my energy. My memory began fading, sometimes I stuttered, and I had difficulty calculating. My doctors recommended surgery. However, after viewing my X-rays, they couldn't identify any problem with my muscle tissue. They offered only tests and medication. I went to two other practitioners who were physical therapists, but they could not significantly improve my condition.

Then, through a friend of my wife who had wonderful healing experiences, I found Dr. Liu. So I began my stroke recovery journey with Dr. Jason Liu and his Brainwave-Meridian (needle-free acupuncture) Therapy.

After my first session, the swelling in my swollen right arm was reduced by about 70%, so I could move my arm and fingers much more easily. I could close my fist, which was something I could not do before. After four sessions, I stopped all my medication (4 kinds for high blood pressure and 1 for blood sugar). Without medication, my blood pressure this morning, for example, was 118/76 (before it was over 160 without medications), and my blood sugar was 108 (it was over 140 without medication before). They are now normal and stable after Dr. Liu's therapy. All these changes occurred in less than two months with Dr. Liu's therapy.

BMT Healed my Bladder and Kidney Infection from the Root

- Mary A.

Nobody loves being sick. Especially, when you don't even know what the problem is, and neither do the doctors. This was my case. My journey to wellness began in late March 2003, when I began a series of illnesses that lasted for over a month. What began, as a bladder infection, or so I thought, then moved into a full blown flu, with terrible back aches and the list goes on, was really, in fact, a virus in my kidneys. I saw three Western medical doctors in three different areas of expertise. No matter what tests they did, they could not find something tangible to diagnose me with. Even the urologist that I saw, scratched his head and said, "You have had so many things going on, I don't know where to begin, so we will just begin a series of tests and go from there." This was in mid-April 2003. After my initial appointment with the urologist, I had to wait two weeks to see him again. Let's just say, that the idea of going through two more weeks of not going to the bathroom without pain and discomfort was not an option anymore! That's when I began seeing Dr. Jason Liu.

I never heard about Acupuncture-Music Therapy. I knew what Acupuncture was. But Dr. Liu's technique did not use needles. In my first session, he pinpointed my disease as low energy in my kidney meridian as well as in my liver. He even found out my physical illness was actually caused from stress and relationship related emotional blocks including anxiety, anger and depression. I was amazed at how clearly he was able to diagnose me by just listening to my pulse! From there the transformation began. The music was mesmerizing. It started with a guided meditation and then the music took over. Our sessions not only included the music and meditation, but Spiritual guidance. Each time, Dr. Jason Liu checked my pulse to see the progress. With each session, I was getting better and better. Little by little the pain was going away in all areas of my body, but the most amazing thing that I began noticing was how I was changing my perception of life, my thought processes, and how my focus shifted to bringing more peace and harmony to my Spirit. The physical challenges are only the manifestation of a Spirit's needs not being met or heard. I had no choice but to listen to my Spirit. What Dr. Liu did for me was heal me from the root. His Acupuncture-Music Therapy broke through the garbage of years of anger, and negative energy blocks and cleared the path to the core so the Light could come in and heal me in mind, body and Spirit. I never met a Doctor or a healer that can do what Dr. Liu does. In my opinion, he does what a traditional Psychologist, a Massage Therapist, and Acupuncturist and Spiritual healer do all in one.

Dr. Jason Liu is also a warm and friendly man, who always emanates a positive energy, strong spirit and stable mentality. It is with these wonderful traits, that he has the ability to encourage people to heal and become whole again. I thank Divine Spirit for bringing Dr. Jason Liu into my life. You will too.

Meridian-Music Gives Back My Life and Soul

- Valerie D

When I decided to meet Dr. Jason Liu, I had reached a desperate point in my life. I'd exhausted my efforts to find relief from my severe angina that had been incapacitating me since March 1997. The angina had escalated to the point that even the slightest physical movement could put me in bed for several hours. I could barely walk; shopping took hours; I had to give up painting (I am a commercial artist); even turning the pages of a magazine could disable me for quite some time. The constriction around my heart was such that I constantly had difficulties. The worst one occurred on September 11, 2001, the day the terrorists attacked. This time the constriction very nearly killed me. I could not move, could not work, and could not live. It was like having a heart attack in slow motion.

I did not obtain the usual Nitroglycerin from any physician or cardiologist, as none of them paid the slightest attention to or showed interest to listen to what I was saying. I consulted different practitioners in the alternative healing arts field. Many were honest, knowledgeable, and did all they could, but still nothing worked. The problem, I think, was an enormous overload of emotional pain that nothing seemed to be able to dislodge, because it was blocked. Dr. Liu was my last hope. From an article I read, I understood that he uses the Chinese Acupuncture theory, but instead of needles, he uses specific musical sounds arranged in beautiful harmonies. Those sounds address the energy blocks that congest the meridians directly, and dissolve them.

The first session really made a difference! Reading my pulse, Dr. Liu detected a huge block in the heart and the liver meridians and a weak kidney, which explained my constant exhaustion. He listened carefully, and chose the right harmonies for me. The music is extraordinary and mysterious: it's like light that can be heard instead of being seen; the genius of it is that it goes to that core of the self we don't even know is there. I came out of this session refreshed and relaxed. The chest pain diminished; the heart rate reduced from 96 to 76. Given the severity of my case, this was quite remarkable for the first session. For the first time in years, I felt more psychic and physical energy during that week.

To my surprise, each following session made a significant improvement to not only the angina, but also the personality, in profound ways. I could sense that the chronic depression that had paralyzed my life for years was leaving me. Something was opening up, creating new shifts in perception, and the ability to trust and create; something that I had never known before.

I had barely mentioned depression to Dr. Liu. The beauty of this therapy is the fact that his approach addresses the whole person - body, feelings, and spirit, not just the illness. His practice combined multiple therapies into one, step by step, systematically to help me to find out the real cause of health problems, and how to practically handle and eliminate them in the future.

I would like to stress that Dr. Liu not only saved my physical health, but he gave my life and my soul back, all in just a few sessions! I am forever grateful to the spirit that allowed me to discover him, grateful to his immense knowledge, and to his beautiful Chinese culture.

Rejuvenated Sex Drive and Overall Health Improvement

- David S.

Being an 84-year old man, I'm not afraid to tell you that I have a girlfriend in her 50's. I love her very much and would do anything to make her happy. But there was one thing I couldn't do because of my age. This really made me feel guilty sometimes.

By accident, I saw Dr. Jason Liu's advertisement on Vision Magazine. I felt a connection with this doctor. I called him to ask if he could help me at my age and was surprised by his positive answer and convincing explanation about his needle-free/drug free energy healing technique, so I immediately made an appointment with him.

After the pulse reading, Dr. Liu very confidently told me that his technique could rejuvenate my lost vital energy and kidney meridian function and may possibly improve sexuality. After he explained about vital life force, energy healing, Oriental medicine, the central neuron system, and the mind-body connection, which are all associated with the sex drive, he started treating me right at the first session. I really enjoyed each session with him. It was so relaxing and comfortable. Sometimes I would fall asleep. After the session, I felt relaxed, refreshed and energetic.

I need to share some surprising results: after the 6th session, my high blood pressure (usually around 180 / 110) returned to normal (118 / 75), and I could stop all five high blood pressure medications. After the 10th session, I was walking much easier and longer without any problem. I used to have weakness in my left leg and knee due to a stroke. After 12 sessions, I started feeling something that I haven't experienced for a long time - my sex drive returned!

I feel younger and happier emotionally, and physically, it's really an improvement to my overall health. I gained a lot of confidence about my relationship.

I Quit Smoking -- And My Shoulder Pain Went Away!

- Mark O.

Amazing! I came to quit smoking, which I did, but what surprised me the most was the fact this therapy also healed my other problems such as shoulder-pain, anxiety, depression and stress…Here is my healing story:

I had a 12-year smoking history. I was having 3/4 pack a day, which exceeded my wife's tolerance level. In order to save my marriage, I had to try my very best to quit smoking. I was skeptical and negative due to the fact that no other techniques were working for me until I met with Dr. Jason Liu. In the very initial session, Dr. Liu read my pulse and diagnosed my energy blocks and emotional blocks, and then he recorded my brainwaves and HeartMath data to find the corrupted frequencies in my neuron system. Based on all these careful researches, he composed a very special series of music sounds for my sessions. His technique, called Brainwave-Meridian Therapy (BMT) is a perfect combination of hypnotherapy, music healing, needle-free acupuncture, physical and mental massages with his very unique and powerful frequencies of therapeutic music sound and melodies. He not only helped me permanently quit smoking, but also healed my other physical conditions at the same time.

During the years, I was also suffering pains in my back and shoulders. I was under lots of stress and anxiety, and of course, my sex drive was low, as I was also addicted to alcohol… After a few sessions with Dr. Liu, I was surprised to find myself no longer craving for drink and smoke, my shoulder pain also stopped! What surprised my wife and me the most was the fact we are a lot closer at bedtime, and I regained my confidence.

Dr. Liu's technology reprogrammed my messed-up neuron system and refreshed me from within. Initially I expect Dr. Liu would use just hypnosis to help me quit smoking, but actually he dealt with all my other problems at the same time and used other integrated techniques. Beyond stress, I believe, this healing art is good for all kinds of things like pain management and weight control, but also for mental and physical issues. I am very happy to recommend Dr. Jason Liu and his drug-free and needle-free therapy, which truly worked for me.

You Gave Me Freedom

- Monica C.

Dear Dr. Liu:

I want to share with you how amazing the results of my sessions have been.

When I first came to see you, my mother had just passed away; my father, after 65 years of marriage, was grieving all day and giving up on wanting to go on. Also at that time, my husband became involved with some Internet activities that were pulling him away from me. I felt grief, anger, and confusion, and was emotionally worn out and physically exhausted.

The sessions with you were delightful! Your heart is so genuine and full of compassion, and your music is indescribable. Your treatments caused me to come back to life! I was able to sort through my marital problems and release all the negativity. Things were getting better, but when my elderly father passed away to reunite with my mother, I looked through my grief over the double loss of both parents, and had a huge revelation.

Without realizing it, I transferred my feelings about my Dad, who was my real life Superman, to my husband. Under the weight of such unspoken expectations, he had to "run away" when he saw me "losing my footing" due to the disintegration of my original family structure. With your help, I once again found within me a strength I didn't know existed, for I had spent all my life being my parents' child. I saw it was time to be a courageous adult, and be the strong one in a relationship. I also learned to set my husband free, in a way, on a psychic level, and be there for him without unexpressed expectations.

I am truly happy to say, "I am back!" Life appears manageable again, and there is a deep acceptance of all that I went through. This is what our sessions gave me: Freedom, with the realization that I am a separate being and no one else is responsible for me. You called on my inner strength to accept this reality by balancing my body, clearing my mind, and "holding my hand" throughout the months it took for me to do the work needed to reach this mountaintop from which I can see clearly.

Thank you for sharing your gifts when I needed them the most and thank you for helping me find this inner peace.

Gratefully,

Monica

My Gallbladder Stones All Gone!

- Larry F.

"I am a very busy professor teaching classes at the Florida International University. My doctor told me that I needed to have surgery to remove my gallbladder stones immediately. I couldn't afford to take much time off, and I was afraid that it would take several months for me to recover. My father-in-law was not happy to hear that I wanted to seek alternative natural healing instead, as he is a doctor himself.

I was very fortunate to find Dr. Jason Liu. His work and healing music removed my energy blocks, and the stones started dissolving from the first day I met him. Three months later, I went to visit my father-in-law. He was surprised to see me so energetic and in such good health. After I assured him that I no longer needed surgery, he dragged me to the hospital for lab testing. To his surprise, we discovered that all of the stones were gone!"

You Are Really A Very Rare "Gem" In This World!

- Connie B.

Dear Doctor Liu:

I will never be able to thank you enough for your wonderful work. You are such a caring and considerate person; you are a rare "gem" in this world. I have waited many years to find a gentle form of therapy to put me back "in the saddle". I wish I could speak and write Chinese to use the very right words…Even so, we understand each other very well, because "healing" is our common concern.

I came to you, as you know, through a lady that I had never met before. She sat next to me for an hour, and must have felt my despair; that special day changed my life forever. I will never forget it.

Doctor, you are a very special person, and I am honored to meet you. Thank you from the bottom of my healed heart.

Yours very sincerely,

Connie B.

【Connie is an immigrant from France with deep French cultural background and respectful manner. Connie had years of conditions with combinations of emotional anxiety, intestine infection, diarrhea, parasites, etc. and could not get help from conventional medicine. By the recommendation of another of Dr. Liu's patients, she visited Dr. Liu's clinic and got healed by BMT treatment. Above is the thank you letter sent from her.】

BMT Has Really Helped Me Immensely

- Christina B.

I hadn't had a good night's sleep for 4 1/2 years. I was sure that part of it was emotional. It began after my sister died very quickly (within a month) in the hospital. The pain in my hip started the day we took her to the hospital; I could hardly get back into the house. Since then, I've been diagnosed with severe arthritis in my left hip and have been taking pain pills. Being an herbalist, I teach about health issues, and advise not taking drugs; however, I was sneaking prescription meds on my own, because the pain was so bad.

After my first treatment with Dr. Liu, I actually slept for nine hours! This therapy worked much better than the pain pills ever did! Nothing else has worked so quickly for me. I had tried a lot of different therapies and seen about 47 different practitioners. Although Dr. Liu scheduled me for the next week, I came back, instead, the very next day! It was doing so much for me, and I was anxious to recover 100%. After the first treatment, the pain was down about 30%, and after the eighth or so, it was down by 95%. It's just amazing, what a difference this made in my life! I was just at a medical supplement conference, where there were many medical doctors, PhDs, medical researchers, and a few herbalists. I was very, very busy, and I didn't really rest all weekend. I was extremely tired yesterday, but this morning I'm feeling great! I know that before my sessions with Dr. Liu, if I had managed to get through three days like that, I would have felt like staying in bed for 3-4 days afterwards. This therapy has helped me immensely.

My friend and I have a small herb company; we grow plants to sell, so we do some manual labor. I had back problems before for trying to lift heavy things (I broke my back in 1983), and to be able to do as much as I am now and not have any pain afterwards is really amazing! I am telling everyone: "You got to try this! It works!! It really has worked for me!!!" To have something that works this well, and all you have do is lie down and listen to music... Hmmm... you can't beat that! "No pain, no Gain" - well, that's baloney! This therapy involves no pain, and I feel so much better.

BMT Saved My Life – My Severe Depression Healed

- Eva C.

When I first came to Dr. Liu for treatment of my severe depression and anxiety, I had already completely stopped menstruating for 3 months. My energy was low, and my circulation was so bad that my hands and feet were always cold. My blood pressure was constantly as low as ~95/55. I felt hopeless in my life. I couldn't work and didn't know what to do. Many times I suddenly started crying uncontrollably.

According to Dr. Liu, all my symptoms were due to a combination of deficiencies in kidney yin, excessive liver fire, hormone imbalance, and mental blocks. My mom saw Dr. Liu's article in the *Epoch Times* newspaper, and made an appointment with him, for me. When I started seeing Dr. Liu, I began to feel better and better each time. I felt energy start flowing within my body; my hands, feet and whole body were growing warmer during the sessions. With each session, I could feel positive changes. I was happier and more peaceful. After the first month, my period resumed, but I still had some emotional frustration, which Dr. Liu indicated was a positive reaction, as emotional blockages were being released.

We continued sessions for another month, and now my depression and anxiety are completely gone. My period returned to normal, with no discomfort. My blood pressure is normal, and my circulation is much better; my hands and feet are no longer cold. I feel very peaceful, and am very appreciative for Dr. Liu's help. He brought light and hope into my life. Right after I finished my sessions, I got a new job.

My Brother's ADHD Healed

- Ivy W.

My brother, Simon (age 16), came to Dr. Liu with ADD/ADHD (Attention Deficit and Hyperactivity Disorder) and some other behavior problems that teenagers sometimes experience. He could not concentrate on his schoolwork, could not communicate with anyone (including family members), and it was difficult for him to understand people's questions. He could hardly make eye contact or smile when talking or listening to people.

After two months of treatment with BMT, the changes were dramatic. He is now able to communicate normally with people and is more aware of the things around him. He can concentrate while studying, and greet friends, teachers and family members politely. He can also participate in conversations without any problems now.

My Bartholin Gland Cyst Healed!

- Ann S.

Six years ago, I was diagnosed with a Bartholin Gland Cyst (an unnatural lump on one side of the labia). It was as big as an egg, causing very much discomfort in my daily life. I knew it was an emotional reaction to some difficulty I had encountered with my boyfriend, and I was broken-hearted when the relationship ended. My doctor suggested I undergo surgery, which I did, but later regretted having made the wrong decision. It was very painful surgery in which the doctor cut the cyst, and left it open, bleeding and draining. I had to lie in bed for 3 full weeks. The surgery left me in pain and with an ugly scar on the skin.

Six years later, at the exact same spot, the cyst came back again. This time, I was in a very similar situation: breaking up with my boyfriend. We had arguments that caused me a lot of anxiety, anger and stress. The cyst grew to the size of an egg, just like the last time. I was scared and wondered what to do this time. I did not want to go through the painful experience of surgery again, so I started researching to see if any alternative method could heal me in a natural way.

I was very, very lucky to have found Dr. Liu, through my friend's referral. She told me about Dr. Liu and how his Brainwave Meridian therapy had helped her greatly. I decided to try my luck. December 2nd was a day I will never forget. I came in for my first session with Dr. Liu. Right after the session, my Bartholin cyst was reduced to half its original size! I was very surprised and excited. It was really an amazing session! I am a scientist; I know that 12% of all women in the US are suffering from this type of problem, and since my experience, I believe this therapy can do miracles!

I continued my sessions with Dr. Liu for about 2 months. As the sessions progressed, the cyst grew smaller and smaller each time, its color turned from its original dark brown to white. Not only the cyst, the flesh also turned from a dull, dark color to pink. What surprised me the most was that the scar from the last surgery completely disappeared! It was unbelievable!!

On another note, I also saw tremendous overall improvement of my dry skin. Everyone said I looked much younger and more attractive. My previously injured left foot healed completely; my emotions became very stable and positive, and I no longer experienced much stress from my work. Recently, I went to interview for a higher paying job, and I was the only one chosen out of 45 applicants. I know that without this therapy I wouldn't have had the courage and energy to do this.

I thank Dr. Jason Liu for being so kind and compassionate, and for his good advice about my life, work, research, relationships and mind-body wellness.

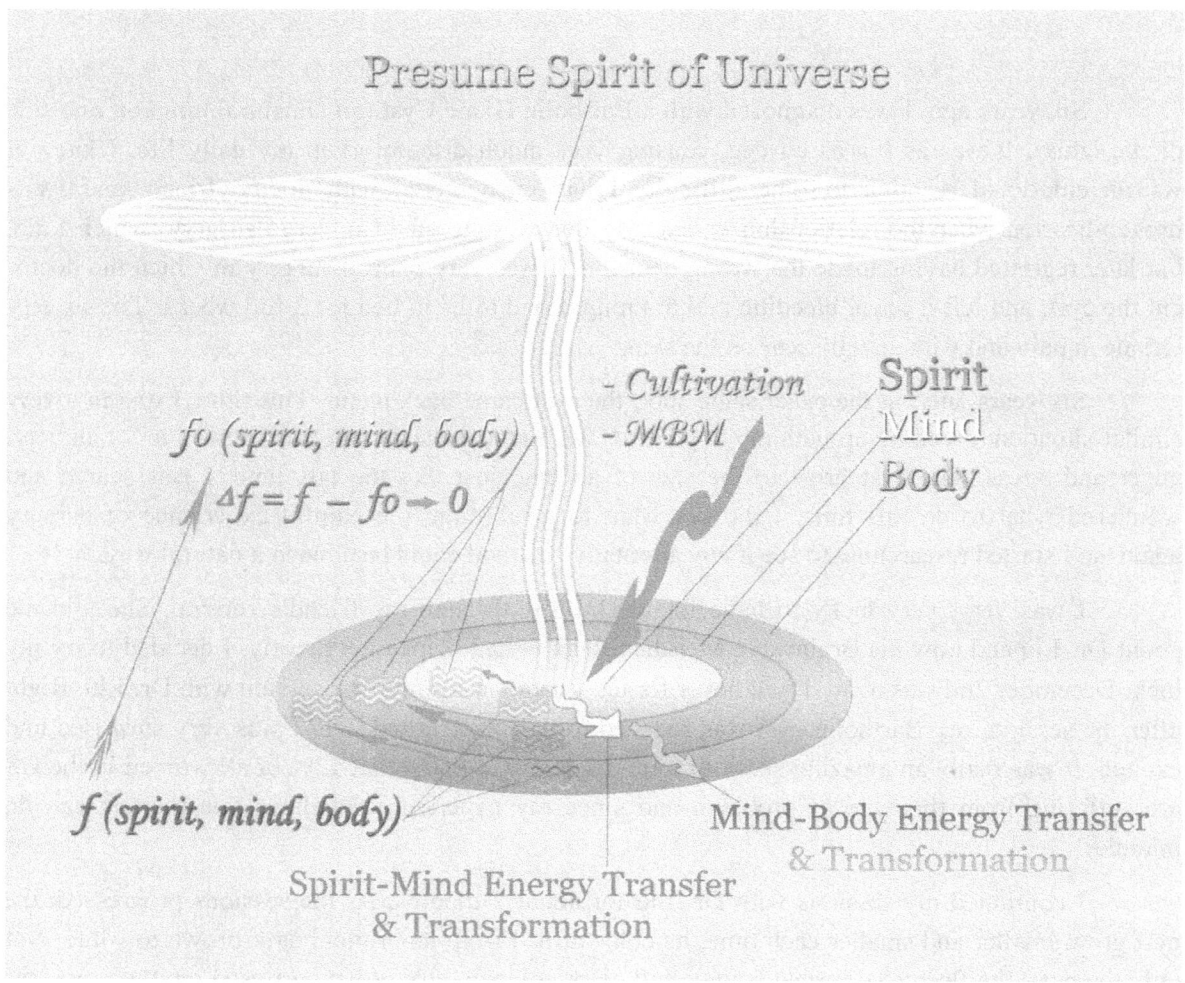

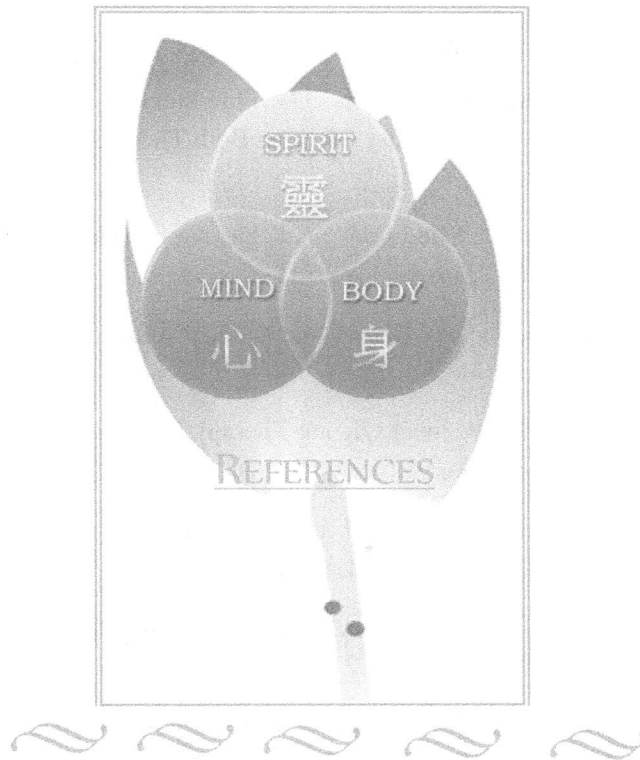

References

[1] Yellow Emperor's Classic of Internal Medicine (475-221 BC)

[2] http://en.wikipedia.org/wiki/Antonie_van_Leeuwenhoek.

[3] Feinstein S (2008): *Louis Pasteur: The Father of Microbiology*. Enslow Publishers, Inc. pp. 1–128. ISBN 9781598450781.

[4] Campbell, D. M. (January 1915). "The Pasteur Institute of Paris". *American Journal of Veterinary Medicine* (Chicago, Ill.: D. M. Campbell) 10 (1): 29–31.

[5] McPherson RA, Pincus MR (Sep 6, 2011): Henry's Clinical Diagnosis and Management by Laboratory Methods, 22nd Edition. Elsevier Health Sciences, ISBN 978-1-4377-0974-2.

[6] WHO (2003): Global cancer rates could increase by 50% to 15 million by 2020. WHO Media Centr. http://www.who.int/mediacentre/news/releases/2003/pr27/en/.

[7] Gallo JJ, Lebowitz BD (1999): The Epidemiology of Common Late-life mental disorders in the Community: Themes for the New Century. *Psychiatric Services* 50:1158–1166, 1999.

[8] Reinberg S (2007): "Depression May Be World's Most Disabling Disease" HealthDay News, HealthDay, Sept. 7, 2007.
http://abcnews.go.com/Health/Healthday/story?id=4508589&page=1#.UdxmsVNqBd4.

[9] Weiss BL (1988): Many Lives, Many Masters: The True Story of a Prominent Psychiatrist, His Young Patient, and the Past-Life Therapy That Changed Both Their Lives. *Fireside* (July 15, 1988), ISBN-13: 978-0671657864.

[10] Barrows KA, Jacobs BP (2002): Mind-body medicine. An introduction and review of the literature. *Med Clin North Am.* 2002 Jan; 86(1): 11-31.

[11] Michelle A (2003): BMT Healed My Kindey and Bladder Infection From the Root. Vision Magazine, Jun. 2003, San Diego.

[12] Chen K, Yeung R (2002): A Review of Qigong Therapy for Cancer Treatment. *Journal of International Society of Life Information Science* (ISLIS). Vol 20 (2). 2002 532

[13] Zent R, Pozzi A (2010): *Cell-Extracellular Matrix Interactions in Cancer.* Springer; 2010 edition (December 14, 2009), ISBN-13: 978-1441908131.

[14] Labat-Robert J, Robert L. (2007): The effect of cell-matrix interactions and aging on the malignant process. *Adv Cancer Res.* 2007, 98:221-59.

[15] Andrei Thomas-Tikhonenko (2010): *Cancer Genome and Tumor Microenvironment.* Springer Science+Business Meida, 2010, ISBN 978-1-4419-0710-3: pp. 3.

[16] Dong Zhongshu (179 BC – 104 BC): "Spring Autumn Fan Lu · Yin Yang Yi"

[17] Lao Tzu (206 BC ~): Tao Te Ching (Lao Tzu), Chapter 25. 206 BC ~.

[18] Li Hongzhi (1992): Zhuan Falun, Yih Chyun Book Co., Ltd. Taipei, Taiwan (Feb. 2003, North America), ISBN: I-59068-013-8. pp. 13. http://www.falundafa.org/book/eng/pdf/zfl_new.pdf

[19] Li Hongzhi (1992): Zhuan Falun, Yih Chyun Book Co., Ltd. Taipei, Taiwan (Feb. 2003, North America), ISBN: I-59068-013-8. pp. 71-72.

[20] Li Hongzhi (1992): Zhuan Falun, Yih Chyun Book Co., Ltd. Taipei, Taiwan (Feb. 2003, North America), ISBN: I-59068-013-8. pp. 77.

[21] Planck, M. (1914): *The Theory of Heat Radiation.* Masius, M. (transl.) (2nd ed.). P. Blakiston's Son & Co. OL 7154661M.

[22] Staley R (2009): *Einstein's generation. The origins of the relativity revolution*, Chicago: University of Chicago Press, ISBN 0-226-77057-5

[23] Gates E (2009): {Einstein's Telescope} The Hunt For Dark Matter And Kark Energy in the Universe. *W.W. Norton & Company, New York London*, 2009, pp 266. ISBN 978-0-393-06238-0.

[24] Hubble E (1929): A relation between distance and radial velocity among extra-galactic nebulae, *Proceedings of the National Academy of Science, USA* 15, no. 3 (March 15, 1929), 168-173.

[25] Moskowitz C (2012): Speed of Universe's Expansion Measured Better Than Ever. *Space On NBCnews.com*. http://www.nbcnews.com/id/49279077/ns/technology_and_science-space/#.Ueddl sqknTo

[26] Wheeler M (2013): Be happy: Your genes may thank you for it. *UCLA Newsroom* (July 29, 2013). http://newsroom.ucla.edu/portal/ucla/don-t-worry-be-happy-247644.aspx

[27] Hawkins DR (2002): Power vs. Force, *Hay House*; 1 edition (March 5, 2002). ISBN-13: 978-1561709335.

[28] http://www.ted.com/talks/jill_bolte_taylor_s_powerful_stroke_of_insight.html

[29] Ungless J (2013): A Stroke Of Enlightenment. May 2013. http://www.prevention.com/mind-body/emotional-health/how-stroke-led-one-brian-scientists-enlightenment?page=2

[30] Taylor JB (2006): My Stroke of Insight: A Brain Scientist's Personal Journey. Bloomington, IN, 2006: 111. ISBN 978-1-4303-0061-8.

[31] Life and Hope Renewed: The Healing Power of Falun Dafa. *Yih Chyun Corporation*, 2005. ISBN-13: 978-1590681022.

[32] Cheng PP, Liu L. (2009): Five elements of music therapy research on the influence of emotion and meridian. *Stud Health Technol Inform*. 2009;146:818-9.

[33] Bankovskii, N. G.; Korotkov, K. G. (1986): "Physical processes of image formation during gas-discharge visualization (the Kirlian effect) (Review)". Petrov, N. N. (Apr 1986). *Radiotekhnika i Elektronika* 31: 625–643.

[34] CV6000 Tesla Coil Electrobiographic Power Unit: http://cebunet.com/kirlian/6000.htm

[35] Quan A, Leung SW, Lao TT, Man RY (December 2003). "5-hydroxytryptamine and thromboxane A2 as physiologic mediators of human umbilical artery closure". *J. Soc. Gynecol. Investig*. 10 (8): 490–5. doi:10.1016/S1071-5576(03)00149-7. PMID 14662162.

[36] Mungan T, Ugur M, Yalcin H, Alan S, Sayilgan A. Treatment of Bartholin's cyst and abscess: excision versus silver nitrate insertion. *Eur J Obstet Gynecol Reprod Biol*. 1995 Nov; 63(1): 61-3.

[37] Ergeneli MH. Silver nitrate for Bartholin gland cysts, *Eur J Obstet Gynecol Reprod Biol*. 1999 Feb; 82(2): 231-2.

[38] Cho JY, Ahn MO, Cha KS. Window operation: an alternative treatment method for Bartholin gland cysts and abscesses. *Obstet Gynecol*. 1990 Nov; 76(5 Pt 1): 886-8.

[39] Yuce K, Zeyneloglu HB, Bukulmet O, Kisnisci HA. Outpatient management of Bartholin gland abscesses and cysts with silver nitrate. *Aust NZ J Obstet Gynaecol*. 1994 Feb; 34(1): 93-6.

[40] Liu G. Acupuncture-music therapy heals mental/physical chronic diseases by enhancing and balancing bio-energy and heart-brain-mind synchronization. *J Altern Complement Med.* 2004 Aug; 10(4, C3): 731

[41] Liu G. Energy field produced by meditation and acupuncture-music therapy enhanced cardiac functionality, bio-Energy and heart-brain-mind synchronization. *J Altern Complement Med.* 2004 Aug; 10(4, B2): 729-730

[42] Basmajian JV. Biofeedback in medical practice. *Can Med Assoc J.* 1978 July 8; 119(1): 8–10.

[43] Borkovec TD, Grayson JB, O'Brien GT, Weerts TC. Relaxation treatment of pseudoinsomnia and idiopathic insomnia: an electroencephalographic evaluation. *J Appl Behav Anal.* 1979 Spring; 12(1): 37–54. doi: 10.1901/jaba.1979.12-37.

[44] McCraty R, Barrios-Choplin B, Atkinson M, Tomasino D. The effects of different types of music on mood, tension, and mental clarity. *Altern Ther Health Med.* 1998 Jan;4(1):75-84.

[45] McCraty R, Barrios-Choplin B, Rozman D, Atkinson M, Watkins AD. The impact of a new emotional self-management program on stress, emotions, heart rate variability, DHEA and cortisol. *Integr Physiol Behav Sci.* 1998 Apr-Jun; 33(2):151-70.

[46] Creath K, Schwartz GE. Measuring effects of music, noise, and healing energy using a seed germination bioassay. *J Altern Complement Med.* 2004 Feb; 10(1): 113-22.

(47) Marzano DA, Haefner HK. The bartholin gland cyst: past, present, and future. J Low Genit Tract Dis. 2004 Jul;8(3):195-204.

(48) Perolo F, De Marchi C, Zauli F. Treatment of Bartholin gland cysts using marsupialization. Minerva Ginecol. 1978 Jun; 30(6): 575-7.

(49) Kim YC, Jeong MD, Lee MS. An examination of the relationship between five oriental musical tones and corresponding internal organs and meridians. Acupunct Electrother Res. 2004; 29(3-4): 227-33.

(50) Legge MF. Music for health: the five elements tonal system. IEEE Eng Med Biol Mag. 1999 Mar-Mpr; 18(2):80-8.

[51] Li QZ, Li P, Garcia GE, Johnson RJ, Feng L. Genomic profiling of neutrophil transcripts in Asian Qigong practitioners: a pilot study in gene regulation by mind-body interaction. J Altern Complement Med. 2005 Feb; 11(1): 29-39.

[52] Natarajan K, Acharya U R, Alias F, Tiboleng T, Puthusserypady SK. Nonlinear analysis of EEG signals at different mental states. Biomed Eng Online. 2004; 3: 7.

[53] Brady B, Stevens L. Binaural-beat induced theta EEG activity and hypnotic susceptibility. Am J Clin Hypn. 2000 Jul; 43(1): 53-69.

[54] Ferrarelli F, Smith R, Dentico D, Riedner BA, Zennig C, et al. (2013) Experienced Mindfulness Meditators Exhibit Higher Parietal-Occipital EEG Gamma Activity during NREM Sleep. PLoS ONE 8(8): e73417. doi:10.1371/journal.pone.0073417

[55]. Massachusetts General Hospital. "Meditation appears to produce enduring changes in emotional processing in the brain." ScienceDaily. ScienceDaily, 12 November 2012.

[56]. Ott, U., Hölzel, B.K., & Vaitl, D. (2011). Brain structure and meditation. How spiritual practice shapes the brain. In H.Walach, S.Schmidt, & W.B.Jonas (Eds.), *Neuroscience, Consciousness and Spirituality. Proceedings of the Expert Meeting in Freiburg/Breisgau 2008.* Berlin: Springer.

[57] Gaëlle Desbordes, Lobsang T. Negi, Thaddeus W. W. Pace, B. Alan Wallace, Charles L. Raison, Eric L. Schwartz. (2012) "Effects of mindful-attention and compassion meditation training on amygdala response to emotional stimuli in an ordinary, non-meditative state." *Frontiers in Human Neuroscience*, 2012; 6 DOI: 10.3389/fnhum.2012.00292

[58] Britta K Holzel, James Garmody, Mark Vangel, Christina Congleton, Sita M, Yerramsetti, Tim Gard, Sara W. Lazar: 2011: "Mindfullness practice leads to increases in regional brain gray matter density." Psychiatry Research: Neuroimaging, 191 (2011) 36-43

[59] Newsweek Magazine (Oct. 2012). "Heaven Is Real: A Doctor's Experience With the Afterlife" http://www.thedailybeast.com/newsweek/2012/10/07/proof-of-heaven-a-doctor-s-experience-with-the-afterlife.html

[60] Eben Alexander, MD (2012): Proof of Heaven: A Neurosurgeon's Journey into the Afterlife. Simon & Schuster, 1ST edition (2012) ASIN: B00B624Z52.

[61] Fadel Zeidan, Katherine T. Martucci, Robert A. Kraft, Nakia S. Gordon, John G. McHaffie, and Robert C. Coghill: "Brain Mechanisms Supporting the Modulation of Pain by Mindfulness Meditation." *The Journal of Neuroscience*, 6 April 2011, 31(14): 5540-5548; doi: 10.1523/JNEUROSCI.5791-10.2011

[62] Wolfson AB, ed. (2005): *Harwood-Nuss' Clinical Practice of Emergency Medicine* (4th ed.). p. 400. ISBN 0-7817-5125-X.

[63] Hempel, S; Newberry, SJ; Maher, AR; Wang, Z; Miles, JN; Shanman, R; Johnsen, B; Shekelle, PG (2012 May 9): "Probiotics for the prevention and treatment of antibiotic-associated diarrhea: a systematic review and meta-analysis.". *JAMA: the Journal of the American Medical Association* 307 (18): 1959–69. doi:10.1001/jama.2012.3507. PMID 22570464.

[64] Pillai, A; Nelson, R (2008 Jan 23). "Probiotics for treatment of Clostridium difficile-associated colitis in adults." *Cochrane database of systematic reviews (Online)* (1): CD004611. doi:10.1002/14651858.CD004611.pub2. PMID 18254055.

[65] Hanahan, D. & Weinberg, R. A (2000): The hallmarks of cancer. *Cell* 100, 57–70 (2000).

[66] Kinzler, K. W. & Vogelstein, B. Lessons from hereditary colorectal cancer. *Cell* 87, 159–170 (1996).

[67] Ming Wu, Jose Carlos Pastor-Pareja and Tian Xu (2010): "Interaction between Ras^{V12} and scribbled clones induces tumour growth and invasion." *Nature*, Vol 463, 28 January 2010| doi: 10.1038/nature08702

[68] Richardson B. (2003): "Impact of aging on DNA Methylation." *Ageing Res. Rev.* 2003, Jul; 2(3): 245-61.

[69] E Unternaehrer, P Luers, J Mill, E Dempster, A H Meyer, S Staehli, R Lieb, D H Hellhammer, G Meinlschmidt (2012): "Dynamic changes in DNA methylation of stress-associated genes (OXTR, BDNF) after acute psychosocial stress." *Translational Psychiatry*, 2012; 2 (8): e150 DOI: 10.1038/tp.2012.77.

[70] Horvath1 S, Zhang Y, Langfelder P, Kahn RS, Boks MPM, Eijk KV, Berg L.H.V.D, Ophoff RA (2012): "Aging effects on DNA methylation modules in human brain and blood tissue." *Genome Biology* 2012, 13:R97 doi:10.1186/gb-2012-13-10-r97.

[71] Suzuki H, Toyota M, Sato H, Sonoda T, Sakauchi F, Mori M. (2006): Roles and causes of abnormal DNA methylation in gastrointestinal cancers. *Asian Pac J Cancer Prev.* 2006 Apr-Jun;7(2):177-85.

[72] Kim YI (2004): Folate and DNA Methylation: A Mechanistic Link between Folate Deficiency and Colorectal Cancer?" Cancer Epidemiol Biomarkers Prev April 2004 13:511-519

[73] Kim YI (1999): Folate and carcinogenesis: evidence, mechanisms, and implications. *J Nutr Biochem*, 1999;10:66–88.

[74] Bailey LB, Rampersaud GC, Kauwell GP (2003): Folic acid supplements and fortification affect the risk for neural tube defects, vascular disease and cancer: evolving science. *J Nutr*, 2003;133:1961S–8S.

[75] Giovannucci E. Epidemiologic studies of folate and colorectal neoplasia: a review. J Nutr, 2002;132:2350S–5S.

[76] Lashner BA, Heidenreich PA, Su GL Kane SV, Hanauer SB. Effect of folate supplementation on the incidence of dysplasia and cancer in chronic ulcerative colitis. A case-control study. Gastroenterology, 1989;97:255–9.

[77] Lashner BA, Provencher KS, Seidner DL, Knesebeck A, Brzezinski A. The effect of folic acid supplementation on the risk for cancer or dysplasia in ulcerative colitis. Gastroenterology, 1997;112:29–32.

[78] Figueiredo JC, Grau MV; Haile RW; Sandler RS; Summers RW; Bresalier RS; Burke CA; McKeown-Eyssen GE; Baron JA (2009). Folic Acid and Risk of Prostate Cancer: Results From a Randomized Clinical Trial. *Journal of the National Cancer Institute*, Volume 101, Issue 6, pp. 432-435.

[79] Cool L.C. (2012): Harmful Side Effects of Antibiotics, Sep 24, 2012. http://health.yahoo.net/experts/dayinhealth/harmful-side-effects-antibiotics.

[80] Science News (2008): Adverse Reactions To Antibiotics Send Thousands Of Patients To The ER. Aug. 13, 2008. http://www.sciencedaily.com/releases/2008/08/080812135515.htm

[81] McFarland LV (1998): Epidemiology, risk factors and treatments for antibiotic-associated diarrhea. *Dig Dis* 1998;16:292-307.

[82] Scientists sound new warning for rising arsenic in rice.
http://tribune.com.pk/story/580689/scientists-sound-new-warning-for-rising-arsenic-in-rice/

[83] Cardillo J (2013): "The Five Seasons: Tap Into Nature's Secrets for Health, Happiness, and Harmony." New Page Books; First Edition (June 24, 2013), ISBN-10: 1601632584

[84] Cardillo J (2013): "Be Like Water: Practical Wisdom from the Martial Arts." Grand Central Publishing (September 1, 2003), ISBN-10: 0446690317

[85] Mindlin G; DuRousseau D; Cardillo J (2012): "Your Playlist Can Change Your Life." Sourcebooks (January 1, 2012), ISBN-10: 1402260245; ASIN: B008W3IVNU

[86] Cardillo J (2009): "Can I Have Your Attention?: How to Think Fast, Find Your Focus, and Sharpen Your Concentration." Career Press (August 1, 2009), ISBN-10: 1601630638

[87] Cardillo J (2006): "Bow to Life: 365 Secrets from the Martial Arts for Daily Life." Da Capo Press (May 19, 2006), ISBN-10: 1569243085

[88] Liu JG, Cooper G. A study at cellular level on the psychological and physical healing effects of advanced Qigong meditation. International Council of Psychologists, 65th Annual Convention, August 11-14, 2007.

[89] Dong YH, Shapiro L, Chen YL and Hsu KH. A Literature Review and Pooled Analysis of the Beneficial Effects of Falun Gong Meditative Practice on Physical and Mental Health. Journal of Evidence-Based Complementary & Alternative Medicine, Submitted, May 27, 2014.

[90] Feng W, Liu G, Allen PD and Pessah IN. Transmembrane redox sensor of calcium release channel ryanodine receptor. J Biol Chem. 2000 Nov 17;275(46):35902-7

[91] Feng W, Liu G, Xia RH, Abramson JJ, and Pessah IN. Site-selective modification of hyperreactive cysteines of ryanodine receptor complex by quinones. Molec. Pharm. 55:821-831 (1999).

[92] Liu G, Pessah IN. Molecular interaction between ryanodine receptor and glycoprotein triadin involves redox cycling of functionally important hyperreactive sulfhydryls. J. Biol. Chem. 269:33028-33034 (1994).

[93] Liu G, Abramson JJ, Zable AC, and Pessah IN. Direct evidence for existence and functional role of hyperreactive sulfhydryl on ryanodine receptor/triadin Ca2+ channel complex selectively labeled by the coumarin maleimide CPM. Molec. Pharm. 45:189-200 (1994).

[94] Liu G and Oba T. Effects of tetraphenylboron-induced increase in inner surface charge on Ca2+ release channel in sarcoplasmic reticulum. Jpn. J. Physiol. (1990), 40, 723-736.

[95] Liu G and Oba T. Negative surface charges provoke conformational change of membrane proteins and release of calcium from sarcoplasmic reticulum. In 'Frontiers in Smooth Muscle Research', Ed. N. Sperelakis and J. D. wood, Alan R. Liss, Inc., Prog. Clin. Biol. Res. (1990), 327, 779-784.

[96] Liu G and Oba T. Change in surface charge of sarcoplasmic reticulum membrane may elicit conformational change in sulfhydryl groups of membrane proteins to release calcium. Jpn. J. Physiol. (1989), 39, 412-417.

[97] Oba T and Liu G. Chemical modification of sulfhydryl groups inhibits skeletal muscle contraction in frog. In 'Frontiers in Smooth Muscle Research', Ed. N. Sperelakis and J. D. Wood, Alan R. Liss, Inc., Prog. Clin. Biol. Res. (1990), 327, 779-784.

[98] Oba T, Aoki T, Liu G and Hotta K. A local anesthetic, tetracaine, similarly inhibits Ag+ and K+ contracture in frog skeletal muscle. Jpn. J. Physiol., 37 (1987), 995-1003.

[99] TIME magazine: CHINA: Tortoise-Pigeon-Dog. May 15, 1933
http://content.time.com/time/magazine/article/0,9171,745510,00.html

Library of Congress Cataloging-in-Publication Data:

© Jason G. Liu, 2014 ~
Mind-Body Medicine & Healthology

*   *   *

July 18, 2014 published in the United States of America
Mind-Body Science Publishing
Mind-Body Science Institute, USA
ISBN-13: 978-0692257913
ISBN-10: 0692257918

Available in Print Book (Paperback and Hardcover), Kindle Book and Audiobook on Amazon.com & Publisher Website www.mbmu.org/books

www.ingramcontent.com/pod-product-compliance
Lightning Source LLC
Chambersburg PA
CBHW081143270326
41930CB00014B/3016